*A*dvanced Concepts in *A*RRHYTHMIAS

THIRD EDITION

HENRY J.L. MARRIOTT, MD, FACP, FACC

Clinical Professor of Medicine (Cardiology),
Emory University School of Medicine,
Atlanta, Georgia;

Director, Shick Cardiac Education Center,
Naples Community Hospital,
Naples, Florida

MARY BOUDREAU CONOVER, RN, BS

Arrhythmia Consultant and Lecturer,
Director of Education, Critical Care Conferences,
Santa Cruz, California

with 335 illustrations

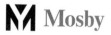

St. Louis   Baltimore   Boston   Carlsbad
Chicago   Minneapolis   New York   Philadelphia   Portland
London   Milan   Sydney   Tokyo   Toronto

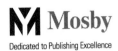

Mosby
Dedicated to Publishing Excellence

A Times Mirror
Company

THIRD EDITION

Publisher: Nancy L. Coon
Editor: Barry Bowlus
Managing Editor: Lisa Potts
Developmental Editor: Cynthia Anderson
Project Manager: Deborah L. Vogel
Production Editor: Jodi M. Willard
Designer: Pati Pye
Manufacturing Manager: Linda Ierardi
Cover Image: Phototake

Printed in the United States of America
Composition by Top Graphics
Lithography by Top Graphics
Printing/binding by Maple-Vail Book Manufacturing Group

Mosby, Inc.
11830 Westline Industrial Drive
St. Louis, Missouri 63146

Library of Congress Cataloging in Publication Data

Marriott, Henry J.L. (Henry Joseph Llewellyn)
    Advanced concepts in arrhythmias / Henry J.L. Marriott, Mary
Boudreau Conover. — 3rd ed.
        p.   cm.
    Includes bibliographical references and index.
    ISBN 0-8151-2090-7 (hardcover)
    1. Arrhythmia.   I. Conover, Mary Boudreau.   II. Title.
    [DNLM: 1. Arrhythmia.   WG 330 M359a 1998]
RC685.A65M369   1998
616.1′28—dc21
DNLM/DLC
for Library of Congress   97-15127
                                                       CIP

97 98 99 00 01 / 9 8 7 6 5 4 3 2 1

To
Garrett Andrew Conover
Welcome to this world!

Preface

In this third edition we have covered the important advances made in electrocardiography during the last decade. The chapters on membrane channels; the action potential; the autonomic nervous system, cardiac rhythms, and drugs; and arrhythmogenic mechanisms have been completely rewritten. We have added an important chapter on atrial fibrillation, a common arrhythmia about which new data are being rapidly accumulated and for which a cure is being aggressively sought. Radiofrequency ablation now provides a safe transvenous cure for arrhythmias sustained by an accessory pathway, as well as for atrial flutter, some types of atrial tachycardia, paroxysmal supraventricular tachycardia caused by AV nodal reentry, and certain types of ventricular tachycardia. Therefore we have devoted several chapters to explaining the mechanisms, ECG recognition, emergency treatment, and cure of these arrhythmias. We have also updated the chapter on polymorphic ventricular tachycardia, differentiating among its three forms.

This book will bring the reader up-to-date regarding the value of the surface ECG as a superior, reproducible, noninvasive, and economical diagnostic tool. For those who are involved in emergency response and care of the critically ill, this new information is vital to patient safety and personal professional adequacy, especially because of new, enlightened treatment protocols and cures.

Henry J.L. Marriott
Mary Conover

Contents

1 *Development and Functions of the Cardiac Conduction System, 1*
Development of the SA node, 1
The AV node, its approaches, and the His bundle, 3
   Compact AV node, 4
   AV nodal approaches, 6
   His bundle, 7
Bundle branches, 7
   Left bundle branch, 7
   Right bundle branch, 9
   Terminal Purkinje fibers, 10
Innervation of the cardiac conduction system, 11

2 *Membrane Channels, 13*
Overview, 13
Normal cell function, 13
Selective permeability and the resting membrane potential, 14
Depolarization, 14
Repolarization, 15
Threshold potential, 15
Automaticity, 15
Membrane pumps, 15
   Na^+-K^+ ATPase (sodium) pump, 15
   ATP-dependent Ca^{2+} pump, 16
Membrane channels, 17
   Sodium channels (I_{Na}), 17
   Calcium channels (I_{Ca}), 19
   Potassium rectifying channels, 21
   Pacemaker current (I_f), 23
Gap junctions, 24

3 *The Action Potential, 29*
Fast- and slow-response action potentials, 29
Recording the action potential, 30
SA and AV nodal action potentials, 32
Phase 4 depolarization, 33
Phase 0, 33
Phase 1, 35
Phase 2, 35
Phase 3, 35

Refractory periods, 36
Conduction velocity, 36
Overdrive suppression, 37

4   *The Autonomic Nervous System, Cardiac Rhythms, and Drugs,* 41
β-Adrenergic receptor-effector coupling system, 41
    β-Adrenergic stimulation, 41
    Modulation of the sodium current by β-adrenergic stimulation, 42
    β-Adrenergic blockade, 42
Muscarinic receptor-effector coupling system, 42
    Vagal stimulation, 42
Effects of drugs on cardiac function, 43
    Drug-channel interactions, 43
    Use-dependent antiarrhythmic drugs, 43
    Voltage-dependent antiarrhythmic drugs, 43
    Prolonged repolarization, 43
    Drug competition and potentiation, 44
Other drugs or conditions that act on the heart, 44

5   *Arrhythmogenic Mechanisms and Their Modulation,* 47
Arrhythmia or dysrhythmia?, 47
Altered automaticity, 47
    Enhanced normal automaticity, 47
    Abnormal automaticity, 48
    Differentiating between the two types of altered automaticity, 49
Triggered activity, 49
    Early afterdepolarizations, 53
    Delayed afterdepolarizations, 54
Reentry, 56
    Anatomic reentry, 57
    Functional reentry, 57
    Anisotropic reentry, 58
    Reflection, 58
    Vulnerable parameters, 60
    Terminating a reentry circuit, 60
Summation, 61
Inhibition, 62
Mechanisms of ischemia-induced arrhythmias, 63

6   *Concealed Conduction,* 69
Silent zones on the surface electrocardiogram, 69
SA nodal electrogram, 69
    Clinical value, 69
    SA conduction time, 69
His bundle electrogram, 70
    Deflections, 71
    Intervals and normal values, 71
    Indications, 71

The ECG related to activation of the conduction system, 72
Concealed conduction, 72
  Historical background, 73
  Concealed conduction in atrial fibrillation, 73
  Aberrant ventricular conduction caused by retrograde concealed
    conduction, 74
  Interpolated ventricular extrasystoles with concealed retrograde
    conduction, 75
  Concealed junctional extrasystoles, 76
  Concealed conduction affecting impulse formation, 81

7   *Sinoatrial Node Dysfunction,* *85*
The SA node, 85
  Anatomy, 85
  Physiology, 85
  Blood supply, 87
  Nerve supply, 87
  Temperature, 88
  Diagnostic evaluation of SA node function, 88
  SA conduction time, 88
24-hour heart rate variability, 88
  Clinical value, 88
  History, 88
  Methods of evaluation, 88
Increased heart rate, 89
SA nodal reentrant tachycardia, 89
  ECG features, 90
  ECG documentation, 90
  Differential diagnosis, 90
  History, 91
  Symptoms, 91
  Mechanism, 91
  Incidence, 91
  Treatment, 91
SA exit block, 92
  First-degree SA block, 92
  Second-degree SA block, 92
  Third-degree SA block, 93
Sick sinus syndrome, 94
  History, 94
  ECG features, 94
  Pediatrics, 94
  Mechanisms, 95
  Causes, 95
  Treatment, 96

8   *Atrial Fibrillation,* *99*
Classification, 99
Descriptive designations, 99

Electrocardiogram recognition, 99
  Heart rate, 99
  Rhythm, 101
  Fibrillatory line, 101
  QRS complexes, 101
  Warning arrhythmias, 101
  Distinguishing features, 102
Mechanism, 102
  Concealed conduction, 104
Tachycardia-induced cardiomyopathy and electrical remodeling, 104
  Cardiomyopathy, 104
  Electrical remodeling, 104
Symptoms, 104
Physical findings, 104
Incidence, 105
Pediatrics, 106
Thromboembolism, 106
Treatment, 106
  DC cardioversion, 106
  Surgery, 106
  Cure by catheter?, 107

9   *Atrial Flutter,* 109
Historical perspective in humans, 109
Electrophysiologic classification, 110
Pertinent atrial structures, 110
ECG findings common to all forms of atrial flutter, 112
Pediatrics, 113
Typical atrial flutter (type I), 115
  Counterclockwise typical atrial flutter, 115
  Clockwise typical atrial flutter, 121
True atypical atrial flutter (type II), 122
  Mechanism, 122
  Genesis of flutter waves, 122
  ECG recognition, 123
  Acute treatment, 123
  Long-term treatment, 123
Incisional reentrant atrial tachycardia, 124
Differential diagnosis, 124
Physical signs, 124
Clinical setting and incidence, 125
Ablation of automatic and reentrant atrial tachycardia, 126
Chemical ablation in the future?, 126
Anticoagulation, 126

10   *Atrial Tachycardia,* 131
Classification and mechanisms, 131
Clinical implications, 131

Incisional reentrant atrial tachycardia, 132
  Mechanism, 132
  Long-term treatment, 132
Focal atrial tachycardia, 134
Chaotic or multifocal atrial tachycardia, 135
Nonparoxysmal atrial tachycardia, 135
Nonsustained paroxysmal atrial tachycardia, 138
Differential diagnosis, 138
Location of focal atrial tachycardias, 139
P' wave configuration as a guide to locations of atrial foci, 139
Pediatrics, 140
Postoperative atrial warning arrhythmias, 140
Incidence, 142
Medical treatment, 142
Radiofrequency catheter ablation for a cure, 142

11   *Reciprocal (Echo) Beats, 145*
AV junction (V-A-V sequence), 145
Ventricles (V-A-V sequence), 145
RP' interval in V-A-V sequences, 147
Atria (A-V-A sequence), 147

12   *Narrow QRS Paroxysmal Supraventricular Tachycardia, 153*
Terminology, 153
Classification (narrow and broad QRS types of paroxysmal supraventricular
  tachycardia), 153
  Common forms (narrow QRS), 153
  Uncommon forms (narrow QRS), 153
  Uncommon forms (broad QRS), 153
Relative incidence (narrow QRS paroxysmal supraventricular
  tachycardia), 154
Maintenance and interruption of a reentry circuit, 154
Emergency response, 155
  Hemodynamically stable patient, 155
  Hemodynamically unstable patient, 155
Importance of recording multiple leads during tachycardia, 155
Methods of vagal stimulation, 156
Carotid sinus massage, 156
  Caution, 157
  Procedure for carotid sinus massage, 157
Bedside diagnosis, 157
AV nodal reentrant tachycardia, 157
  Definition, 157
  Anatomy, 157
  Mechanism, 158
  ECG recognition, 160
  Clinical implications, 160
  Treatment, 160

Orthodromic circus movement tachycardia, 160
    Definition, 160
    Anatomy, 160
    Mechanism, 162
    ECG recognition, 163
    Clinical implications, 165
    Treatment, 171
Atypical AV nodal reentrant tachycardia, 171
    Definition, 171
    Mechanism, 171
    ECG recognition, 171
    Clinical implications, 173
    Treatment, 173
Incessant junctional tachycardia (atypical orthodromic circus movement
    tachycardia), 173
    Definition and mechanism, 173
    ECG recognition, 173
    Clinical implications, 174
    Treatment, 174
Differentiating the reciprocating supraventricular tachycardias, 174
Pediatrics, 176
    Neonate and infant, 176
    Fetus, 176

13   *Digitalis Dysrhythmias,* *179*
Digitalis glycosides, 179
Mortality in undiagnosed digitalis toxicity, 179
Cellular basis for digitalis dysrhythmias, 179
Triggered activity, 180
Digitalis and K^+ derangements, 180
    Hypokalemia, 180
    Hyperkalemia, 181
Factors that interact with digoxin, 182
    Factors that may require a decrease in digoxin dosage, 182
    Factors that may require an increase in digoxin dosage, 182
Serum digoxin concentration, 182
ECG effects of therapeutic digoxin, 183
Systematic approach to the ECG, 183
    Evaluating the events in the atria first, 183
    Monitoring, 184
    Evaluating for AV conduction, 184
Clinical alert to digitalis toxicity, 184
ECG recognition of digitalis dysrhythmias, 185
    Sinus bradycardia and junctional tachycardia, 185
    SA block, 185
    AV block, 185
    Atrial tachycardia, 186
    Junctional tachycardia, 188
    Fascicular ventricular tachycardia, 192

Bifascicular ventricular tachycardia, 192
Double tachycardia, 194
Ventricular bigeminy, 195
Concealed ventricular bigeminy, 197
Treatment, 198
Early stages, 198
Life-threatening digitalis toxicity, 198

14 *Exacerbation of Arrhythmias by Antiarrhythmic Drugs, 203*
History of awareness of proarrhythmia in the postinfarction period, 204
Clinical manifestations, 205
Predictors of arrhythmia aggravation, 205
Drugs that are proarrhythmic, 206
Mechanisms, 206
Slow conduction, 206
Prolonged refractory period, 206
The membrane channel, 207
Fast sodium channel blockade by local anesthetic antiarrhythmics, 208
Abnormal conduction, 210
Sodium channel blockade, 210
Prolonging the refractory period, 211

15 *Aberrant Ventricular Conduction, 215*
Mechanisms, 215
Phase 3 aberration, 215
Phase 4 aberration, 217
Rate-dependent and critical rate bundle branch block, 220
Patterns of aberration, 223
RBBB aberration, 223
LBBB aberration, 223
Additional helpful clues, 226
QRS duration, 226
Preceding atrial activity, 227
Initial deflection identical with that of conducted beats, 227
Second-in-the-row anomaly, 229
Aberrancy in atrial fibrillation, 230
Ashman's phenomenon, 230
Aberrancy in atrial tachycardia, 231
Alternating aberrancy, 233
Clinical implications, 233

16 *Aberrancy Versus Ectopy, 237*
Prevalence of misdiagnosis in broad QRS tachycardia, 237
When in doubt use procainamide, 237
What cannot be used in the differential diagnosis, 238
Value of a baseline 12-lead ECG, 238
Steps in the differential diagnosis, 238
Importance of obtaining a history, 238

Physical signs of AV dissociation, 240
   The jugular pulse, 240
   The first heart sound, 240
   Systolic blood pressure, 240
ECG signs of AV dissociation, 240
   Finding the Ps, 241
ECG signs of VA conduction, 241
QRS configuration, 243
   V_1-positive broad QRS tachycardia, 245
   V_1-negative broad QRS tachycardia, 247
   Clinical correlations of axis, 252
QRS width, 253
Capture beats and fusion beats, 253
Concordant pattern, 253
Other findings, 256

17   *The Other Broads,* 261

Accesory pathways, 261
   Mahaim fibers, 262
Supraventricular tachycardias that look like ventricular tachycardia, 262
   Atrial fibrillation with an accessory pathway, 262
   Atrial fibrillation with multiple accessory pathways, 269
   Atrial flutter with an accessory pathway, 269
   Antidromic circus movement tachycardia, 269
   Circus movement tachycardia with two accessory pathways, 274
   Broad QRS paroxysmal supraventricular tachycardia using
     nodoventricular fibers, 274
Ventricular tachycardias that look like supraventricular tachycardia, 276
   Idiopathic ventricular tachycardia, 276
   Idiopathic right ventricular tachycardia, 279
   Idiopathic left ventricular tachycardia, 281
   Bundle branch reentrant ventricular tachycardia, 282
   Fascicular ventricular tachycardia, 286

18   *Polymorphic Ventricular Tachycardia,* 293

Classification, 293
Acquired long QT syndrome, 294
   ECG warning signs, 294
   ECG recognition of the tachycardia itself, 294
   Potassium channel blockers and torsades de pointes, 296
   Common clinical causes, 298
   Clinical characteristics, 298
   Latent long QT syndrome, 298
   Symptoms, 298
   Emergency treatment, 298
   Possible outcomes, 299
   Contraindications for magnesium, 299
   Advantages of magnesium for torsades de pointes, 299
   Prevention, 300

Congenital long QT syndrome, 300
  Chromosomal defects, 300
  ECG recognition, 300
  Abnormal T waves, 302
  The corrected QT interval, 302
  Treatment, 302
  Screening, 302
Polymorphic ventricular tachycardia (without QT prolongation), 303
  Chronic coronary artery disease, 303
  Acute myocardial ischemia, 304

19   *AV Block,* 311
The PR interval, 311
Nonconducted beats, 311
Type I and type II block, 312
Anatomy versus behavior, 312
Wenckebach periodicity and RP/PR reciprocity, 314
2:1 AV block, 316
"Skipped" P waves, 317
High-grade (or advanced) AV block, 318
Complete AV block, 319
Ventricular asystole, 320
Need to reclassify, 320
  Definitions are wanting, 320
  Nondegrees of block, 321
  Misconceptions are rife, 323
Remedial measures, 326

20   *Parasystole,* 329
ECG in parasystole, 329
  No fixed coupling, 329
  Fusion beats, 329
  Interectopic intervals, 330
Modulated parasystole, 330
Exit block, 331
Classic ventricular parasystole, 333
  Interectopic intervals as simple multiples of a common denominator, 333
  Fusion beats, 333
Classic parasystole without exit block, 334
Classic parasystole with exit block, 337
Concealed parasystole, 337
Intermittent parasystole, 337
Parasystolic accelerated idioventricular rhythm, 338
Fixed coupling in parasystole, 338
Clinical significance, 338
Atrial parasystole, 340

21   *Supernormal Conduction, 345*

The supernormal period, 345
Concealed supernormal conduction, 346
Mimics of supernormal conduction, 348
   Concealed junctional extrasystoles, 349
   Phase 4 (paradoxical critical rate), 349
   Concealed reentry, 349
   The gap phenomenon, 349

22   *An Approach to Arrhythmias, 355*

Principles of monitoring, 355
   Monitor according to the clinical setting, 355
   One lead is not enough, 356
   Electrode postions for MCL$_1$ and MCL$_6$, 356
A systematic approach, 358
   Know the causes, 358
   Milk the QRS, 359
   Cherchez le P, 359
   Who's maried to whom?, 363
   Pinpoint the primary disturbance, 363

23   *Signal-Averaged ECG, 367*

Historical background, 367
Clinical application of the signal-averaged ECG, 367
Problems in analyzing small ECG signals, 368
Signal averaging, 368
Spatial averaging, 369
Ensemble averaging (signal averaging), 369
Time domain analysis of the signal-averaged ECG, 369
Interpreting the time domain signal-averaged ECG, 370
Frequency domain analysis of the signal-averaged ECG, 372
   Method, 372
   Interpreting the frequency domain signal-averaged ECG, 375
Limitations, 376
Other analytic methods, 376

Advanced Concepts in ARRHYTHMIAS

CHAPTER **1**

Development and Functions of the Cardiac Conduction System

Development of the SA
  node 1
The AV node, its
  approaches, and the His
  bundle 3
Bundle branches 7
Innervation of the cardiac
  conduction system 11

THE CARDIAC CONDUCTION SYSTEM IS COMPOSED OF HIGHLY SPECIALIZED MUSCLE tissue that is unique to the heart. The function of this system is to generate the cardiac impulse, transport it across the fibrous ring of the atrioventricular (AV) junction, and deliver it throughout the ventricles. The cardiac conduction system is composed of the sinus (sinoatrial [SA]) node, the AV node, and the His-Purkinje system (penetrating His bundle, ventricular bundle branches, and Purkinje fibers). Because of the speed with which an impulse is conducted through the His-Purkinje system, conduction tissue is often falsely equated with nerve tissue. The cardiac conduction system is decisively myocardial in nature.

The cardiac impulse originates within the SA node and is conducted through the two atria via working atrial myocytes. After activating the right atrium, the impulse enters the approaches to the AV node and is delayed within the compact AV node. After traversing the AV node, the impulse is rapidly delivered to the endocardium through the bundle branches and their Purkinje fibers. The ventricular myocardium is then activated from endocardium to epicardium; the right and left ventricles are activated simultaneously. The amount of time necessary for right ventricular activation is small compared with that required for the much larger left ventricle.

DEVELOPMENT OF THE SA NODE

After 11 weeks of intrauterine life the SA node can be recognized. Its formation begins with a thickening of the junction between the superior vena cava and the sinus venosus in the region of the sinus nodal ring cells. This thickening is confined to the anteromedial quadrant of the junction between the superior vena cava and the atrium and, in most hearts, aggregates around a prominent artery. The embryonic origin of the SA node is illustrated in Figure 1-1.

Location

The SA node lies less than 1 mm from the epicardial surface. It lies within the sulcus terminalis (terminal groove) where the trabeculated right atrial appendage meets the

1

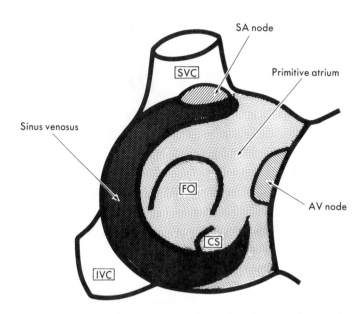

FIGURE 1-1 SA node begins with a thickening of the junction between the superior vena cava and sinus venosus. *SVC*, Superior vena cava; *IVC*, inferior vena cava; *FO*, fossa ovalis; *CS*, coronary sinus. (From Anderson RH, Becker AE, Wenick ACG: The development of the conducting tissues. In Roberts NK, Gelband H, editors: *Cardiac arrhythmias in the neonate, infant, and child*, New York, 1977, Appleton-Century-Crofts.)

smooth tissue of the superior vena cava. In most people, the SA node runs along the crest of the atrial appendage, with its tail extending toward the opening of the superior vena cava (Figure 1-2). However, in 10% of the population the head of the SA node extends across the crest of the atrial appendage and into the interatrial groove in the shape of a horseshoe ("horseshoe" node).

Structure

The SA node is an oval, spindle-shaped structure approximately 10 to 20 mm long and 5 mm thick. It is composed of small cells set in a dense matrix of fibrous tissue that increases with age. Transitional cells extend from the borders of the SA node into the musculature of the crista terminalis. In the heart of a rabbit, the pacemaking function of the SA node arises rhythmically in a large number of small nodal cells (approximately 5000) that discharge simultaneously.[1,2]

Blood supply

The large central SA nodal artery is usually a branch of either the right coronary artery or the circumflex coronary artery. However, occasionally it may originate distally or from the crux of the heart.[1]

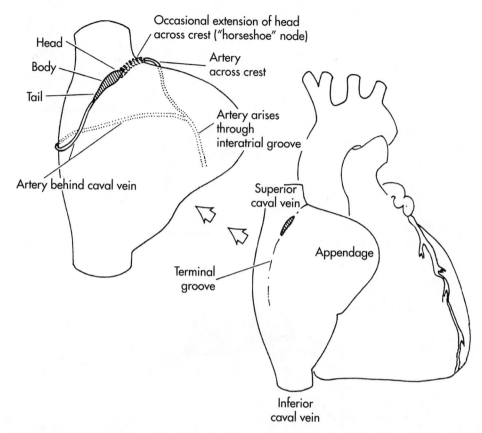

FIGURE 1-2   The usual location of the SA node. Inset shows the "horseshoe" variation and possible pathways for the artery to the node. (From Anderson RH, Becker AE: Anatomy of the conduction tissues and accessory atrioventricular connections. In Zipes DP, Jalife J, editors: *Cardiac electrophysiology from cell to bedside,* Philadelphia, 1990, WB Saunders.)

SA nodal dysfunction

One of the causes of sick sinus syndrome is that SA nodal cells are dominated and overcome by the fibrous matrix in which they are set. Sinus exit block may result when the transitional cells become fibrosed.

THE AV NODE, ITS APPROACHES, AND THE HIS BUNDLE

The AV node, its approaches, and the His bundle make up the conductive tissue of the AV junction. These structures are located within the triangle of Koch, which is formed by the tricuspid annulus and the tendon of Todaro (Figure 1-3).

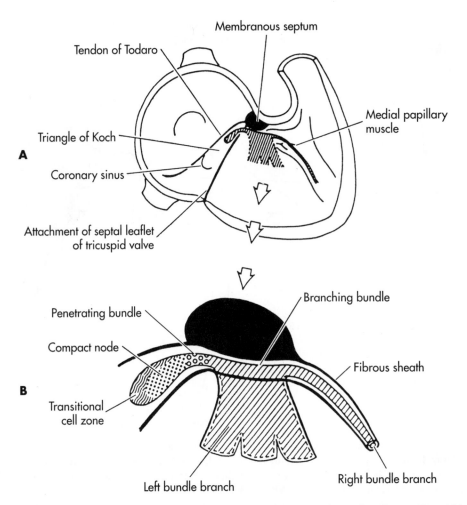

FIGURE 1-3 A, Schematic illustration of the position of the AV node–His bundle complex within the triangle of Koch. **B,** AV node–His bundle complex. (From Anderson RH, Becker AE: Anatomy of the conduction tissues and accessory atrioventricular connections. In Zipes DP, Jalife J, editors: *Cardiac electrophysiology from cell to bedside,* Philadelphia, 1990, WB Saunders.)

Compact AV Node
Location

The compact AV node is located just beneath the endocardium on the muscular septum that separates the right atrium from the left ventricle. It lies directly above the insertion of the septal leaflet of the tricuspid valve and at the apex of the triangle of Koch. The compact AV node is isolated from the ventricular myocardial fibers by the annulus fibrosus and is usually far removed anteriorly from the coronary sinus.

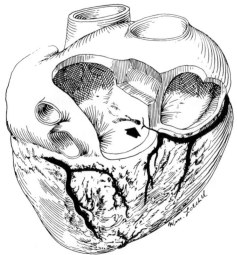

FIGURE 1-4 Arterial blood supply to the inferior wall of the human heart as it occurs in approximately 90% of the population. (From James TN: *Anatomy of the coronary arteries*, New York, 1961, Harper & Row.)

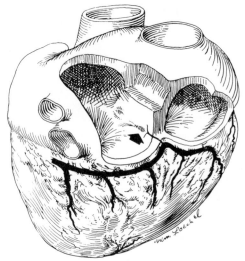

FIGURE 1-5 Arterial blood supply to the inferior wall of the human heart as it occurs in approximately 10% of the population. (From James TN: *Anatomy of the coronary arteries*, New York, 1961, Harper & Row.)

Structure

A cross section of the AV node reveals an elongated half oval. The cells of the compact portion are similar in appearance to those of the SA node. Around the compact region of the node is a transitional layer that circles the compact node and terminates at the base of the tricuspid valve. The transitional cell zones extend backward and superiorly from the compact node but are contained within the boundaries of the triangle of Koch.

Blood supply

In 90% of the population the AV node receives its blood supply from the right coronary artery (Figure 1-4). In the remaining 10% of the population the circumflex artery supplies the AV node (Figure 1-5).

AV Nodal Approaches

The mammalian AV node has a complex structure with anatomic limits that are not easily defined.[3] This is especially true of the anatomically irregular proximal portion of the AV node, called the *transitional node*. Parallel strands of fibers emanate from the floor of the coronary sinus and are directed inferiorly along the tricuspid annulus toward the compact AV node. These strands are separated by fibrous tissue and form a "slow" conduction pathway that is posterior and inferior to the compact AV node.[4] Another set of fibers are located anteriorly and superiorly along the compact AV node and exit into the atrial septum near the tendon of Todaro, forming a "fast" conduction pathway. Thus the fibers of the fast and slow pathways run along opposite edges of the compact AV node and into the atrium in a fanlike fashion. A block in the slow pathway has no impact on the PR interval during sinus rhythm.[5]

Figure 1-6 represents an important ice-mapping study by Keim, Werner, and Jazayeri et al,[5] which was performed on six patients who were having surgery to cure AV nodal reentrant tachycardia (see Chapter 12). During surgery the slow and fast pathways emanating from the compact AV node were demonstrated. In most patients the slow pathway was found along the tricuspid annulus, posterior (inferior) to the compact AV

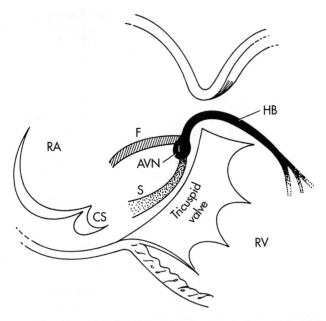

FIGURE 1-6 The slow *(S)* and fast *(F)* pathway approaches to the compact AV node *(AVN)* are shown in the process of supporting an AV nodal reentrant mechanism. This schematic drawing demonstrates that atrial and nodal fibers form an eccentric continuum as they converge into the compact AV node. The fast conducting fibers are superior; slow conducting fibers are inferior. *RA*, Right atrium; *CS*, coronary sinus; *HB*, His bundle; *RV*, right ventricle. (From Keim S, Werner P, Jazayeri M et al: Localization of the fast and slow pathways in atrioventricular nodal reentrant tachycardia by intraoperative ice mapping, *Circulation* 86:919, 1992.)

node; in two patients it was superior along the tendon of Todaro. The fast pathway was anterior (superior) to the compact AV node. Both pathways were anatomically distinct from the compact AV node.

His Bundle
Location

At the apex of the triangle of Koch, the compact AV node becomes the penetrating His bundle, which crosses through the central fibrous body (annulus fibrosus) while encased in its insulating tissues and passes into the ventricular septum posterior to the membranous septum.[6] Normal cardiac conduction depends on the isolation of the atrial musculature from the ventricular musculature (except at the point at which the His bundle penetrates the annulus fibrosus). The His bundle has longitudinal strands of Purkinje-like cells with loosely arrayed mitochondria and few myofibrils.

In some hearts the penetrating His bundle may continue and thus warrant the title of nonbranching bundle. In other hearts, branching begins as soon as the bundle has penetrated the annulus fibrosus.[1]

Blood supply

The upper muscular ventricular septum (wherein the His bundle lies) receives its blood supply from branches of the left anterior and posterior descending coronary arteries.[7] This double blood supply makes this important link of the conduction system less vulnerable to ischemic damage.[8]

BUNDLE BRANCHES

At approximately 6 weeks of gestation the bundle branches in the embryonic heart can be seen cascading down both sides of the septum, with ramifications into the trabeculated pouches. At 18 weeks of gestation the left bundle branch (LBB) is recognizable as a fanlike structure and the right bundle branch (RBB) as a cordlike structure.[9]

The bundle branches begin on the crest or on the left side of the muscular intraventricular septum. Throughout their course through the ventricles, the bundle branches are encased in sheaths of fibrous tissue, which insulate them from the ventricular myocardium.[1] Ventricular activation occurs once the impulses emerge from the Purkinje fibers. The cells of the bundle branches are called Purkinje cells and are large and vacuolated. The major intercellular connection of Purkinje fibers involves an end-to-end structure through gap junctions (p. 24); this structure enhances conduction velocity.

Left Bundle Branch
Location

The LBB, originally described by Tawara[10] in 1906, begins as a single structure and fans out into three divisions (Figure 1-7). This fan of conductive fibers streams down the left ventricular septum in a "virtual sheet" to form large posterior, smaller anterior, and midseptal radiations (Figure 1-8).[1] The third midseptal radiation was also noted by Demoulin and Kulbertus[11,12] in 33 out of 49 normal hearts (type I in Figure 1-9). This lesser-known fascicle was readily identified by these investigators and was found to originate either from the common left bundle or from the anterior or posterior fascicle. In

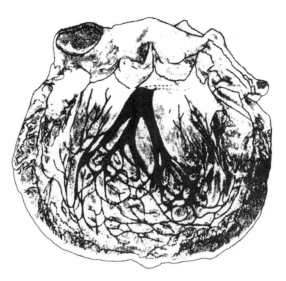

FIGURE 1-7 Human left bundle branch anatomy as depicted by Tawara in 1906, showing three divisions of the left bundle branch.

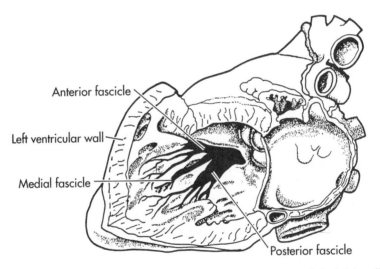

FIGURE 1-8 Left ventricle opened to show a simplified representation of the left bundle branch with its anterior (superior), medial (septal), and posterior (inferior) divisions.

the remaining 16 cases the septum was supplied by radiations from the posterior fascicle or by combined radiations from both the anterior and posterior fascicles.

Demoulin and Kulbertus observed the following[11,12]:

1. There are three, not two, main interconnecting fascicles in the left ventricle. One fascicle supplies the anterior (superior) wall, another the posterior (inferior) wall, and a third the midseptum.

Type I

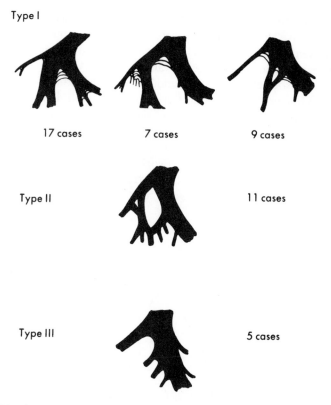

17 cases   7 cases   9 cases

Type II   11 cases

Type III   5 cases

FIGURE 1-9 Distribution of left bundle branch fibers in 49 human hearts. (From Kulbertus HE, Demoulin J: Pathological basis of concept of left hemiblock. In Wellens HJJ, Lie KI, Janse MJ, editors: *The conduction system of the heart,* Hingnamma, 1976, Martinus Nijhoff.)

2. The electrocardiographic pattern of left anterior hemiblock reflects LBB disease and is hardly ever confined entirely to the anterior fascicle.

Blood supply

The posterior fascicle of the LBB receives its blood supply from both the left anterior descending and posterior descending coronary arteries. The anterior and medial fascicles of the LBB are supplied mainly by septal perforators from the left anterior descending coronary artery.

Right Bundle Branch

The RBB descends in its sheath subendocardially to the bases of the medial and anterior papillary muscles; it becomes a subendocardial structure in the middle and lower third of the ventricular septum. At its origin it is a direct continuation of the penetrating bundle along the right side of the ventricular septum; it remains unbranched until it reaches the apex of the right ventricle. It descends as a cordlike structure and emerges from its septal subendocardial course to continue beneath the medial papillary muscle of the tricuspid valve (Figure 1-10). It proceeds down the septal band, where it penetrates the right ventricular apex and sends a branch through the moderator band to the anterior papillary muscle of the tricuspid valve.

The difference in size between the right and left bundle branches is striking and explains why the RBB can be compromised by a lesser lesion than can the larger LBB. This fact may account for the common clinical innocence of right bundle branch block (RBBB).

Terminal Purkinje Fibers

The bundle branches terminate in a network of fibers on the endocardial surfaces of the ventricles. This network is very difficult to trace. The terminal Purkinje fibers tend to be concentrated at papillary muscles and tend to penetrate the subendocardial and myocardial tissue.[8]

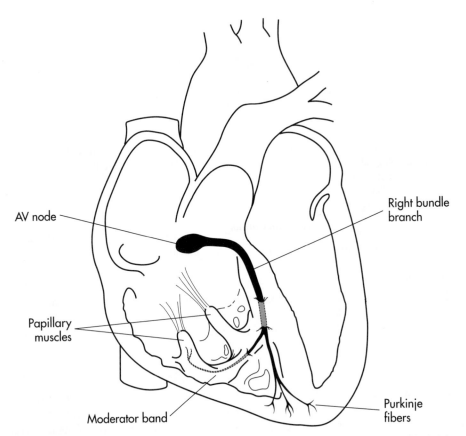

FIGURE 1-10 Right bundle branch. Note its cordlike structure as opposed to the fanlike bundle branch.

INNERVATION OF THE CARDIAC CONDUCTION SYSTEM

In keeping with its important role of pacing and regulating the heart rhythm, the nerve supply to the conduction system of the heart is more generous than to the myocardium. Within the conduction system itself, the *SA node* is the most densely innervated region, with the nerve fibers and fascicles distributed between nodal cells in the fibrous tissue matrix. Within the SA node, the central region around the nodal artery is more densely innervated than the nodal periphery. The opposite is true in the *AV node*, where the density of nerve fibers and nerve trunks is greater in the transitional region than in the compact node. In the penetrating *His bundle* and *bundle branches*, the density of nerves is significantly higher than that in the ventricular myocardium but is much lower than that in the AV node. As shown by Crick, Wharton, Sheppard et al,[4] the vagal inhibitory dominance of the heart is confirmed by the predominance of acetylcholinesterase-positive activity in the SA node and transitional region of the AV node.

REFERENCES

1. Anderson RH, Becker AE: Anatomy of the conduction tissues and accessory atrioventricular connections. In Zipes DP, Jalife J, editors: *Cardiac electrophysiology from cell to bedside,* Philadelphia, 1990, WB Saunders.
2. Bleeker WK, Mackay AJC, Masson-Pevet M et al: Functional and morphological organization of the rabbit sinus node, *Circ Res* 46:11, 1980.
3. Racker DK: Atrioventricular node and input pathways: a correlated gross anatomical and histological study of canine atrioventricular junctional region, *Anat Rec* 224:336, 1989.
4. Crick SJ, Wharton J, Sheppard MN et al: Innervation of the human cardiac conduction system: a quantitative immunohistochemical and histochemical study, *Circulation* 89:1697, 1994.
5. Keim S, Werner P, Jazayeri M et al: Localization of the fast and slow pathways in atrioventricular nodal reentrant tachycardia by intraoperative ice mapping, *Circulation* 86:919, 1992.
6. Ferguson TB Jr, Cox JL: Surgical treatment of arrhythmias. In Willerson JT, Cohn JN, editors: *Cardiovascular medicine,* New York, 1995, Churchill Livingstone.
7. James TN: Anatomy for the conduction system of the heart. In Hurst JW, editor: *The heart,* New York, 1982, McGraw-Hill.
8. Waller BF, Gering LE, Branyas NA, Slack JD: Anatomy, histology, and pathology of the cardiac conduction system. Part I, *Clin Cardiol* 16:249, 1993.
9. Anderson RD, Davies MJ, Becker AM: The development of the cardiac specialized tissue. In Wellens HJJ, Lie KI, Janse MJ, editors: *The conduction system of the heart,* Philadelphia, 1976, Lea & Febiger.
10. Tawara S: *Das Reizleitungssystem des Saugetierherzens,* Jena, 1906, Gustav Fischer.
11. Demoulin JC, Kulbertus HE: Histopathological examination of concept of left hemiblock, *Br Heart J* 34:809, 1972.
12. Kulbertus HE, Demoulin J: Pathological basis of concept of left hemiblock. In Wellens HJJ, Lie KI, Janse MJ, editors: *The conduction system of the heart,* Philadelphia, 1976, Lea & Febiger.

CHAPTER 2

Membrane Channels

Overview 13
Normal cell function 13
Selective permeability and
 the resting membrane
 potential 14
Depolarization 14
Repolarization 15
Threshold potential 15
Automaticity 15
Membrane pumps 15
Membrane channels 17
Gap junctions 24

C ARDIAC CELLULAR ELECTROPHYSIOLOGY HAS EXPANDED DRAMATICALLY DURING the last decade. The development of new techniques has provided an opportunity to study molecular structures of single ion channels, pumps, and receptors, which has enhanced the ability to identify drug targets and understand the nature of drug-target interaction.[1,2] This chapter reviews normal cellular electrophysiology and membrane channels. Subsequent chapters discuss action potentials and molecular targets for antiarrhythmic drugs (i.e., channels, pumps, and receptors), as well as physiologic drug action.

OVERVIEW

A cardiac muscle fiber is a complex electrochemical entity that, when stimulated, propagates electrical impulses and contracts. These actions are made possible by the cyclic changes in the transmembrane potential gradient *(membrane potential)* that occur within each cardiac cell with each heartbeat. All cells in the heart are electrically active, with different cell groups responsible for specialized activity. The electrical signal that is generated and propagated in the heart is also thought to be responsible for the release of atrionaturetic factor (ANF), or atrionaturetic peptide.[3] During the electrical cardiac cycle, nonpacemaker cells (atrial and ventricular muscle cells) do not respond until they are driven to *threshold potential* by an outside stimulus. This period of electrical stability occurs during *electrical diastole* and is called the *resting membrane potential.*

In contrast, pacemaker cells, which are found in the sinoatrial (SA) and atrioventricular (AV) nodes and in His-Purkinje fibers, do not "rest" in this way. Near the onset of electrical diastole they briefly reach their *maximum diastolic potential,* after which they become less and less negative *(slow diastolic depolarization)* as they spontaneously depolarize toward threshold potential. In normal hearts the SA node reaches threshold first and initiates the propagated action potential. All other cells are stimulated by this propagated action potential, which constitutes the required outside source.

NORMAL CELL FUNCTION

Normal cell function depends on many mechanisms, including the following:
1. Selective permeability of the sarcolemma. During diastole, for example, potassium ions (K^+) diffuse more readily through the sarcolemma than do sodium ions (Na^+).
2. Specialized molecular pumps. For example, the Na^+-K^+ adenosine triphosphatase (ATPase) pump transports Na^+ out of the cell and K^+ into the cell. This pump

maintains the low intracellular concentration of Na^+ and high intracellular concentration of K^+.

3. Maintenance of ion gradients across the sarcolemma. These ion gradients underlie the resting potential, the action potential, and *excitation-contraction coupling*, in which contractions are triggered by the influx of calcium ions (Ca^{2+}) through channels in the sarcolemma.

4. Specialized channels. Specialized channels allow the selective passage of ions across the cell membrane and permit the control of electrical activity of the heart.

5. Muscle contractions. Rapid changes in intracellular calcium ($[Ca^{2+}]_i$) underlie the "triggering" of muscle contractions.

SELECTIVE PERMEABILITY AND THE RESTING MEMBRANE POTENTIAL

Resting membrane potential is the voltage that exists across the cell membrane when a point of equilibrium is reached between the pull of the electrical gradient to keep K^+ in the cell and the push of the concentration gradient for K^+ to leave the cell.

To visualize this concept, imagine a cell with a membrane that is highly permeable to K^+ and relatively impermeable to Na^+. This cell is filled with a solution that has a high concentration of K^+ and a low concentration of Na^+. The extracellular fluid is just the opposite; it has a high concentration of Na^+ and a low concentration of K^+. The membrane is permeable to chloride ions (Cl^-), which makes both the intracellular and extracellular solution electrically neutral.

Driven by the concentration gradient across the cell membrane, K^+ tends to leave the cell. Na^+ on the outside of the cell is also driven by the concentration gradient but is stopped by the membrane, which is impermeable to Na^+. The result is a positive ionic current carried by the efflux of K^+ from the cell. Because of this movement, there is a slight deficit of positive charge, and the inside of the cell becomes negatively charged relative to the outside. As this membrane potential becomes more negative, the electrical field generated inside the cell exerts more pull to keep K^+ in the cell. Eventually, the electrical field and the concentration gradient exert equal but opposing influences on K^+, and the current flow stops. This equilibrium point is called the *resting membrane potential* and is approximately -90 mV in atrial and ventricular muscle cells.[4] During electrical activation, Na^+ pours into the cell through transiently open Na^+ channels. An active pump (the Na^+-K^+ ATPase pump) is required to rid the cell of Na^+ and replace the lost K^+.

DEPOLARIZATION

Depolarization is the process by which the negativity of a cell is reduced. During diastole, the maximum negative potential of the membrane of an atrial or ventricular myocardial cell or a His-Purkinje cell is approximately -90 mV. If this potential is reduced to a less negative voltage, depolarization has occurred.

There are two types of normal depolarization: (1) slow "pacemaker" diastolic (phase 4) depolarization, which was discussed previously; and (2) rapid (phase 0) depolarization.

Rapid depolarization is the sudden reversal of membrane potential that occurs when a normal atrial or ventricular cell reaches threshold potential. This abrupt process depends on the availability of a large number of Na^+ and Ca^{2+} channels (p. 17), which in turn depends on the negativity of the resting membrane potential. The greater the negativity, the greater the number of Na^+ and Ca^{2+} channels available for activation.

REPOLARIZATION

Repolarization is the process by which the cell returns to its resting state after excitation. It is accomplished by several mechanisms, the most prominent of which are the closing of Ca^{2+} channels, the exodus of K^+ from the cell, and the ongoing activity of the Na^+-K^+ pump. The process of repolarization is explained in more detail in Chapter 3.

THRESHOLD POTENTIAL

The threshold potential is the voltage to which the cell membrane must be reduced before it can be activated regeneratively. Normally only the pacemaker cells of the SA node achieve threshold potential without outside help. In the remainder of the heart the cells are driven to threshold potential by a propagating regenerative action potential, which originates in the SA node. The threshold potential in the healthy atrial and ventricular muscle cells of the heart lies between -65 and -75 mV; the threshold potential of the cells in the SA and AV nodes is approximately -50 mV.

AUTOMATICITY

Automaticity is the capability of a cell to depolarize spontaneously, reach threshold potential, and initiate a propagated action potential. Normally this property is exercised only by the SA node and held in reserve by the latent pacemaker cells of the AV node and His-Purkinje system.

MEMBRANE PUMPS

Within the sarcolemma there are at least two pumps that depend on adenosine triphosphate (ATP) for their energy: the Na^+-K^+ ATPase pump and the ATP-dependent Ca^{2+} pumps. These pumps are able to transport ions against their electrochemical gradients (upstream).

Na^+-K^+ ATPase (Sodium) Pump

The sodium pump is an electrogenic transporter. For each enzyme cycle one molecule of ATP is hydrolyzed; in a ping-pong fashion three sodium ions are transported to the outside of the cell in exchange for two potassium ions (Figure 2-1). This process depends on ATP hydrolysis and uses the energy released to move Na^+ and K^+ against their electrochemical gradients. There are two basic subunits of the Na^+-K^+ ATPase protein: alpha and beta. The alpha subunit spans the sarcolemma and is on the extracellular side of the sarcolemma. When present, ouabain competes with K^+ for a binding site. The ATP binding site (beta subunit) is on the cytoplasmic side of the membrane.[5]

The following is a partial list of sodium pump functions:

1. Ensures a large negative resting potential. A negative resting potential is indirectly created by Na^+-K^+ pumping. It guarantees a large K^+ gradient by continually restoring K^+ to the inside of the cell and by removing the Na^+ that enters during depolarization and via background currents.

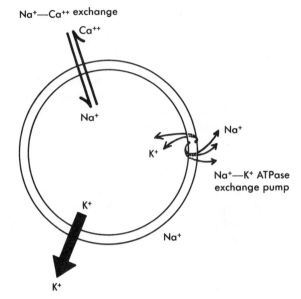

FIGURE 2-1 The Na$^+$-K$^+$ ATPase pump removes three sodium ions from the cell for every two potassium ions, creating an electrogenic current with a net positive flow to the outside. The cell is permeable to K$^+$ but not to Na$^+$; therefore K$^+$ leaves the cell down its concentration gradient, which is always being replenished by the Na$^+$-K$^+$ ATPase pump. This exodus of K$^+$ from the cell produces a net positive current to the outside. Together the pump and the K$^+$ gradient create and maintain the resting membrane potential. The lack of Na$^+$ in the cell allows the cell to rid itself of free Ca^{2+} by the Na$^+$-Ca^{2+} exchange. (From Conover M: *Understanding electrocardiography,* ed 5, St Louis, 1988, Mosby.)

2. Ensures excitability. The Na$^+$-K$^+$ pump ensures excitability because activation of the cell involves a large influx of Na$^+$ (rapid depolarization). If Na$^+$ were already in the cell, this large influx could not occur.
3. Contributes negativity to the resting membrane potential. The Na$^+$-K$^+$ pump has a direct electrogenic effect because it removes three sodium ions from the cell for every potassium ion restored, which creates a net negative electrical current to the inside (up to 10 mV during the resting state of the cell).[5] The term *electrogenic* refers to the generation of a current that directly contributes to the cell membrane potential.[6] This electrogenic pump current figures importantly in the mechanism termed *overdrive suppression* (p. 37).
4. Produces the Na$^+$ gradient that provides the energy for the removal of free Ca^{2+} and hydrogen ions (H$^+$) (indirect function).

ATP-dependent Ca^{2+} Pump

The sarcolemmic Ca^{2+} pump transports free intracellular Ca^{2+} out of the cell. However, this transfer removes only a small fraction of the Ca^{2+} that leaks into the cell. Almost all of the Ca^{2+} that enters heart cells is removed by the Na$^+$-Ca^{2+} exchange. A different ATP-dependent Ca^{2+} pump transports Ca^{2+} back into the sarcoplasmic reticulum following contraction.[5]

MEMBRANE CHANNELS

There are four major time-dependent and voltage-gated membrane channels[3]:

- I_{Na}: The ionic sodium current responsible for rapid depolarization in atrial and ventricular muscle and in Purkinje fibers
- I_{Ca}: The ionic calcium current responsible for depolarization in the SA and AV nodes and for triggering contraction in all cardiomyocytes
- I_K: The ionic repolarizing potassium current responsible for the repolarization of all cardiomyocytes
- I_f: The ionic pacemaker current, which is partly responsible for pacemaker activity in SA and AV nodal cells and in Purkinje fibers

The SA and AV nodes are controlled by the interaction of I_{Ca}, I_K, and I_f. Atrial and ventricular muscle fibers are controlled by the interaction of I_{Na}, I_{Ca}, and I_K. Purkinje fibers are controlled by all four channels.

Membrane channels (depicted by Rosen and Wit[7] in Figure 2-2), can be visualized as protein pores that traverse the cell membrane from outside to inside.[8] They are composed of a channel protein, a selectivity filter, and gating proteins. When appropriately stimulated, they permit ions to pass rapidly across the membrane and are often highly selective for either Na^+, Ca^{2+}, or K^+.

As shown in Figure 2-2, the channel protein (white area) separates the portal itself from the lipid bilayer of the cell membrane (shaded area). The selectivity filter is situated near the outer surface of the channel and has a diameter specific for certain ions; it guards the channel and is ion-specific. For example, the selectivity filter for the fast channel is specific for Na^+ with its waters of hydration, but hydrogen ions may also pass through.[9]

The stimuli for opening the membrane channels include voltage, receptor occupation, chemical signals, and mechanical deformation. *Voltage-operated channels* open in response to a certain voltage; *receptor-operated channels* open when specific substances such as norepinephrine, histamine, acetylcholine, and adenosine interact with specific receptors on the surface of the cell. Once open, such channels may either inactivate (i.e., close despite a maintained stimulation) or stay open until a different signal causes them to close. Channels that inactivate must first recover from the inactive state before they can again respond to a stimulus. The inactive state is time-dependent and sometimes voltage-dependent. The magnitude of the currents through some channels (e.g., K_{ATP}, p. 23) varies with physiologic and pathophysiologic conditions.

Gating is the process whereby channels change their conformation in response to an external stimulus.[2] Gating kinetics can be rapid (<1 ms) or slow (seconds). The channels that carry Na^+ and Ca^{2+} are activated by depolarization and undergo inactivation. *Permeation* is the ability of a channel to conduct ions once it is open.

Sodium Channels (I_{Na})

Sodium channels carry a large Na^+ current into the cell to produce rapid depolarization. Sodium current is the largest current in heart muscle because of the number of

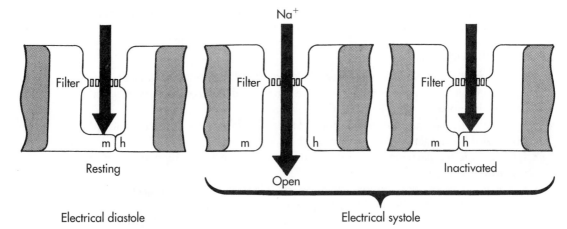

FIGURE 2-2 The fast sodium channel during its resting, open, and inactivated states. Note the selectivity filter toward the extracellular surface of the membrane. The gates are voltage-dependent. (Modified from Rosen MR, Wit AL: Arrhythmogenic actions of antiarrhythmic drugs, *Am J Cardiol* 59(11):10E, 1987.)

channels involved (possibly as many as 200 channels per square micron).[3] The rapid upstroke of the action potential and the robust impulse conduction is a result of the large Na^+ current in atrial, ventricular, and His-Purkinje cells. In the SA and AV nodes, sodium channels are sparse or absent; the conducted action potential depends on calcium channels (see the following section).

Features

The most important features of Na^+ channels are their large number, voltage-dependent gating, and ability to open quickly.[10] Together these features permit rapid depolarization and fast conduction velocity. Another feature of fast Na^+ channels is a binding spot between the selectivity filter and the gates where certain anesthetic agents such as lidocaine may bind, partially blocking I_{Na} (see Chapter 14).

Gates

Na^+ channels have two gates, which are designated as "m" and "h" and can assume one of three states (see Figure 2-2):
1. Resting state. The channel is closed but excitable ("m" is closed and "h" is open).
2. Open state. The channel is open briefly (hundreds of microseconds) when the "m" gate opens. After being activated by the local depolarization produced by the conducted action potential, the channel moves briefly to an *open* position when its threshold potential of -70 mV is reached. In response to the high concentration gradient and the electrical gradient, sodium enters through the open channel, which results in phase 0 depolarization of the action potential (see Chapter 3).
3. Inactivated state. The channel is closed but not excitable. The "h" gate is voltage-dependent and closes in response to the positive voltage caused by the Na^+ influx. The channel is now *inactivated* and remains so until the cell repolarizes to approximately

−60 to −70 mV. At this time the "m" gate closes and the "h" gate opens to return the cell to its resting state (closed but excitable). The initiation of the inactivated state is partially responsible for phase 1 of the action potential (rapid repolarization), after which a very small but important component of I_{Na} is maintained to help prolong the refractory period (phase 2 of the action potential).[3]

Calcium Channels (I_{Ca})

Like sodium channels, calcium channels carry currents into the cell. Relatively small amounts of Ca^{2+} enter the cell during the cardiac cycle, whereas much larger amounts move into and out of the sarcoplasmic reticulum.[11]

I_{Ca} currents serve the following functions[3]:
1. To activate the release of Ca^{2+} from the sarcoplasmic reticulum in atrial and ventricular muscle cells by the process known as Ca^{2+}-induced Ca^{2+} release (CICR)
2. To contribute to pacemaker activity in the SA node
3. To provide the regenerative action potential in the SA and AV nodes
4. To prolong the refractory period by maintaining a small I_{Ca} during phase 2 of the action potential
5. To provide an electrical delay between atrial and ventricular contractions, with a smaller current during phase 0 of the action potential in the AV node and thus a slower conduction and slower discharge of membrane capacitance of neighboring cells
6. To contribute to phase 0 of the action potential (along with I_{Na}) in atrial, ventricular, and Purkinje fibers, thus increasing conduction velocity in these fibers

As with Na^+ channels, the gates of Ca^{2+} channels are closed (resting state) at very negative potentials. They rapidly activate (in approximately 1 ms) and, while the membrane is still positive, inactivate.

There are at least four types of channels that normally carry Ca^{2+} in cardiac cells—two on the cell membrane (L-type and T-type) and two within the cell itself (the ryanodine receptor [RyR] and inositol triphosphate receptor [IP$_3$R] channels).[12] Within the SA and AV nodes, conduction of the cardiac impulse depends on inward current through Ca^{2+} channels, which explains why Ca^{2+} channel blockers preferentially slow AV conduction.

The intracellular Ca^{2+} channels (i.e., the RyR and IP$_3$R) are located in the sarcoplasmic reticulum and mediate the release of Ca^{2+} from that intracellular store. In heart muscle the RyR is the dominant Ca^{2+} release channel.

The L- and T-type channels differ from each other in the voltage range of activation and inactivation, in the manner in which they open and close, in their numbers in the sarcolemma, and in their responses to drugs. The L-type Ca^{2+} channels are referred to clinically; they predominate in all cardiac tissues, and they have receptors for and are partially blocked by verapamil, diltiazem, and nifedipine.

An increase in Ca^{2+} current through L-type channels speeds conduction in the AV node and in all cardiac cells, prolongs the action potential, and increases the height of its plateau. In contrast, blockade of Ca^{2+} current reduces conduction velocity in the AV node and shortens the action potential duration in all cardiac myocytes. The L-type Ca^{2+} channels are thought to interact with regulatory proteins, which allows them to be controlled by a number of intrinsic and extrinsic factors. This modulation of I_{Ca} thus influences the electrical behavior of the heart and also can influence the force of contraction (see the following paragraphs).[13]

The L-type Ca^{2+} channels mediate the effects of sympathetic stimulation, producing an increase in Ca^{2+} current during each action potential. L-type channels are also modulated by the actions of magnesium (Mg^{2+}). Magnesium can change the amount of Ca^{2+} that goes through Ca^{2+} channels, and it has other important actions. For example, each step in the complicated process of phosphorylation of channel proteins requires Mg^{2+} and/or a magnesium nucleotide.

T-type Ca^{2+} channels are smaller than the L-type Ca^{2+} channels, and their function is not fully defined. They are found at a lower density than L-type channels and may play a role in pacemaker activity.

Contraction, relaxation, and removal of calcium from the cell

Ca^{2+} enters the cell most strikingly during phase 0 of the action potential through voltage-activated L-type Ca^{2+} channels. The close proximity of RyR to L-type Ca^{2+} channels permits the influx of Ca^{2+} through the L-type Ca^{2+} channels, which triggers RyRs to open through CICR.[14,15] This amplification of the triggering Ca^{2+} influx raises Ca^{2+} sufficiently so that Ca^{2+} can bind to the contractile protein troponin C and initiate contraction.

Following contraction most of the intracellular Ca^{2+} is pumped back into the sarcoplasmic reticulum (the intracellular stores) by the Ca^{2+} ATPase or extruded from the cell by the Na^+-Ca^{2+} exchanges. If the sodium gradient is reduced, Ca^{2+} accumulates inside the cell.

Both the toxic and the therapeutic effects of digitalis are related to an excess (toxic) and an increase (therapeutic) of intracellular Ca^{2+}. The normal intracellular handling of Ca^{2+} is illustrated in Figure 2-3. Relaxation is initiated by the separation of Ca^{2+} from the binding spots on the contractile proteins and by the removal of Ca^{2+} from the cytoplasm during diastole through four main mechanisms[16]:

1. It is pumped back into the sarcoplasmic reticulum by an ATPase-dependent pump.[17]
2. It is extruded from the cell by the Na^+-Ca^{2+} exchange (see the following section).[18,19]
3. It is pumped out of the cell by an ATPase-dependent pump.[20]
4. It binds to intracellular calcium buffers.

Na^+-Ca^{2+} exchanger

The Na^+-Ca^{2+} exchanger is an electrogenic transporter that normally moves three sodium ions into the cell and extrudes one calcium ion. It serves the following functions[3]:

1. To contribute an inward depolarizing current
2. To prolong the plateau phase of the action potential
3. To contribute to depolarization during diastole

The relative absence of Na^+ in the cell provides an inward sodium gradient across the sarcolemma and an energy source that can be used to rid the cell of Ca^{2+}. The sodium/calcium countertransport system uses this Na^+ gradient to extrude Ca^{2+} by transporting three sodium ions into the cell for each calcium ion pumped out of the cell. This transporter is the chief means of Ca^{2+} efflux through the sarcolemma and is responsible for extruding the Ca^{2+} that enters the heart cells during I_{Ca}.[2]

Potassium Rectifying Channels

Currents through potassium channels are complementary to sodium currents; sodium currents depolarize, whereas potassium currents repolarize. Potassium rectifying channels conduct ions across the membrane more effectively in one direction than in the other.[2] For example, a strong rectifying current occurs when the channel is open at some membrane potentials and closed at others.[9] There are also other means of rectification.

Outward K^+ rectifier currents can both prolong and shorten the refractory period according to heart rate. They may also mediate physiologic reactions. For example, they enable the parasympathetic nervous system to inhibit cardiac functions and the sympathetic nervous system to enhance them.

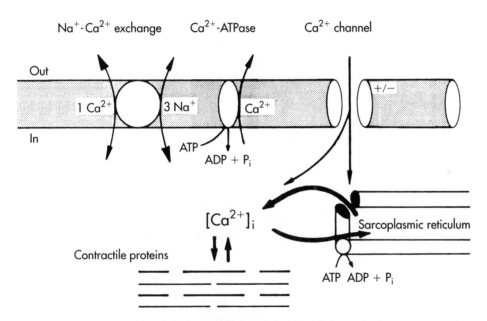

FIGURE 2-3 Schema of intracellular calcium (Ca^{2+}) handling in a ventricular myocyte. Ca^{2+} enters the cell through voltage-activated calcium channels and triggers the release of calcium from the sarcoplasmic reticulum. Intracellular calcium increases and binds to troponin C, initiating contraction. Relaxation is initiated by the separation of Ca^{2+} from the calcium-binding contractile proteins and removal from the cytoplasm by sarcolemmic Ca^{2+}-ATPase, extrusion via the Na^+-Ca^{2+} exchange system, calcium reuptake by Ca^{2+}-ATPase of the sarcoplasmic reticulum, and binding to intracellular calcium buffers. (From Beuckelmann DJ, Näbauer M, Krüger C, Erdmann E: Altered diastolic [Ca^{2+}]$_i$ handling in human ventricular myocytes from patients with terminal heart failure, *Am Heart J* 129:684, 1995.)

In cardiac tissue, there are at least seven relevant K^+ channels through which K^+ moves across the cell membrane. In all cases K^+ channels carry outward currents during the action potential and thus tend to shorten the action potential. Five of the relevant K^+ channels are discussed in the following sections[21]:

1. Delayed rectifier (I_K)
2. Inward K^+ rectifier (I_{K1})
3. Transient outward K^+ current (I_{to})
4. Acetylcholine-activated inward K^+ rectifier ($I_{K(ACh)}$)
5. ATP-activated K^+ current (K_{ATP})

Delayed rectifier current (I_K)

The delayed rectifier current, also called the repolarizing K^+ current, is the K^+ current with the largest effect on ventricular repolarization. It activates long after phase 0, thus ensuring that the refractory period is long enough at normal heart rates to protect the heart from premature excitation and early beats yet short enough during tachycardia to allow for repolarization and a resting, diastolic phase between beats.

I_K has two components: rapidly activated (I_{Kr}) and slowly activated (I_{Ks}). Most of the currently available potassium channel blockers (e.g., D-sotolol) block I_{Kr}; isoproterenol activates I_{Ks}.[22] Blockade of I_{Ks} prolongs action potential duration according to the density of the channels, the heart rate, and the neurohormonal status of the heart. β-Adrenergic stimulation may augment I_{Ks} and its effect on repolarization; an increase in heart rate may enhance the ability of I_{Ks} to prolong action potential duration.[23] Some available I_{Ks} blockers are tedisamil, amiodarone, quinidine, clofilium, and dofetilide.

The effects of drugs on the components of I_K are further discussed in Chapter 14.

DURING NORMAL RHYTHMS. Following rapid depolarization of the cell the outward flow of K^+ slowly increases with time until eventually it exceeds the inward positive currents (Ca^{2+} and Na^+) and thus terminates the plateau phase of the action potential.

DURING TACHYCARDIA. During rapid heart rates the time between action potentials is insufficient to fully deactivate the outward flow of K^+. As a result, a fraction of the action potential continues during the cardiac cycle. It thus contributes to the progressive shortening of the action potential, which is reflected in the decreasing duration of the QT interval during tachycardia.

Inward K^+ rectifier current (I_{K1})

The steady-state inward K^+ current (I_{K1}) is seen in atrial, AV nodal, His-Purkinje, and ventricular cells.[2,24] It is called an inward rectifier because the channel current decreases during depolarization and increases with membrane hyperpolarization.

I_{K1} contributes critically to the maintenance of the resting membrane potential and maintains it near the potassium equilibrium potential. It is small or absent in SA nodal cells, which permits the small SA nodal currents to control the heart rate.[2]

An important feature of I_{K1} current is that it allows inward current more readily than outward current. I_{K1} current is confined functionally to a small voltage range between the resting potential and -30 mV. Therefore it contributes to the terminal part of phase 3 (repolarization).

Blockage of the I_{K1} channel may prolong action potential duration slightly. Inhibiting this channel may induce membrane depolarization when there is an increase of inward currents and may produce arrhythmia.[23]

Transient outward K+ current (I_{to})

After rapid depolarization, a transient outward K+ current (I_{to}) rapidly activates and inactivates. It is voltage-activated and plays a role in modifying action potential duration. Because it is present in subepicardial but not subendocardial muscle cells, I_{to} contributes to the heterogeneity of repolarization.[2] This current contributes to the notch (phase 1) that immediately follows the upstroke of the action potential in Purkinje and ventricular cells.

Blockage of I_{to} decreases the rate of repolarization during the plateau and elevates the early plateau voltage. Suppression of I_{to} by pharmacologic agents can prolong the duration of the action potential.[23]

Acetylcholine-activated K+ currents ($I_{K(ACh)}$; $I_{K(Ado)}$)

In SA and AV nodal cells, stimulation of the parasympathetic nervous system leads to the release of acetylcholine. This release activates an outward K+ current ($I_{K(ACh)}$) during phase 3 and phase 4 of the action potential. The exodus of K+ from the cell during repolarization drives the cell to a more negative maximum diastolic potential than it could otherwise achieve. From this "super-negative" position, it takes longer for the cell to depolarize during diastole and to reach threshold potential. This and the reduction of I_{Ca} by acetylcholine accounts for the negative chronotropic action of vagal stimuli.

Acetylcholine-activated K+ channels are also opened by activation of the adenosine receptor and therefore are also called $I_{K(Ado)}$. Thus adenosine (Adenocard) has a dramatic slowing action on the rate of the SA node and AV node conduction.

Studies have also shown that the heart rate will decrease even when the level of acetylcholine is ineffective in activating the $I_{K(ACh)}$ current. This decrease can occur because of the strong inhibiting effect that acetylcholine has on the pacemaker current (I_f) and on I_{Ca} (Figure 2-4).[25,26]

Adenosine triphosphate–activated potassium current (K_{ATP})

ATP-sensitive potassium channels (K_{ATP}) are inhibited by physiologic levels of intracellular ATP and are activated during ischemia or anoxia. This activation possibly contributes to shortening of the action potential during ischemia. This K+ current can be made to increase or decrease with experimentally available antiarrhythmic drugs.[2] Lederer and Nichols[27] have found that K_{ATP} channel activity becomes more and more intense during contractile failure, which reflects the decline of intracellular ATP. These channels close when contractile activity returns.

Pacemaker Current (I_f)

The pacemaker current (I_f) is found in SA and AV nodal cells and in Purkinje fibers. I_f is unique in that it does not activate at positive potentials as do other currents but instead is activated when the cell *hyperpolarizes*. That is, at the end of phase 3 of the action potential—when the cell is at its most negative potential (maximal diastolic potential)—

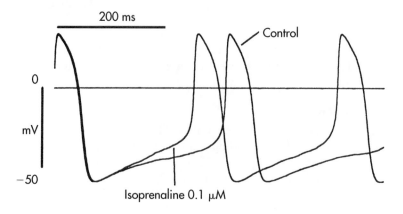

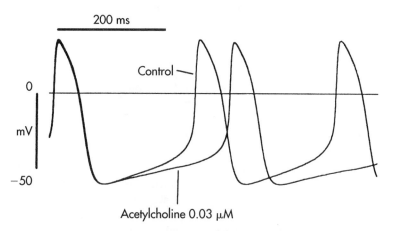

FIGURE 2-4 Rate modulation by low adrenergic and cholinergic agonist concentrations in isolated SA nodal myocytes. Note that both the acceleratory action of isoprenaline *(top panel)* and the slowing action of acetylcholine *(bottom panel)* occur with no appreciable alteration of the shape or duration of the action potential. (From DiFrancesco D, Mangoni M, Maccaferri G: The pacemaker current in cardiac cells. In Zipes DP, Jalife J, editors: *Cardiac electrophysiology from cell to bedside,* ed 2, Philadelphia, 1995, WB Saunders.)

I_f "turns on," opposing the repolarization process and contributing to the onset of diastolic depolarization. At diastolic potentials it slowly begins to produce an inward positive current carried by Na^+ and K^+. Equally important to pacemaker depolarization are I_{Ca} and the time-dependent deactivation of I_K.

It is well known that the rate of the SA nodal discharge is controlled by the opposing actions of sympathetic (acceleration) and parasympathetic (deceleration) inputs. As previously stated, these neurohormones have opposing actions on I_{Ca}, I_K, and I_f.

GAP JUNCTIONS

Much has been learned about gap junctions and more is being learned on an almost-daily basis. Gap junctions were previously defined simply as highly specialized cell-to-

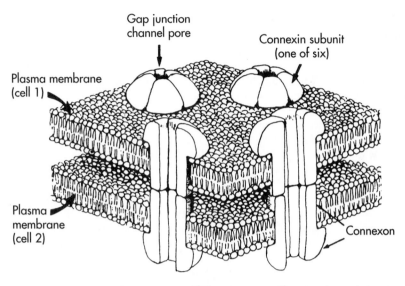

FIGURE 2-5 Gap junction channels consist of two connexons aligned end to end, forming a cytoplasm-filled connection between the interior of two juxtaposed cells. Each connexon consists of six hexagonally arranged protein subunits, or connexins. (From Jongsma HJ, Rook MB: Morphology and electrophysiology of cardiac gap junction channels. In Zipes DP, Jalife J, editors: *Cardiac electrophysiology from cell to bedside,* ed 2, Philadelphia, 1995, WB Saunders.)

cell low resistance channels that permit the direct exchange of ions and small metabolites, coupling cardiac cells electrically and chemically. The discovery of the patch clamp technique has generated an incredible amount of information about cellular electrophysiology. Jogsma and Rook[28] provide a detailed review of the morphology and electrophysiology of cardiac gap junction channels.

It is now known that cardiac gap junctions form cell-to-cell connections and consist of arrays of intercellular channels that are subdivided into small groups of approximately 40 channels. Each gap junction channel is halved so that two opposing cells are directly connected (Figure 2-5). *Connexons* is the name given to these hemichannels; the connexon is composed of six identical subunits called *connexins.* Connexins are under intense investigation using connexin-specific antibody and DNA probes, recombinant expression techniques, and electrophysiologic techniques. It is through the intercellular channels contained within gap junctions that the cardiac current is transferred from one cell to another. This unique pathway permits very rapid propagation of the cardiac action potential. Because of the larger number of gap junctions at the ends of cardiac myocytes compared with the number on the sides, the electrical impulse velocity is much greater along the length of the fiber *(isotropic conduction)* than across the fiber bundle *(anisotropic conduction).*[29]

REFERENCES

1. Hamill OP, Martz A, Neher E et al: Improved patch clamp techniques for high-resolution current recording from cells and cell-free membrane patches, *Pflugers Arch* 391:85, 1981.
2. Task Force of the Working Group on Arrhythmias of the European Society of Cardiology: The Sicilian gambit: a new approach to the classification of antiarrhythmic drugs based on their actions on arrhythmogenic mechanisms, *Circulation* 84:1831, 1991.
3. Lederer WJ: Regulation and function of adenosine triphosphate–sensitive potassium channels in the cardiovascular system. In Zipes DP, Jalife J, editors: *Cardiac electrophysiology from cell to bedside,* ed 2, Philadelphia, 1995, WB Saunders.
4. Hanna MS, Dresdner KP Jr, Wit AL: Cellular mechanisms of cardiac arrhythmias. In El-Sherif N, Samet P, editors: *Cardiac pacing and electrophysiology,* ed 3, Philadelphia, 1991, WB Saunders.
5. Kléber AG: Sodium-potassium pumping. In Rosen MR, Janse MJ, Wit AL, editors: *Cardiac electrophysiology: a textbook,* Mount Kisco, NY, 1990, Futura.
6. Thomas RC: Electrogenic sodium pump in nerve and muscle cells, *Physiol Rev* 52:563, 1972.
7. Rosen MR, Wit AL: Arrhythmogenic actions of antiarrhythmic drugs, *Am J Cardiol* 59:10E, 1987.
8. Rosen MR: Fast response action potential. In Podrid PJ, Kowey PR, editors: *Cardiac arrhythmia mechanisms, diagnosis, and management,* Baltimore, 1995, Williams & Wilkins.
9. Hille B: *Ionic channels of excitable membranes,* Sunderland, Mass, 1984, Sinauer Associates.
10. Hanck DA: Biophysics of sodium channels. In Zipes DP, Jalife J, editors: *Cardiac electrophysiology from cell to bedside,* Philadelphia, 1995, WB Saunders.
11. Opie LH: Mechanisms of cardiac contraction and relaxation. In Braunwald E, editor: *Heart disease: a textbook of cardiovascular medicine,* ed 5, Philadelphia, 1997, WB Saunders.
12. Marban E, O'Rourke B: Calcium channels: structure, function, and regulation. In Zipes DP, Jalife J, editors: *Cardiac electrophysiology from cell to bedside,* Philadelphia, 1995, WB Saunders.
13. Sperelakis N, Xiong Z, Haddad G, Masuda H: Regulation of slow calcium channels of myocardial cells and vascular smooth muscle cells by cyclic nucleotides and phosphorylation, *Mol Cell Biochem* 140:103, 1994.
14. Cheng H, Lederer WJ, Cannell MB: Calcium sparks: elementary events underlying excitation-contraction coupling in heart muscle, *Science* 262:740, 1993.
15. Cannell MB, Cheng H, Lederer WJ: The control of calcium release in heart muscle, *Science* 268:1045, 1995.
16. Beuckelmann DJ, Näbauer M, Krüger C, Erdmann E: Altered diastolic $[Ca^{2+}]_i$ handling in human ventricular myocytes from patients with terminal heart failure, *Am Heart J* 129:684, 1995.
17. Carafoli E: Membrane transport of calcium: an overview. In Fleischer S, Fleischer B, editors: Methods in enzymology, *Biomembranes,* vol 157, San Diego, 1988, Academic Press.
18. Mullins LJ: A mechanism for Na^+/Ca^{2+} transport, *J Gen Physiol* 70:681, 1977.
19. Caroni P, Carafoli E: The regulation of the Na^+-Ca^{2+} exchanger of heart sarcolemma, *Eur J Biochem* 132:451, 1983.
20. Jencks WP: How does a calcium pump pump calcium? *J Biol Chem* 264:18855, 1989.
21. Pennefather P, Cohen IS: Molecular mechanisms of cardiac K^+ channel regulation. In Zipes DP, Jalife J, editors: *Cardiac electrophysiology,* Philadelphia, 1990, WB Saunders.
22. Vanoli E, Priori SG, Nakagawa H et al: Sympathetic activation, ventricular repolarization and I_{Kr} blockade: implications for the antifibrillatory efficacy of potassium channel blocking agents, *J Am Coll Cardiol* 25:1609, 1995.
23. Gea-Ny T: Potassium channels: their modulation by drugs. In Zipes DP, Jalife J, editors: *Cardiac electrophysiology from cell to bedside,* ed 2, Philadelphia, 1995, WB Saunders.

24. Irisawa H, Giles WR: Sinus and atrioventricular node cells: cellular electrophysiology. In Zipes DP, Jalife J, editors: *Cardiac electrophysiology,* Philadelphia, 1990, WB Saunders.

25. DiFrancesco D, Tromba C: Inhibition of the hyperpolarization-activated current, I_f, induced by acetylcholine in rabbit sino-atrial node myocytes, *J Physiol* 405:477, 1988.

26. DiFrancesco D, Ducouret P, Robinson RB: Muscarinic modulation of cardiac rate at low acetylcholine concentrations, *Science* 243:669, 1989.

27. Lederer WJ, Nichols CG: Regulation and function of adenosine triphosphate–sensitive potassium channels in the cardiovascular system. In Zipes DP, Jalife J, editors: *Cardiac electrophysiology from cell to bedside,* ed 2, Philadelphia, 1995, WB Saunders.

28. Jogsma HJ, Rook MB: Morphology and electrophysiology of cardiac gap junction channels. In Zipes DP, Jalife J, editors: *Cardiac electrophysiology from cell to bedside,* Philadelphia, 1995, WB Saunders.

29. Lesh MD, Spear JF, Moore EN: Myocardial anisotropy: basic electrophysiology and role in cardiac arrhythmias. In Zipes DP, Jalife J, editors: *Cardiac electrophysiology,* Philadelphia, 1990, WB Saunders.

CHAPTER 3

The Action Potential

Fast- and slow-response
    action potentials 29
Recording the action
    potential 30
SA and AV nodal action
    potentials 32
Phase 4 depolarization 33
Phase 0 33
Phase 1 35
Phase 2 35
Phase 3 35
Refractory periods 36
Conduction velocity 36
Overdrive suppression 37

THE ACTION POTENTIAL IS THE SIGNAL THAT TRIGGERS CONTRACTION. A RECORDING of the action potential is a graph of the time and voltage course of the transmembrane potential of a single cell during electrical excitation. It consists of four successive phases: (1) phase 0 depolarization (rapid in atrial, ventricular, and His-Purkinje cells; slower in sinoatrial [SA] and atrioventricular [AV] nodal cells), (2) phase 1 (initial rapid repolarization), (3) phase 2 (the plateau), and (4) phase 3 (rapid repolarization). Phase 4 is the resting membrane potential (see Chapter 2). These phases reflect the rapid sequence of voltage changes that occurs across the cell membrane during the electrical cardiac cycle. As shown in Figure 3-1, all phases are well defined in the His-Purkinje and ventricular myocardial cells, whereas in nodal and atrial cells only two phases are seen. The distinctive shapes and durations of action potentials from different parts of the heart reflect the functions of these different parts.

The cardiac cycle begins in the SA node with depolarization. This electrical signal passes through the entire heart, with currents flowing intracellularly through the gap junctions and extracellularly in response to the differences in electrical potential generated during the action potential. This flow of extracellular current is recorded by the electrocardiogram. Figure 3-2 illustrates the microstructure of the cardiac cell and the intercalated disk. As explained in Chapter 2, cardiac cells are electrically connected to each other via gap junctions. These gap junctions are mostly located in the end-to-end intercalated disks, but there are also some lateral locations.[1]

The major time-dependent and voltage-gated membrane currents were discussed in Chapter 2 and are reviewed in the following list:
- I_{Na}: The ionic sodium current responsible for rapid depolarization in atrial and ventricular muscle and in Purkinje fibers
- I_{Ca}: The ionic calcium current responsible for depolarization in the SA and AV nodes and for triggering contraction
- I_K: The repolarizing potassium current
- I_f: The pacemaker current

FAST- AND SLOW-RESPONSE ACTION POTENTIALS

A *fast-response* action potential is recorded from a cell that has a high rate of depolarization because of the presence of many Na^+ channels. Such cells possess the property of fast conduction and may or may not be automatic. His-Purkinje cells possess the property of automaticity, whereas atrial and ventricular cells do not.

A *slow-response* action potential is recorded from a cell that has a slow rate of depolarization because of the absence of Na^+ channels. This type of action potential is de-

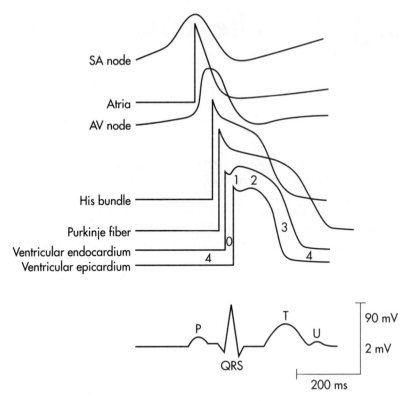

FIGURE 3-1 Transmembrane potentials in atrial and ventricular tissues during normal sinus rhythm as compared with each other and with the surface ECG.

pendent on I_{Ca}. Cells with a slow-response action potential possess the properties of slow conduction and automaticity. In the normal heart, such cells are found in the SA and AV nodes. Abnormally, they can be found anywhere in the heart, usually secondary to ischemia, injury, or an electrolyte imbalance.

RECORDING THE ACTION POTENTIAL

Figure 3-3 illustrates and explains the general technique for recording an action potential and resting membrane potential. The action potential shown is from a Purkinje cell, which has a fast-response action potential (steep phase 0), the longest refractory period, and the fastest conduction velocity in the entire heart. The long refractory period of a Purkinje cell is evident in Figure 3-1.

With the exception of phase 4 and the longer refractory period of His-Purkinje cells, the action potentials of His-Purkinje and ventricular cells are similar. They, along with atrial action potentials, have steep upstrokes (phase 0). The remarkable feature of the atrial action potential is its short refractory period, which consists of only phase 3; phases 1 and 2 are absent. This short refractory period and the steep, quick downstroke of phase 3 is dramatically noted when compared with other action potentials (see Fig-

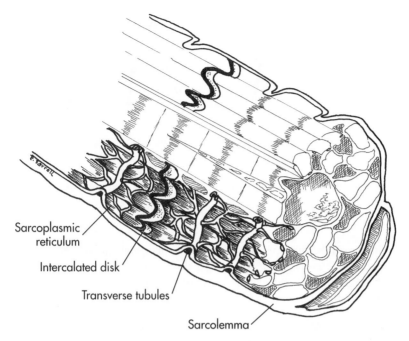

FIGURE 3-2 Microstructure of a cardiac cell. (Modified from Conover M: *Understanding electrocardiography*, ed 5, St Louis, 1988, Mosby.)

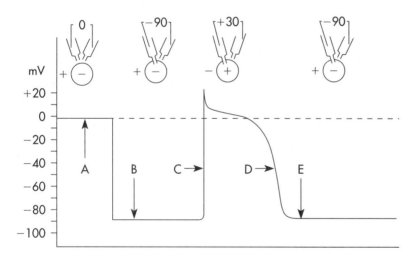

FIGURE 3-3 Recording the action potential. The upper row of diagrams shows a cell and two microelectrodes. Before the recording begins, both electrodes are in the extracellular fluid *(A)*. Phase 4 *(B)* is recorded when one electrode penetrates the cell membrane; the inside of the cell is approximately −90 mV compared with the outside. Phase 0 *(C)* is the upstroke of the action potential. Phase 1 is the sharp initial downstroke; phase 2 is the plateau. Phase 3 *(D)* is the phase of rapid repolarization. The membrane then returns to its resting potential *(E)* (From Cranefield PF: *The conduction of the cardiac impulse*, Mount Kisco, NY, 1975, Futura.)

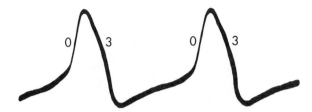

FIGURE 3-4 Action potential of the SA node. A large influx of Ca^{2+} (I_{Ca} and I_{Na}) is responsible for phase 0. The delayed outward K^+ current (I_K) is the main current responsible for repolarization (phase 3) and hyperpolarization (the most negative point). With hyperpolarization of the cell the small inward positive current (I_f) is activated and in turn triggers an inward Ca^{2+} current. (Modified from Sano T, Yamagishi S: *Circ Res* 16:423, 1965.)

ure 3-1). The short refractory period of the atria explains why it is capable of faster rates than the ventricles. Nevertheless, atrial fibers do not normally possess the property of automaticity. In both atrial and ventricular myocardial cells, phase 4 is flat; these cells are maintained at equilibrium during phase 4 and wait for a stimulus.

SA AND AV NODAL ACTION POTENTIALS

The following are the most notable features of cells in the SA and AV nodes:
1. Slow conduction
2. Aggressive pacemaker activity (steep phase 4); this activity is slower in the AV node than in the SA node and is therefore secondary
3. Virtual absence of Na^+ channels
4. Virtual absence of the inward K^+ rectifier current (I_{K1})
5. Absence of phases 1 and 2 of the action potential

I_{Ca}, I_K, and I_f are three major time-dependent and voltage-gated channels that interact in the electrophysiology of the SA node. There are also two major background currents: the Na^+-K^+ pump current and an Na^+ background current.

The membrane currents of the SA and AV nodes are affected by acetylcholine, which slows the heart rate; epinephrine and norepinephrine, which speed the heart rate; and by therapeutic agents such as calcium channel blockers and β-adrenergic blockers.

Typical action potentials from the SA node are seen in Figure 3-4. Individual current components are as follows[2]:
1. Initiation of depolarization. As soon as the SA nodal cells repolarize, they begin to depolarize again to reach the threshold potential for the T- and L-type Ca^{2+} channels. By the time the I_K current has decayed, the cell is hyperpolarized to approximately -70 mV. The onset of hyperpolarization activates I_f, which is finely tuned by the opposing actions of the autonomic nervous system, increasing with epinephrine and decreasing with acetylcholine.[3]
2. Phase 0. The absence of I_{Na} in the SA node action potential is reflected in the slow upstroke of phase 0, which is entirely generated by I_{Ca}.
3. Phase 3. Repolarization is generated by the inactivation of I_{Ca} and the simultaneous activation of I_K.

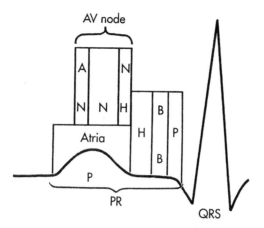

FIGURE 3-5 AV nodal activation is not seen on the ECG. It begins as the P wave crests and ends on its downslope (midway in the PR interval). *AN,* Atrionodal; *N,* nodal; *NH,* nodal-His bundle; *H,* His bundle; *BB,* bundle branches; *P,* Purkinje fibers.

Although less is known about the AV node, it appears to be electrophysiologically similar to the SA node. The main functions of the AV node are (1) to provide time for ventricular filling with a delay between atrial and ventricular activation, and (2) to protect the ventricles from being activated by excessively rapid atrial rates. The AV node accomplishes these functions by prolonging its conduction time when the atria increase their rate. In addition, the refractoriness of the AV node outlasts the action potential duration (postrepolarization refractoriness). The AV node is activated from approximately the peak of the P wave to the midportion of the PR segment and therefore is a major contributor to the PR interval (Figure 3-5).

PHASE 4 DEPOLARIZATION

As illustrated in Figure 3-6, His-Purkinje fibers exhibit phase 4 depolarization (automaticity). At the end of phase 3 (when the cells are hyperpolarized) I_f is activated, which causes the cell to slowly become less negative. The currents thought to be responsible for phase 4 depolarization in Purkinje fibers are I_f, I_{Ca}, I_{K1}, a steady-state inward Na^+ window current, and the Na^+-K^+ pump.[4]

The difference between excitability and automaticity is illustrated in Figure 3-7. All normal myocardial cells are excitable; that is, they are all capable of producing an action potential when driven by an adequate stimulus. However, only pacemaker cells possess the property of automaticity and can reach threshold potential without an outside stimulus.

PHASE 0

In the normal heart, myocardial cells are driven to threshold potential by an impulse from the SA node. After reaching this threshold (approximately -65 mV), the Na^+ channels abruptly open and close. This event is the main cause of the steep spike of phase 0 and is a feature of all healthy cardiac cells (except those of the SA and AV nodes).

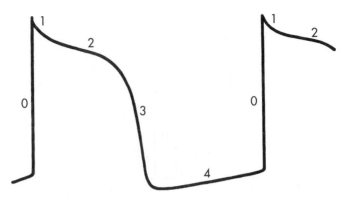

FIGURE 3-6 Action potential of the His-Purkinje system. Note the normal automaticity of phase 4 (it becomes less and less negative). (Modified from Conover M: *Understanding electrocardiography,* ed 5, St Louis, 1988, Mosby.)

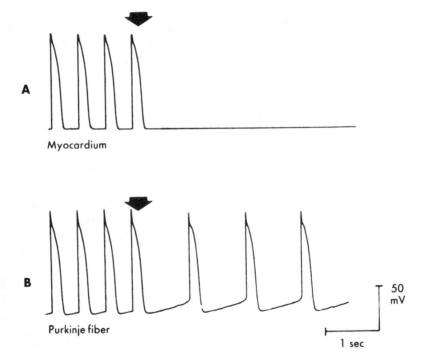

FIGURE 3-7 Excitability and automaticity in excitable fibers that are being driven by an extracellular electrode. The arrows indicate the discontinuation of the stimulus. The myocardial fiber (**A**) will not begin to fire again until the stimulus is reinstated, but the Purkinje fiber (**B**) can depolarize spontaneously during phase 4 until threshold potential is attained and an action potential is initiated (automaticity). (From Rosen MR, Hordof AJ: Mechanisms of arrhythmias. In Roberts NK, Gelband H, editors: *Cardiac arrhythmias in the neonate, infant, and child,* New York, 1977, Appleton-Century-Crofts.)

The more negative the membrane potential at activation and the more Na$^+$ channels available, the steeper phase 0 and the faster the conduction. A strong Na$^+$ current is possible from a membrane potential negative to -70 mV.

Na$^+$ channels also contribute to the plateau or slow repolarization phase of the action potential (phase 2). Thus they have at least two types of opening sequences: a brief (1 to 2 ms) opening and closing (without again opening), and a burst of openings and slow closings that result in a late sodium current that makes an important contribution to phase 2 of the action potential.[5] The sum of these bursts resembles slow channel activity.[6]

A second inward current is initiated when the T-type Ca^{2+} channels briefly open during phase 0 (at approximately -60 to -50 mV). At approximately -30 to -10 mV the L-type (slow) Ca^{2+} channels open in clustered bursts and remain open during phase 2.

A third inward current is initiated during phase 0 in the range of -30 mV to -10 mV. At this time the Ca^{2+} channels open and close in a very complex pattern of clustered bursts. The opening of these channels is also a major contributor to the plateau of the action potential and causes the sarcoplasmic reticulum to release calcium for cardiac contraction.

PHASE 1

Phase 1 is the rapid, brief beginning of repolarization immediately following phase 0. It results from the inactivation of I$_{Na}$ and/or I$_{Ca}$.

PHASE 2

Phase 2 is the plateau phase and is most notable in the Purkinje fibers. During this time there is a balance of inward and outward ion fluxes across the membrane to maintain an equilibrium. This balance occurs in the following steps:

1. Ca^{2+} and Na$^+$ continue to flow into the cell through the L-type calcium channels.
2. K$^+$ leaves the cell (I$_K$ current), with its exodus increasing with time until the efflux of K$^+$ exceeds the influx of Ca^{2+} and Na$^+$. At this point, phase 2 and contraction terminate, and rapid repolarization begins.
3. The increasing exodus of K$^+$ from the cell is regulated by a steady-state inward K$^+$ rectifier current (I$_{K1}$), which ensures that the refractory period is long enough to be protective.
4. The sodium channels also contribute to the plateau with bursts of Na$^+$ into the cell and with a steady-state flow of Na$^+$ through sodium channels that do not inactivate.

PHASE 3

Phase 3 is the phase of late and rapid repolarization. In ventricular myocardial cells, the T wave on the ECG is completed during this time (see Figure 3-1). The following major currents are active during phase 3:

1. The onset of phase 3 is triggered when both the gradually increasing outward I$_K$ current that is active during the plateau and the Na$^+$-K$^+$ ATPase current exceed the inward positive current.
2. At this point the slow calcium channels close, accelerating the process of repolarization.

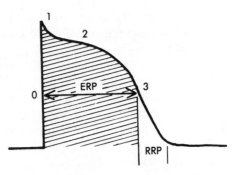

FIGURE 3-8 Refractory periods. The effective refractory period *(ERP)* extends from phase 0 to approximately −60 mV in phase 3. The remainder of the action potential is the relative refractory period *(RRP)*. (Modified from Conover M: *Understanding electrocardiography,* ed 5, St Louis, 1988, Mosby.)

3. The activity of the Na^+-K^+ pump increases with the increased intracellular Na^+ concentration, which helps the cell reach a more negative level.
4. The continued background inward steady-state K^+ current (I_{K1}) is also active during this phase.

REFRACTORY PERIODS

Refractoriness is the inability of a cell or fiber to respond normally to a stimulus because it has been too recently activated by a previous stimulus. The *refractory period* is the interval during which the cell remains unresponsive (effective refractory period [ERP]) or responds inadequately (relative refractory period [RRP]) (Figure 3-8). The refractory period itself is determined by the level of transmembrane potential; a depolarized cell is not capable of responding to a stimulus.

During ERP (from phase 0 to −60 mV in phase 3), no stimulus can evoke a propagated response. During RRP (−60 mV in phase 3 to −70 mV), only a strong stimulus can evoke a propagated response. During the ERP of the AV node it is impossible for a stimulus to activate and penetrate the node; during the RRP of the AV node, a strong stimulus can penetrate the node.

CONDUCTION VELOCITY

The speed of conduction is determined by the negativity of cardiac cells at the time of excitation. Optimal negativity, (−85 to −95 mV), ensures a huge influx of Na^+ into the cell during phase 0, a strong stimulus (large current flow) for neighboring cells, and maximal conduction velocity. The larger the current passed from cell to cell, the faster the conduction. Because this requirement is fulfilled in the cells of the His-Purkinje system, it is here that the tallest amplitude upstroke in the heart is found. In addition, there are many low-resistance connections to neighboring Purkinje cells, which facilitates conduction and a larger cellular radius than other cells in the heart. Conduction velocity is proportional to the square root of the fiber radius.

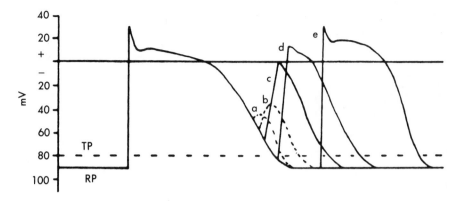

FIGURE 3-9 Normal action potential and responses elicited by stimuli applied at various stages of repolarization. The amplitude and upstroke velocity of such responses are related to the level of membrane potential from which they arise. The earliest responses (*a* and *b*) are slow-response action potentials that arise from low levels of membrane potential; they do not propagate. Response *c* is a depressed response action potential and represents the earliest propagated action potential; it propagates slowly because of its slow upstroke velocity and low amplitude. Response *d* is elicited just before complete repolarization; this rate of rise and amplitude is greater than *a*, *b*, and *c* because it arises from a higher membrane potential. However, it propagates more slowly than normal. Response *e* is elicited after complete repolarization and therefore has a normal rate of depolarization and amplitude and propagates rapidly. *TP,* Threshold potential; *RE,* resting potential. (From Singer DH, Ten Eick RE: Pharmacology of cardiac arrhythmias, *Prog Cardiovasc Dis* 11:488, 1969.)

Figure 3-9 illustrates the action potentials elicited when stimuli are applied during phase 3 when the membrane potential has not achieved optimal negativity. Note that phase 0 of the resulting action potential becomes steeper and taller as the stimulus is applied at a more negative level. The first two stimuli result in slow-response action potentials because no fast sodium channels are available. Stimuli *c* and *d* result in depressed fast-response action potentials. When a stimulus is delivered at maximum diastolic potential, the action potential has a steep, tall phase 0 and the possibility for fast conduction velocity.

OVERDRIVE SUPPRESSION

Overdrive suppression is the inhibitory effect of a faster pacemaker on a slower one. This suppression, along with the successful race to threshold potential exhibited by the SA node, normally assures the SA node of its role as the dominant pacemaker of the heart and makes it more difficult for a subsidiary pacemaker to emerge and compete with it.

The mechanism of overdrive suppression is hyperpolarization. Rapid pacing causes an increase in extracellular K^+ and an increased influx of Na^+ into the cells through the sodium channels. The increase in intracellular Na^+ is in turn a stimulus to Na^+-K^+ pumping, which empties the cell of Na^+ and eventually renders it more negative than normal (hyperpolarization) and depresses pacemaker activity.[7]

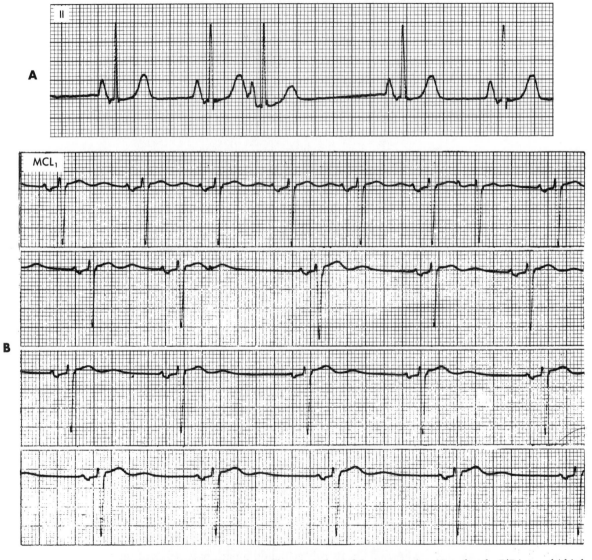

FIGURE 3-10 A, Normal manifestation of overdrive suppression. Note that the P'P interval (third complex) is longer than the PP interval that precedes it. Instead of resetting the SA node, the atrial premature beat has suppressed it. **B,** Abnormal response by the SA node to overdrive suppression by two atrial premature beats. The first one is in the top strip (seventh complex); the second one is not conducted and is seen in the second strip after the second QRS complex.

The rate-dependent suppression of the subsidiary pacemakers is reduced during sinus bradycardia. These subsidiary pacemakers can thus become active without much delay if the SA node slows sufficiently or fails. This action is in contrast to the effects of a sudden suppression of the SA node or the sudden development of complete AV heart block. In such cases it takes several seconds for the overdrive suppression to subside and the escape pacemaker to assume its intrinsic rate. Although vagal stimulation inhibits the SA node, the resulting bradycardia secondarily removes an inhibition from subsidiary pacemakers, which allows escape beats to appear more promptly.

Figure 3-10 illustrates overdrive suppression as exerted on the SA node by atrial extrasystoles. In Figure 3-10, *A*, the lengthening of the cycle after the premature atrial beat is a manifestation of normal overdrive suppression; however, in Figure 3-10, *B*, the exaggerated slowing that occurs after the atrial premature beats is clearly indicative of sinus node dysfunction.

SUMMARY

The initial phase of the action potential (phase 0) is defined by rapid depolarization. This depolarization is caused by a rapid increase in Na^+ permeability and is mediated by the voltage-sensitive Na^+ channels. It is this influx of Na^+ into the cell that largely determines cardiac excitability and the conduction velocity of the cardiac impulse.[8] Rapid depolarization is followed by a rapid, incomplete early repolarization (phase 1) caused by a rapid K^+ efflux through transiently active channels. Phase 2 is the plateau of the action potential during which there is an inward movement of Ca^{2+} through voltage-sensitive slow (L-type) Ca^{2+} channels and a rising K^+ permeability that ultimately repolarizes the cell. The Ca^{2+} that enters the cell at this time stimulates the sarcoplasmic reticulum to release its stores of Ca^{2+}, thus initiating excitation-contraction coupling. Phase 3 begins the termination of the action potential (repolarization) and is mediated by voltage-sensitive K^+ channels.

REFERENCES

1. Lederer WJ: Regulation and function of adenosine triphosphate–sensitive potassium channels in the cardiovascular system. In Zipes DP, Jalife J, editors: *Cardiac electrophysiology from cell to bedside*, ed 2, Philadelphia, 1995, WB Saunders.
2. Noble D, DiFrancesco D, Denyer JC: Ionic mechanisms in normal and abnormal cardiac pacemaker activity. In Jacklet JW, editor: *Cellular and neuronal oscillators*, New York, 1989, Dekker.
3. DiFrancesco D: Current I_f and the neuronal modulation of heart rate. In Zipes DP, Jalife J, editors: *Cardiac electrophysiology*, Philadelphia, 1990, WB Saunders.
4. Gintant GA, Cohen IS: Advances in cardiac cellular electrophysiology: implications for automaticity and therapeutics, *Ann Rev Pharmacol Toxicol* 28:61, 1988.
5. Kirsch GE, Brown AM: Cardiac sodium channels. In Zipes DP, Jalife J, editors: *Cardiac electrophysiology*, Philadelphia, 1990, WB Saunders.
6. Gintant GA, Datyner N, Cohen IS: Slow inactivation of a tetrodotoxin-sensitive current in canine cardiac Purkinje fibers, *Biophys J* 45:509, 1984.
7. Kléber AG: Sodium-potassium pumping. In Rosen MR, Janse MJ, Wit AL, editors: *Cardiac electrophysiology: a textbook*, Mount Kisco, NY, 1990, Futura.
8. Fozzard HA, Hanck DA: Sodium channels. In Fozzard HA, Haber E, Jennings RB et al, editors: *The heart and cardiovascular system*, New York, 1991, Raven Press.

CHAPTER 4

The Autonomic Nervous System, Cardiac Rhythms, and Drugs

β-Adrenergic receptor-
  effector coupling
  system 41
Muscarinic receptor-
  effector coupling
  system 42
Effects of drugs on cardiac
  function 43
Other drugs or conditions
  that act on the heart 44

THE AUTONOMIC NERVOUS SYSTEM IS COMPOSED OF THE SYMPATHETIC AND parasympathetic nervous systems. These systems are important modulators of cardiac rhythm and can be affected by certain drugs and physical maneuvers. Much is known about the receptor-effector coupling system that results in the physiologic responses of the autonomic nervous system[1]:

- **Receptors.** The α- and β-adrenergic receptors of the sympathetic nervous system and the muscarinic and nicotinic receptors of the parasympathetic nervous system act on membrane channels and pumps to influence the formation of normal and abnormal impulses. The β-adrenergic and the M_2-muscarinic are the best understood receptor-effector coupling systems.
- **Effectors.** Receptors are coupled to effector systems by G proteins, which then translate the results of an external stimulus into a physiologic response.
- **Physiologic response.** An external stimulus (such as vagal stimulation) causes a receptor to be occupied. This receptor occupancy is changed by the G proteins into a physiologic response such as the activation of membrane channels; the receptor may also be linked (by the G proteins) to second messenger systems and pumps.

β-ADRENERGIC RECEPTOR-EFFECTOR COUPLING SYSTEM
β-Adrenergic Stimulation

β-Adrenergic receptor stimulation affects currents that are modulated by the cyclic adenosine monophosphate (cAMP)–dependent protein kinase, such as the L-type calcium current, the I_f current, and the I_K current.

The tachycardias and QT shortening that follow β-adrenergic stimulation may result from the following cellular effects[1]:

1. An increase in L-type Ca^{2+} currents, which causes an increase in contractility; an increase in free intracellular Ca^{2+} could also result in delayed afterdepolarizations and arrhythmias because of triggered activity

2. An increase in I_K currents, which accelerates repolarization and shortens refractoriness and, along with the increase in intracellular Ca^{2+}, may accelerate AV nodal conduction and shorten AV nodal refractoriness
3. An increase in I_f currents, which may increase not only the rate of SA nodal discharge but also the rate of the subordinate pacemakers

Modulation of the Sodium Current by β-Adrenergic Stimulation

In addition to its well-known cardiac stimulatory effect, β-adrenergic stimulation has a direct cellular depressant effect. β-Adrenergic stimulation prolongs the inactivation state of the sodium channel, which inhibits the sodium current in depressed cells and causes slow conduction. Both depressed cells and catecholamines are present in ischemia, with the depression resulting from the release of K^+ into the extracellular fluid. The resultant slowed conduction can cause reentrant arrhythmias and ventricular fibrillation. This explains the correlation between high levels of catecholamines and an increased risk of arrhythmias in myocardial infarction.[1,2]

β-Adrenergic Blockade

β-Adrenergic blocking agents have the following antiarrhythmic actions[1]:
1. Decrease of conduction velocity and prolongation of refractoriness in the AV node. This action is accomplished by blocking the effect of catecholamines on Ca^{2+} and K^+ channels.
2. Reduction of ventricular arrhythmias in a limited subset of patients. Such arrhythmias include exercise-induced ventricular tachycardias, some ventricular tachycardias inducible by programmed stimulation, adenosine-sensitive ventricular tachycardias, and some ventricular premature beats.
3. Reduction of sudden cardiac death following myocardial infarction (MI) and in patients with long QT syndrome. The mechanism of protection in post-MI patients is not yet understood.

MUSCARINIC RECEPTOR-EFFECTOR COUPLING SYSTEM

The dominant cardiac muscarinic receptor has been pharmacologically identified as M_2. It is more abundant in atrial than in ventricular tissue, and it is coupled to the $I_{K(ACh)}$ channel by the protein G_I.

Vagal Stimulation

There is indirect evidence that activation of the muscarinic receptors by vagal stimulation plays an important role in protecting post-MI patients from ventricular arrhythmias and sudden death.[3,4]

Clinically, vagal activation terminates AV reentry mechanisms (paroxysmal supraventricular tachycardia) because it slows AV conduction. The action and inhibition of automaticity in the SA node involves at least three mechanisms:
1. Activation of the acetylcholine-activated inward K^+ rectifying current ($I_{K(ACh)}$)
2. Inhibition of the inward positive I_f current
3. Inhibition of the inward Ca^{2+} current

These effects hyperpolarize the membrane (make it more negative). As a result, it takes longer to reach threshold potential, which slows SA nodal impulse formation and AV nodal conduction velocity.

EFFECTS OF DRUGS ON CARDIAC FUNCTION

Pharmacology involves the use of many experimental and clinical indexes. These indexes include ionic currents and activity, action potentials, extracellular electrograms, excitability, conduction, refractoriness, impulse initiation, pharmacodynamics, drug and ion competition and interaction, receptor-mediated modulation, contractility, vascular tone, cardiac disease, and pharmacokinetics.[1]

Drug-Channel Interactions

Membrane channels exist in three states: resting, open, and inactivated. In the resting state ions cannot pass; in the open state ions can pass; in the inactivated state the channel is in transition back to the resting state, and ions cannot pass.

Antiarrhythmic drugs that act on channels block ionic currents, but some activators such as vagal stimulation and adenosine cause channels to increase ionic currents.

Use-Dependent Antiarrhythmic Drugs

A use-dependent drug is one that is more effective at faster heart rates. Antiarrhythmic drugs act by binding at a specific location in channels. Access to these channels is determined by how many times per minute the channel is open. Hence, a use-dependent drug such as lidocaine is more effective at faster heart rates since there is more blocking during tachycardia than during bradycardia. Other variables that influence channel blockade are membrane potential (voltage), pH, and the molecular weight and structure of the drug.[5]

Voltage-Dependent Antiarrhythmic Drugs

Lidocaine is both use-dependent and voltage-dependent. When the resting voltage of cardiac cells is reduced by a depolarizing current, such as in ischemia, the sodium channels become accessible to the blocking action of lidocaine. Thus lidocaine slows conduction in ischemic tissue without having a marked effect on normal tissue.

Prolonged Repolarization

The prolongation of repolarization by antiarrhythmic drugs involves a complicated interplay between heart rate, channel blockade, and the competition of the sympathetic nervous system.

Rate dependency

The prolongation of repolarization (QT interval) is usually mediated by the action of the drug on K^+ channels in a rate-dependent fashion; the degree of rate dependency varies among drugs. Thus the prolongation of refractoriness is more marked at slow heart rates than at fast heart rates.

Sodium channels

The effect of a drug on refractoriness is also determined by sodium channels (i.e., their availability at excitation and residual block during phases 3 and 4 of the action potential).

Potassium channel blockade and the sympathetic nervous system

As discussed in Chapter 3, the delayed rectifier potassium current (I_K) has two components: one rapidly activated (I_{Kr}) and one slowly activated (I_{Ks}). Most of the currently available potassium channel blockers (e.g., D-sotalol) block I_{Kr}. On the other hand, isoproterenol activates and dominates the I_{Ks} component. Therefore potassium channel blockers have little effect in the setting of elevated sympathetic activity.[6]

Erythromycin as a proarrhythmic

Erythromycin blocks I_{Kr}. This blockage causes excessive lengthening of the QT interval and predisposes patients to potentially lethal cardiac arrhythmia and torsades de pointes, especially when erythromycin is combined with other action potential–lengthening drugs.[7-10]

Regulation of potassium channels by nonsedating antihistamines

It has been shown in guinea pig and rat ventricular myocytes that nonsedating antihistamines (e.g., terfenadine and astemizole) have a significant inhibitory action on I_{K1} channels. Such inhibitory actions render the antihistamines potentially arrhythmogenic in conditions of overdose or conditions in which these channels are already compromised.[11]

Drug Competition and Potentiation

Drugs compete with each other by having an affinity for the same binding site or by producing opposite electrophysiologic effects and canceling each other out. Drugs complement each other by having the same physiologic effects. The advantage of such drug summation is to allow lower doses of each drug, with a resultant lower toxicity. Unfortunately there has been no systematic documentation of either this subject or of the interaction of a drug with its metabolite.

OTHER DRUGS OR CONDITIONS THAT ACT ON THE HEART

Calcium and sodium channel blockers and adrenergic receptor modulation can have substantial negative inotropic effects. Drugs that change vascular tone can affect heart rate and metabolic state, and disease may alter channel properties and the action of receptors on pumps.

REFERENCES

1. Wollenberger AM, Shahab L: Anoia-induced release of noradrenaline from the isolated perfused heart, *Nature* 207:88, 1965.
2. Hill JL, Gettes LS: Effects of acute coronary artery occlusion on local myocardial extracellular K+ activity in swine, *Circulation* 61:768, 1980.

3. Kleiger RE, Miller JP, Bigger JT Jr, Moss AJ: The Multicenter Post-Infarction Research Group: decreased heart rate variability and its association with increased mortality after acute myocardial infarction, *Am J Cardiol* 59:256, 1987.

4. LaRovere MT, Specchia G, Mortara A, Schwartz PJ: Baroreflex sensitivity, clinical correlates and cardiovascular mortality among patients with a first myocardial infarction: a prospective study, *Circulation* 78:816, 1988.

5. Rosen MR: Antiarrhythmic drugs. In El-Sherif N, Samet P, editors: *Cardiac pacing and electrophysiology,* ed 3, Philadelphia, 1991, WB Saunders.

6. Vanoli E, Priori SG, Nakagawa H et al: Sympathetic activation, ventricular repolarization and I_{Kr} blockade: implications for the antifibrillatory efficacy of potassium channel blocking agents, *J Am Coll Cardiol* 25:1609, 1995.

7. Daleau P, Lessard E, Groleau MF, Turgeon J: Erythromycin blocks the rapid component of the delayed rectifier potassium current and lengthens repolarization of guinea pig ventricular myocytes, *Circulation* 91:3021, 1995.

8. Brandriss MW, Richardson WS, Barold SS: Erythromycin-induced QT prolongation and polymorphic ventricular tachycardia (torsades de pointes): case report and review, *Clin Infect Dis* 18:995, 1994.

9. Nattel S, Ranger S, Talajic M et al: Erythromycin-induced long QT syndrome: concordance with quinidine and underlying cellular electrophysiologic mechanism, *Am J Med* 89:235, 1990.

10. Farrar HC, Walsh-Sukys MC, Kyllonen K, Blumer JL: Cardiac toxicity associated with intravenous erythromycin lactobionate: two case reports and a review of the literature, *Pediatr Infect Dis J* 12:688, 1993.

11. Berul CI, Morad M: Regulation of potassium channels by nonsedating antihistamines, *Circulation* 91:2220, 1995.

CHAPTER 5

Arrhythmogenic Mechanisms and Their Modulation

Arrhythmia or
  dysrhythmia? 47
Altered automaticity 47
Triggered activity 49
Reentry 56
Summation 61
Inhibition 62
Mechanisms of ischemia-
  induced arrhythmias 63

C ARDIAC ARRHYTHMIAS AND CONDUCTION DISTURBANCES HAVE DIVERSE PATHO-logic causes. However, the ultimate cause is a critical alteration in the electrical activity of the myocyte. This chapter discusses the four known arrhythmogenic mechanisms: altered automaticity, triggered activity, sodium dependent reentry, and calcium dependent reentry. The termination of these mechanisms should be possible by the alteration of one or more of several electrophysiologic properties. The *vulnerable parameter* is that property of a specific arrhythmogenic mechanism that is the easiest to alter and has the least adverse affect on the heart.[1]

ARRHYTHMIA OR DYSRHYTHMIA?

Both *arrhythmia* and *dysrhythmia* are acceptable terms despite the declaration that the traditional term *arrhythmia* be abandoned for *dysrhythmia* on the premise that the a prefix (alpha privative) means "absence of."[2] The original meaning of the alpha privative often implied "imperfection in" or "lack of" rather than the flat, negative "absence of." In addition, the original *rhythmos* had much a broader application than the anglicized word *rhythm*. Apart from original meanings, the most important factor for retaining the term *arrhythmia* is the sovereign role of usage. In this book both terms are accepted: *arrhythmia* because it has tradition and no perceptible flaws, and *dysrhythmia* because it offers variety.[3]

ALTERED AUTOMATICITY

Altered automaticity may be caused by either enhanced normal automaticity in normal Purkinje fibers or abnormal automaticity in severely depressed Purkinje or myocardial fibers.

Enhanced Normal Automaticity

Enhanced normal automaticity is the steepening of phase 4 depolarization in pacemaker cells (e.g., the sinoatrial [SA] node and His-Purkinje system). This mechanism is illustrated in Figure 5-1, *A*. Note that the action potential with enhanced normal automaticity reaches threshold potential prematurely because of a steepening of phase 4 depolarization; it is normal in all other respects. An important cause of enhanced normal automaticity is adrenergic stimulation.

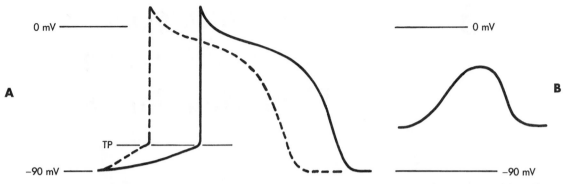

FIGURE 5-1   Enhanced normal automaticity (**A**) compared with abnormal automaticity (**B**). **A,** The solid line depicts normal automaticity, and the broken line, enhanced normal automaticity. In both cases the action potential is normal in shape and has a high membrane potential at the end of phase 3. During enhanced normal automaticity the resting membrane potential has a steeper slope to threshold potential *(TP)*. **B,** Abnormal automaticity occurs in fibers with low membrane potentials (-60 mV) where fast Na^+ channels are not present, guaranteeing automaticity and slow conduction.

Arrhythmias caused by enhanced normal automaticity

- Inappropriate sinus tachycardia
- Atrial tachycardia
- Certain accelerated idioventricular rhythms
- Junctional tachycardia

Vulnerable parameter

The vulnerable parameter for enhanced normal automaticity is phase 4 depolarization.[1] However, modulation of the enhanced diastolic depolarization can also be achieved by changing the voltage of the maximum diastolic potential, the threshold potential, and/or the action potential duration.[4]

Abnormal Automaticity

Abnormal automaticity is the process by which phase 4 depolarization (spontaneous impulses) occurs in pathologically depressed fibers. Such automaticity can occur anywhere in the heart, including in fibers that never possessed the property of automaticity while healthy. When a fiber is depressed, it becomes less negative. If ischemia reduces the maximum diastolic potential of Purkinje or myocardial cells to -55 mV or less, the action potential is like that of the sinus node (i.e., Ca^{2+} dependent and possessing automaticity and slow conduction). Figure 5-1 compares the two mechanisms of altered automaticity.

Arrhythmias caused by abnormal automaticity

- Atrial tachycardias (excluding those caused by digitalis toxicity)
- Accelerated idioventricular rhythms

- Ventricular tachycardias during the first few days post-myocardial infarction (MI)
- Junctional tachycardia

Vulnerable parameter

The vulnerable parameter for abnormal automaticity is the reduced maximum diastolic potential (the period immediately following phase 3); a more practical vulnerable parameter is phase 4 depolarization.[1]

Differentiating Between the Two Types of Altered Automaticity

A parallel relationship exists between the level of membrane potential and the possibility of overdrive suppression. This is one characteristic that distinguishes enhanced normal automaticity (fast sodium channel dependent) from abnormal automaticity (slow calcium channel dependent). As the membrane potential becomes less and less negative, fast sodium channels become less and less available, and overdrive suppression becomes less and less possible. This phenomenon occurs because, unlike fibers with high membrane potentials, depressed fibers are unable to hyperpolarize.

As discussed on p. 37, overdrive suppression depends on the creation of a state of hyperpolarization. Rapid pacing causes an increase in extracellular K^+ and an increased influx of Na^+ into the cells through the fast sodium channels. The increase in intracellular Na^+ stimulates Na^+-K^+ pumping, which empties the cell of Na^+ and eventually renders it more negative than normal (hyperpolarization) and depresses pacemaker activity. Depressed cells cannot achieve the state of hyperpolarization because they have no fast sodium channels to help build this series of events.

Figures 5-2, 5-3, and 5-4 illustrate the use of overdrive suppression to differentiate between the two mechanisms of altered automaticity: one that can be suppressed (enhanced normal automaticity) and one that cannot be suppressed (abnormal automaticity). In Figure 5-2, overdrive stimulation successfully suppresses an idioventricular rhythm in a patient with complete atrioventricular (AV) block, which suggests that the mechanism is enhanced normal automaticity from cells with a high diastolic potential. Figures 5-3 and 5-4 are from the same patient and illustrate an arrhythmia compatible with abnormal automaticity. The patient has an old MI and is in severe heart failure. An accelerated junctional rhythm at a rate of 75 beats/min is present. Neither the overdrive pacing seen in Figure 5-4 nor lidocaine could suppress the junctional rhythm.[5] Thus the mechanism of this arrhythmia is abnormal automaticity caused by severely depressed cells in the AV junction.

TRIGGERED ACTIVITY

Triggered activity consists of propagated action potentials that arise when afterdepolarizations (early or delayed) reach threshold potential. *Afterdepolarizations* are membrane potential oscillations that appear after and are dependent on the upstroke of the action potential. They occur either during the process of repolarization (early afterdepolarization) or after full repolarization (delayed afterdepolarization). Any resultant impulse formation is "triggered" because it does not occur unless preceded by at least one action potential. This mechanism should not be equated with altered automaticity.

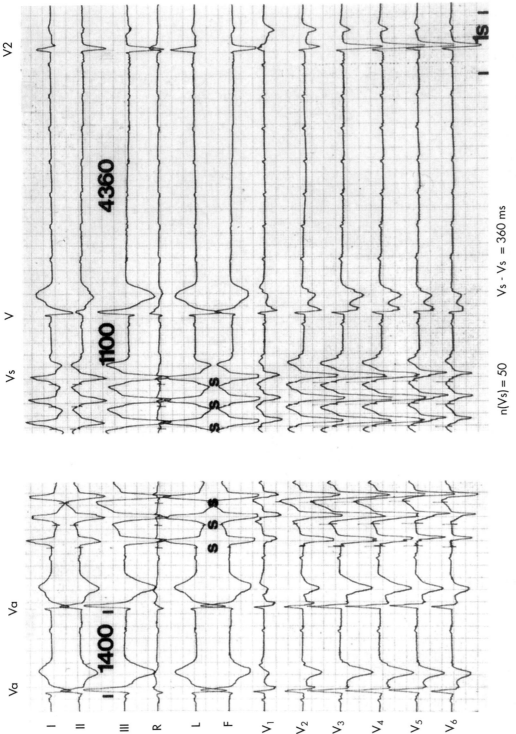

FIGURE 5-2 The effect of overdrive stimulation (S) on enhanced normal (high potential) automaticity. There is complete AV block and an idioventricular rhythm with a cycle length of 1400 ms. This rhythm is overdriven with 50 stimuli (S) at interstimulus intervals of 360 ms. The following should be noted: (1) the original rhythm is overdrive-suppressed, suggesting enhanced normal automaticity from cells with a high diastolic potential; (2) a different QRS complex with a short coupling interval occurs at 1100 ms and is probably caused by triggered activity; and (3) following a pause (4360 ms), ventricular activity resumes from a different focus. (From Gorgels APM, Vos MA, Brugada P, Wellens HJJ: The clinical relevance of abnormal automaticity and triggered activity. In Brugada P, Wellens HJJ, editors: *Cardiac arrhythmias: where to go from here?* Mt Kisco, NY, 1987, Futura.)

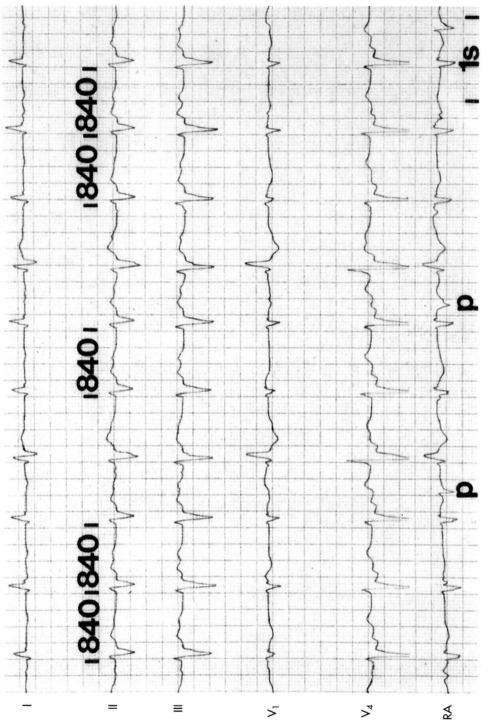

FIGURE 5-3 Clinical manifestation of abnormal automaticity in leads I, II, III, V₁, V₄, and in a right atrial (*RA*) lead in a patient with an old MI and severe heart failure. The two sinus P waves are called out in the RA lead. An accelerated junctional rhythm is present with an interectopic interval of 840 ms. This arrhythmia is interrupted twice (following the P waves) by sinus-conducted beats (ventricular captures) that are conducted with right bundle branch block (best seen in V₁) and left axis deviation (seen in leads I and II), which indicates that conduction is exclusively over the posterior fascicle of the left bundle. (From Gorgels APM, Vos MA, Brugada P, Wellens HJJ: The clinical relevance of abnormal automaticity and triggered activity. In Brugada P, Wellens HJJ, editors: *Cardiac arrhythmias: where to go from here?* Mt Kisco, NY, 1987, Futura.)

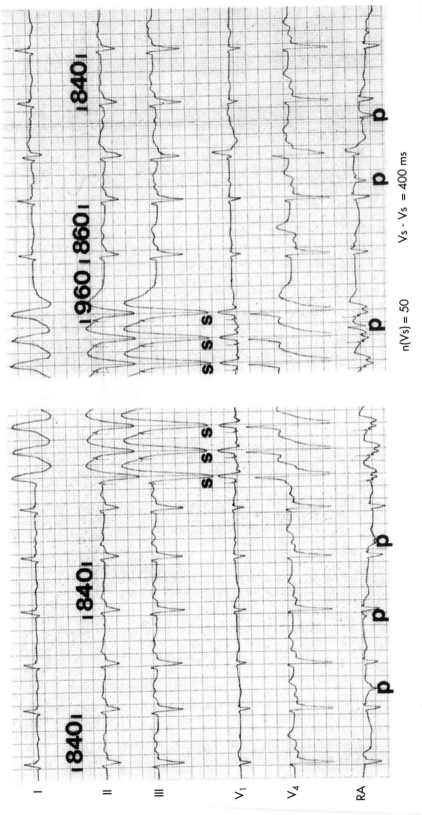

FIGURE 5-4 The effect of overdrive stimulation (*S*) on abnormal (low potential) automaticity (same patient as in Figure 5-3). Following overdrive pacing stimuli (*S*), there is slight lengthening of only the first coupling interval, after which the arrhythmia resumes its original rate. This lack of response to overdrive stimulation is compatible with reduced potential automaticity. (From Gorgels APM, Vos MA, Brugada P, Wellens HJJ: The clinical relevance of abnormal automaticity and triggered activity. In Brugada P, Wellens HJJ, editors: *Cardiac arrhythmias: where to go from here?* Mt Kisco, NY, 1987, Futura.)

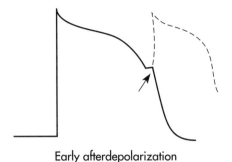

Early afterdepolarization

FIGURE 5-5 An early afterdepolarization *(arrow)* results in a triggered beat *(dotted line)*.

Early Afterdepolarizations

Early afterdepolarizations are oscillations in membrane potential that occur before the completion of phase 3 repolarization. If such an oscillation reaches threshold potential, triggered activity at a low membrane potential may result (Figure 5-5).

Mechanisms

The mechanisms of early afterdepolarizations involve a delay or interruption of repolarization because of a change in net inward membrane currents.[1]

Causes

The causes of early afterdepolarizations include the following[6-9]:
- Hypoxia
- Low pH
- Cesium
- Aconitine
- Sotalol
- *N*-acetylprocainamide (NAPA)
- Quinidine
- Excessive catecholamines

Distinguishing features
- A tendency to occur in salvos
- Termination when full repolarization is reached
- More likely when prevailing heart rate is slow
- Suppressed by rapid pacing
- Occurs at two levels of membrane potential: 0 to -30 mV, and -60 to -70 mV; 0 to -30 mV probably mediated by L-type calcium channels

Arrhythmias caused by early afterdepolarizations

Torsades de pointes is thought to be caused by triggered activity as a result of early afterdepolarizations. Reperfusion arrhythmias may also be caused by this mechanism.

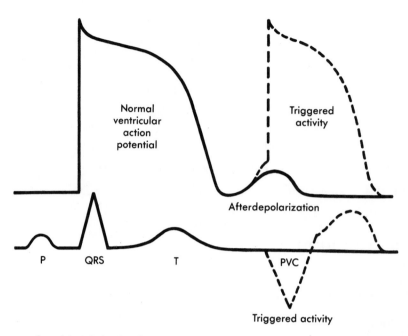

FIGURE 5-6 A delayed afterdepolarization causes a triggered beat *(dotted line)*. This cellular event is compared with the surface ECG. (From Conover M: *Understanding electrocardiography,* ed 5, St Louis, 1988, Mosby.)

Vulnerable parameter

The vulnerable parameter for early afterdepolarization–related triggered activity is the prolonged action potential duration (the QT interval). Treatment may involve the following[1]:

1. Shortening the action potential duration (increasing heart rate or extracellular K^+, action potential–shortening drugs, β-adrenergic activation, and/or withdrawal of the offending drugs)

or

2. Suppressing the triggering inward currents (calcium and sodium current–blocking drugs, α- or β-adrenergic receptor blockers, and Mg^{2+})

Delayed Afterdepolarizations

Delayed afterdepolarizations are oscillations in membrane potential that occur after the completion of phase 3 repolarization. If such an oscillation reaches threshold potential, triggered activity at a high membrane potential may result (Figure 5-6).

Mechanisms

Delayed afterdepolarizations are caused by anything that results in an increased intracellular Ca^{2+} concentration. A Ca^{2+} accumulation in the cell is a stimulus for

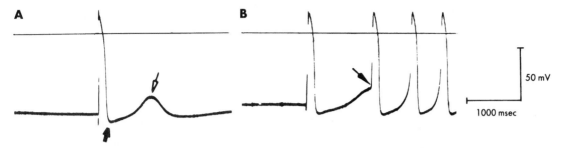

FIGURE 5-7   A, A driven (paced) action potential is followed by hyperpolarization *(solid arrow)* and delayed afterdepolarization *(open arrow).* **B,** A driven action potential is followed by a delayed afterdepolarization that reaches threshold potential. A nondriven action potential *(arrow)* arises from the peak of this delayed afterdepolarization. (From Wit AL, Boyden PA, Gadsby DC, Cranefield PF: Triggered activity as a cause of atrial arrhythmias. In Narula OS, editor: *Cardiac arrhythmias: electrophysiology, diagnosis, and management,* Baltimore, 1979, Williams & Wilkins.)

the repetitive release of even more Ca^{2+} from the sarcoplasmic reticulum.[10] The presence of free Ca^{2+} within the cell at the end of repolarization is a stimulus for the Na^+-Ca^{2+} exchanger, and there is a transient influx of Na^+ in an attempt to rid the cell of Ca^{2+}. It is this transient influx of Na^+ that causes the membrane oscillation during phase 4.

If membrane oscillation reaches threshold potential for the fast Na^+ channels, triggered activity results. Sympathetic stimulation or shortening of the cycle length can exacerbate the situation by causing an afterdepolarization that has not reached threshold potential (no arrhythmias) to increase its height, resulting in tachycardia (atrial, junctional, or fascicular). Figure 5-7 compares a normal action potential that ends in hyperpolarization and a delayed afterdepolarization but no triggered activity with an action potential that is followed by delayed afterdepolarizations and triggered activity.

Causes

Causes of delayed afterdepolarizations include the following:
- Digitalis
- Catecholamines
- Hypercalcemia
- Rapid pacing

Arrhythmias caused by delayed afterdepolarizations

- Extrasystoles and tachycardias related to digitalis excess (atrial, junctional, and fascicular ventricular tachycardia)[11-13]
- Some catecholamine-dependent atrial and ventricular tachycardias[14]
- Perhaps some arrhythmias associated with ischemia and reperfusion[15]
- Perhaps idiopathic ventricular tachycardias originating in the right ventricular outflow tract[16]

Vulnerable parameter

The vulnerable parameter for delayed afterdepolarizations is calcium overload. Treatment may involve the following:

1. Reducing intracellular Ca^{2+}
2. Increasing K^+ conductance, which increases outward current[1]

REENTRY

The cardiac impulse normally moves rapidly through the heart and is extinguished in its first pass because the entire heart becomes refractory; the impulse, having "no place to go," expires.[17] *Reentry* is the propagation of an impulse through tissue already activated by that same impulse. It may be the result of a reentrant loop or, less commonly, reflection. The terms used to describe arrhythmias supported by reentry are circus movement, reciprocal or echo beats, reciprocating tachycardia, and reentry or reentrant tachycardia.

The following are requirements for reentry:

1. An initiating stimulus
2. Slow conduction or a long enough loop to maintain excitability at the tail of the circulating impulse (slow conduction is clinically important to reentry but is not a prerequisite)
3. One-way conduction
4. An activating wave front that circulates around a central inexcitable area (anatomic and/or functional)

A reentry pathway may be sustained because of the following:

1. Slowed conduction along the entire length or a portion of the pathway
2. Shortened effective refractory period along the entire length or a portion of the pathway
3. Depression of Na^+ or Ca^{2+} excitatory currents
4. Inhomogeneous recovery of excitability and responsiveness
5. Changes in membrane or gap junction resistance
6. Any combination of points 1 to 5

An *excitable gap* is said to exist if, during the tachycardia that results from the reentrant loop, a stimulus (overdrive pacing) is delivered that enters the loop in advance of the circulating wave front.

The circus movement reentry (orthodromic and antidromic) seen in patients with Wolff-Parkinson-White (WPW) syndrome is both calcium-channel and sodium-channel dependent and can be interrupted at either site. The *calcium channel–dependent* arm of the circuit is the AV node, with its normal milieu of slow–calcium channel action potentials and slow conduction. The *sodium channel–dependent* arm of the circuit is the accessory pathway, which is composed of myocardial tissue and has fast–sodium channel action potentials. The circuit usually proceeds anterogradely through the AV node and retrogradely up the accessory pathway (orthodromic circus movement tachycardia), but in a small percentage of cases the circuit moves in the opposite direction. This circuit can be interrupted in either arm (i.e., at the AV node with a vagal maneuver, adenosine, or verapamil; or at the accessory pathway with procainamide).

In AV nodal reentry tachycardia, procainamide is used for a different reason; it blocks the retrograde fast pathway in the AV node and thus interrupts the circuit. Following MI the ischemic tissue has slow conduction and so can support a reentry circuit, resulting in ventricular tachycardia.

The most common types of reentry describe a circular pathway (anatomic or functional). Reentry may also depend on fiber orientation, such as anisotropic reentry and reflection. Reentry can also occur using a damaged bundle branch for the slowly conducting arm and an undamaged bundle branch for the return circuit.

Anatomic Reentry

Anatomic reentry is an excitation wave that passes around an anatomic obstacle or obstacles. The earliest and simplest model of reentry, introduced by Mayer in 1906[18,19] and Mines in 1913,[20] shows an impulse that circles a large anatomic obstacle. In Figure 5-8, *A*, the white part within the circle represents fibers that are nonrefractory. This "excitable gap" continues to move around the circle behind the refractory tissue (stippled area). The wave of excitation is thus propagated to produce a regular tachycardia. These descriptions of reentrant excitation around an anatomic obstacle did not include an area of slow conduction. Although not a prerequisite for reentrant circuits, at least one area of slow conduction is thought to be a component of clinically important sustained reentrant rhythms.[21]

In 1920 Lewis[22] introduced a reentry loop in which the pathway involves two anatomic obstacles (e.g., venae cavae). Such a large circuit could result in the impulse crossing at the isthmus to establish a smaller circuit and a faster tachycardia (see Figure 5-8, *B*).[23]

Figure 5-8, *E, F,* and *G* are also models of anatomic reentry. In Figure 5-8, *E*, the impulse wavelength is shortened. Such an impulse may circle an anatomic obstacle and produce a stable reentry circuit. In Figure 5-8, *F*, there is an area of depressed conduction between the two anatomic boundaries, which allows for an excitable gap in the normal myocardium. In Figure 5-8, *G*, note an area of prolonged refractoriness next to an anatomic obstacle; the depolarization wave encircles both areas in a pathway that may be long enough to create an excitable gap in the normal myocardium. Such a circuit may pivot at slightly different points, allowing for different cycle lengths. This type of reentrant tachycardia could last for an extended length of time.[23]

Functional Reentry

Functional reentry does not require circling around an anatomic structure; it depends on the local differences in conduction velocity and is characterized by the "leading circle" (see Figure 5-8, *C* and *D*). In 1980 Moe, Pastelin, and Mendez[24] described a reentry circuit conducted at different velocities through the atria (e.g., on Bachman's bundle and the internodal muscle bands). In 1977 Allessie, Bonke, and Schopman[25] described the "leading circle" type of reentry, in which the length of the pathway was not defined by an anatomic obstacle but by the functional electrophysiologic properties of the myocardium. In this model the reentrant impulse conducts in partially refractory myocardium, with the crest of activation constantly on the refractory tail of the circuit.

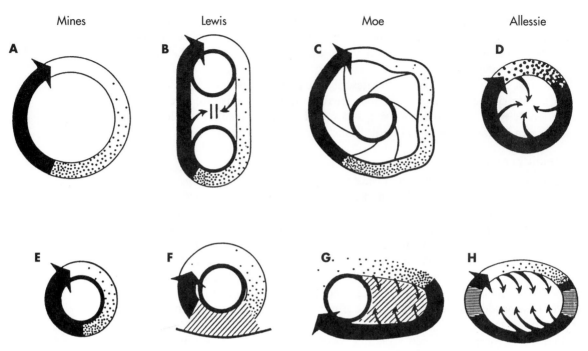

FIGURE 5-8 Schematic representation of various types of reentry. The black arrows represent the crest of a circulating depolarization wave and the tissue that is absolutely refractory. The dotted area indicates the tail of the tissue that is relatively refractory. (From Allessie MA, Rensma W, Brugada J et al: Modes of atrial reentry. In Touboul P, Waldo AL, editors: *Atrial arrhythmias,* St Louis, 1990, Mosby.)

Anisotropic Reentry

Anisotropic reentry is a circuit that is determined by the difference in conduction velocities through the length of the fiber as opposed to across its width. *Isotropic* conduction is uniform in all directions; *anisotropic* is not. Slow conduction in at least part of the reentrant pathway is not required for reentry to occur but facilitates the mechanism and allows recovery time for tissue in the path of the circulating wave front. One-way conduction (unidirectional block) is an essential component of the reentry circuit; without it the impulse would be canceled out by opposing traffic. The anisotropic properties of cardiac muscle (i.e., conduction is faster lengthwise in the fiber than it is across the fiber) contribute to slow conduction and unidirectional block. An anisotropic reentry circuit is diagrammatically illustrated in Figure 5-8, *H* and Figure 5-9.

Reflection

Reflection is another form of reentry that occurs in parallel pathways of Purkinje fibers or myocardial tissue and in which two excitable regions are separated by an area of depressed conduction (Figure 5-10).[26] When the cardiac impulse reaches the severely depressed segment, it is blocked but is transmitted slowly in a less severely depressed

Anisotropic Reentry

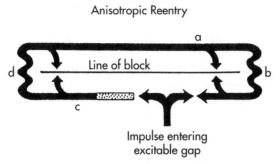

FIGURE 5-9 Schematic representation of an anisotropic reentrant circuit. The line of block is parallel to fiber orientation. Part of the circuit is absolutely refractory *(black)*, part is relatively refractory *(stippled)*, and part is fully excitable *(white)*. Conduction parallel to the long fiber axis (longitudinal conduction) is fast; conduction perpendicular to this axis (transverse conduction) is slow. Only the two longitudinal limbs of the circuit have an excitable gap. (From Task Force of the Working Group on Arrhythmias of the European Society of Cardiology: The Sicilian gambit: a new approach to the classification of antiarrhythmic drugs based on their actions on arrhythmogenic mechanisms, *Circulation* 84:1831, 1991.)

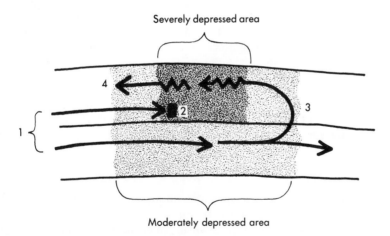

FIGURE 5-10 Reflection. In this form of reentry the impulse *(1)* is at first blocked in the severely depressed fiber *(2)*, but it proceeds slowly in the less depressed fiber (lightly stippled area) to return in the opposite direction *(3)*. It is then able to travel through the severely depressed fiber to reenter its origin *(4)*.

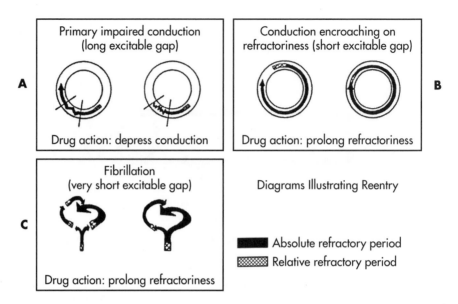

FIGURE 5-11 Schematic representation of methods of terminating reentry. **A,** The left figure shows depressed conduction and depressed excitability in a segment of a reentry circuit (delineated by the two lines). In the right figure, further depression of conduction and excitability results in conduction block. **B,** Conduction during the reentrant tachycardia *(left)* encroaches on the relative refractory period *(right).* If refractoriness is prolonged, the reentrant wave front is blocked in its own refractory tail (or the wave front may merely slow down). **C,** On the left, fibrillation is maintained by the presence of many independent wave fronts. On the right, prolongation of the wavelength of refractoriness reduces the number of wave fronts in a given chamber below a critical number; block and collision of forces terminate the arrhythmia. (From Task Force of the Working Group on Arrhythmias of the European Society of Cardiology: The Sicilian gambit: a new approach to the classification of antiarrhythmic drugs based on their actions on arrhythmogenic mechanisms, *Circulation* 84:1831-1851, 1991.)

neighboring fiber. After reaching the end of the segment, the impulse activates the surrounding tissue and returns in the retrograde direction through the severely depressed segment.

Vulnerable Parameters

The vulnerable parameters of reentry are conduction, refractoriness, and the gap junctions. This unique interface permits very rapid propagation of the stimulus. As a result, the electrical impulse velocity is much greater along the length of the fiber *(isotropic conduction)* than across the fiber bundle *(anisotropic conduction).*[27]

Terminating a Reentry Circuit

Drugs that effectively terminate a reentry circuit either block conduction or prolong the refractory period (Figure 5-11). It is important to note that the same drugs that terminate a reentry circuit by slowing conduction can, by the same mechanism,

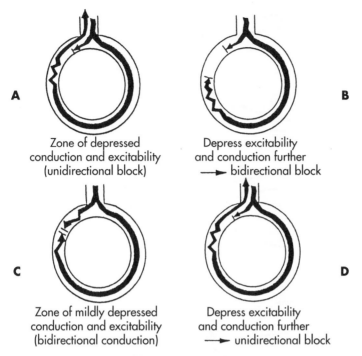

Zone of depressed
conduction and excitability
(unidirectional block)

Depress excitability
and conduction further
⟶ bidirectional block

Zone of mildly depressed
conduction and excitability
(bidirectional conduction)

Depress excitability
and conduction further
⟶ unidirectional block

FIGURE 5-12   Schematic diagram illustrating how depression of excitability and conduction may either prevent or promote the initiation of reentry. **A,** Excitability and conduction in a segment are depressed so that unidirectional block can set the stage for induction of reentry by a premature impulse entering the circuit. **B,** Excitability and conduction are further impaired, creating a zone of bidirectional block so that reentry can no longer be initiated. **C,** The segment is only mildly depressed. Bidirectional conduction is responsible for collision of wave fronts (causing bidirectional block). **D,** Further depression creates the setting for unidirectional block and a completed reentry circuit. (From Task Force of the Working Group on Arrhythmias of the European Society of Cardiology: The Sicilian gambit: a new approach to the classification of antiarrhythmic drugs based on their actions on arrhythmogenic mechanisms, *Circulation* 84:1831-1851, 1991.)

create a reentry circuit in mildly depressed but adequately propagating fibers (Figure 5-12).[1] For example, if there is present in the heart an area of mildly depressed conduction, the sinus impulse will invade this segment from both directions; the impulses will fuse and be annihilated, causing no problems. However, if drugs are given to further depress conduction, unidirectional conduction sets up a reentry circuit, and a reentry tachycardia results.

SUMMATION

Summation has been mentioned by Cranefield[26] as a possible cause of one-way conduction block. It requires a particular arrangement of fibers. If two fibers converge to form one, it is possible that two impulses, both traveling toward the convergence, could meet and form a stronger current. If the segment is depressed, conduction may actually

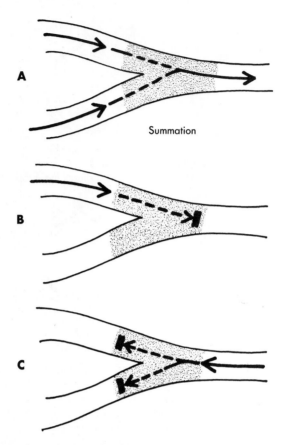

FIGURE 5-13 Summation. **A,** Two impulses converge within a depressed area to form a current strong enough to emerge from the depressed area. **B,** Only one impulse is entering the depressed area and is blocked. **C,** An impulse traveling in the opposite direction through the depressed area divides instead of converging and is blocked.

depend on this convergence and the resulting "summation" (Figure 5-13, *A*). On the other hand, one of the impulses may reach the depressed area at the convergence before the other and be unable to propagate through by itself (Figure 5-13, *B*). In Figure 5-13, *C,* the impulse is traveling in the opposite direction through the depressed area; because it divides instead of uniting, block results.

INHIBITION

The term *inhibition* is used to describe the mechanism by which one impulse that is unable to travel through a depressed segment reaches that segment first and leaves it refractory. As a result, a stronger impulse entering the depressed segment through another fiber is also blocked. In Figure 5-14, *A* and *B,* impulse 1 is able to travel through the depressed segment, whereas impulse 2 is not. However, if impulse 2 reaches the de-

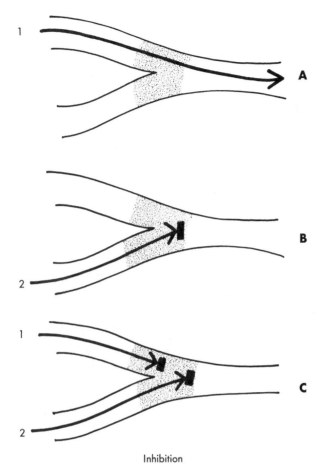

Inhibition

FIGURE 5-14 Inhibition. **A,** The stronger impulse *(1)* can negotiate the depressed *(shaded)* area. **B,** The weaker impulse *(2)* cannot. **C,** The weaker impulse *(2)* reaches the depressed area first and, as a result, blocks the stronger impulse *(1)*.

pressed segment first (Figure 5-14, *C*), it is not only blocked but also leaves refractory tissue in the pathway of impulse 1 and blocks that impulse.

MECHANISMS OF ISCHEMIA-INDUCED ARRHYTHMIAS

During the early phase of myocardial ischemia, reentry is the mechanism of ventricular tachycardia and ventricular fibrillation. Following occlusion of the left anterior descending coronary artery, the first change is depolarization of the resting membrane potential (i.e., it becomes less negative). In the following minutes, the resting membrane potential, upstroke velocity, and amplitude of phase 0 of the action potential decrease further, resulting in slow conduction. Figure 5-15 illustrates the depolarization of

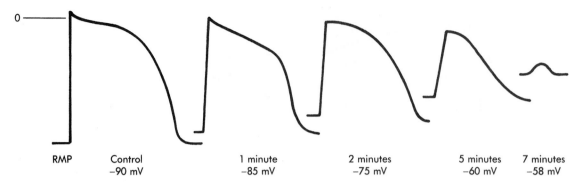

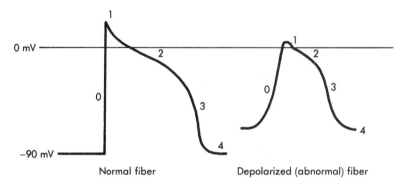

FIGURE 5-15 Effect of ischemia on cardiac action potential. *RMP,* Resting membrane potential.

FIGURE 5-16 Effect of cardiac disease and ischemia on cardiac action potential. A normal Purkinje fiber is compared with the action potential of an abnormal fiber.

a fiber after coronary occlusion. The membrane potential is reduced from its normal of approximately −90 mV to a depressed fast response within 5 minutes and to a slow response within 7 minutes. The slow-response action potential is devoid of all fast sodium channels. Therefore it not only conducts slowly enough to support a reentry circuit but may also be a focus for abnormal automaticity even though it never possessed the capability for automaticity while healthy. An action potential from a normal fiber is compared with that of a depolarized fiber in Figure 5-16.

After approximately 7 minutes, ischemic cells become completely inexcitable at resting membrane potentials of approximately −60 mV. This phase of inexcitability is followed by a transient period of returning electrical activity. After approximately 1 hour, all electrical activity has irreversibly disappeared. Potassium leaves the cell and accumulates in the extracellular space, and there is an abrupt transition from high conduction velocities to inexcitability. Electrical uncoupling occurs over several minutes, and conduction is blocked.

The sympathetic nervous system is also enhanced, and there is local catecholamine release and eventually a massive accumulation of norepinephrine with prolonged ischemia. The effect of sympathetic stimulation on ischemic tissue is the opposite of that on normal cells; the action potential is prolonged instead of shortened. Coupled with all these phenomena is the inhomogeneous distribution of norepinephrine in ischemic tissue, all of which result in an increase in the dispersion of recovery of excitability.[28]

In addition to prolonging conduction of the excitation wave front, ischemia also prolongs the cardiac vulnerable period. Stimulation of fibers during their vulnerable period results in unidirectional block, a condition that increases the probability of a premature beat initiating a reentry circuit.[29,30]

The uncoupling of the cells already mentioned may produce anisotropic conduction, which is capable of supporting a reentry circuit. The low-resistance cell-to-cell connections called *gap junctions* develop a higher resistance during ischemia, which causes them to "uncouple" (i.e., fail to conduct longitudinally). This uncoupling is the result of the elevation of intracellular Ca^{2+} typically associated with myocardial ischemia. Such cells may still retain their high membrane potential and conduct through their transverse margins, where gap junctional density is low. This type of slow discontinuous conduction is anisotropic, in which case slow conduction and reentry can occur in spite of the presence of fast-response action potentials.[31]

SUMMARY

Table 5-1 lists the types of tachycardias and their mechanisms (documented or presumed), location, rate range, and AV or VA conduction characteristics. Arrhythmogenic mechanisms can be deduced with variable certainty from the clinical information and a 12-lead electrocardiogram. The mechanism should in turn imply a particular treatment. An improvement in specific pharmacologic treatment of arrhythmias is linked to an understanding of the mechanisms of arrhythmias and their vulnerable parameters. The future will bring more information on the mechanisms of arrhythmias and the actions of antiarrhythmic drugs, as well as an increase in the number and variety of these drugs.

TABLE 5-1 TACHYCARDIAS, THEIR MECHANISM, AND SELECTED CHARACTERISTICS

TACHYCARDIA	MECHANISM	LOCATION	RATE RANGE (beats/min)	AV OR VA CONDUCTION
Sinus tachycardia	Automatic	SA node	≥100	1:1
SA node reentry	Reentry	SA node and right atrium	(?) 110-180	1:1 or variable
Atrial fibrillation	Reentry	Atria	260-450 (usually >300)	Variable
Atrial flutter	Reentry	Right atrium	240-350 (usually 300 ± 20)	2:1 or variable
Atrial tachycardia	Reentry	Atria	150-240	1:1, 2:1, or variable
	Automatic	Atria	?	?
	Triggered (DADs) secondary to digitalis toxicity	Atria	150-240	1:1, 2:1, or variable
AV nodal reentry tachycardia	Reentry	AV node	120-250 (usually 150-220)	1:1
AV reentry (WPW or concealed accessory AV connection)	Reentry	Circuit includes accessory AV connection, atria, AV node, His bundle, Purkinje system, ventricles	140-250 (usually 150-220)	1:1
Accelerated AV junctional tachycardia	Automatic or (?) triggered	AV junction (AV node and His bundle)	61-200 (usually 80-130)	1:1 or variable
Accelerated idio-ventricular rhythm	Abnormal automaticity	Purkinje fibers	>60-?	Variable, 1:1, or AV dissociation
Ventricular tachycardia	Reentry	Ventricles	120-300 (usually 140-240)	AV dissociation
	Automatic (rare)	Ventricles	?	Variable 1:1, or AV dissociation
Bundle branch reentrant tachycardia	Reentry	Bundle branches and ventricular septum	160-250 (usually 195-240)	AV dissociation, variable, or 1:1
Torsades de pointes	(?) Triggered (EADs)	Ventricles	>200	AV dissociation

Modified from Waldo AL, Wit AL: Mechanisms of cardiac arrhythmias and conduction disturbances. In Schlant RC, Alexander RW, editors: *Hurst's the heart arteries and veins*, ed 8, New York, 1994, McGraw-Hill.

DAD, Delayed afterdepolarization; *EAD,* early afterdepolarization; *WPW,* Wolff-Parkinson-White syndrome.

REFERENCES

1. Task Force of the Working Group on Arrhythmias of the European Society of Cardiology: The Sicilian gambit: a new approach to the classification of antiarrhythmic drugs based on their actions on arrhythmogenic mechanisms, *Circulation* 84:1831, 1991.
2. Trommer PR: Cardiolocution and dysrhythmia (letter), *Am J Cardiol* 50:1198, 1982.
3. Marriott HJL: Arrhythmia versus dysrhythmia, *Am J Cardiol* 53:628, 1984.
4. Whitcomb DC, Gilliam FR III, Starmer CF, Grant AO: Marked QRS complex abnormalities and sodium channel blockade by propoxyphene reversed with lidocaine, *J Clin Invest* 84:1629, 1989.
5. Brugada P, Wellens HJJ, editors: *Cardiac arrhythmias: where to go from here?* Mt Kisco, NY, 1987, Futura.
6. Damiano BP, Rosen M: Effects of pacing on triggered activity induced by early afterdepolarizations, *Circulation* 69:1013, 1984.
7. Wit AL, Rosen MR: Afterdepolarizations and triggered activity. In Fozzard HA, Haber E, Jennings RB et al, editors: *The heart and cardiovascular system,* New York, 1986, Raven Press.
8. Gintant GA: Advances in cardiac cellular electrophysiology: implications for automaticity and therapeutics, *Annu Rev Pharmacol Toxicol* 28:61, 1988.
9. January CT, Riddle JM, Salata JJ: Model for early afterdepolarizations: induction with the Ca^{2+} channel agonist Bay K 8644, *Circ Res* 62:563, 1988.
10. Cranefield PF, Aronson RS: *Cardiac arrhythmias: the role of triggered activity and other mechanisms,* Mt Kisco, NY, 1988, Futura.
11. Rosen MR, Gelband HB, Hoffman BF: Correlation between effects of ouabain on the canine electrocardiogram and transmembrane potentials of isolated Purkinje fibers, *Circulation* 47:65, 1973.
12. Ferrier GR, Saunders JH, Mendez C: A cellular mechanism for the generation of ventricular arrhythmias by acetylstrophanthidin, *Circ Res* 32:600, 1973.
13. Gorgels APM, de Wit B, Beekman HDM et al: Triggered activity induced by pacing during digitalis intoxication, *PACE* 10:1309, 1987.
14. Malfatto G, Rosen TS, Rosen MR: The response to overdrive pacing of triggered atrial and ventricular arrhythmias in the canine heart, *Circulation* 77:1139, 1988.
15. Ferrier GR, Moffat MP, Lukas A: Possible mechanisms of ventricular arrhythmias elicited by ischemia followed by reperfusion: studies on isolated canine ventricular tissues, *Circ Res* 56:184, 1985.
16. Waldo AL, Wit AL: Mechanisms of cardiac arrhythmias and conduction disturbances. In Schlant RC, Alexander RW, editors: *Hurst's the heart arteries and veins,* ed 8, New York, 1994, McGraw-Hill.
17. Zipes DP: Genesis of cardiac arrhythmias: electrophysiological considerations. In Braunwald E, editors: *Heart disease,* ed 4, Philadelphia, 1992, WB Saunders.
18. Mayer AG: *Rhythmical pulsation in scyphomedusae,* publication no 47, Washington, DC, 1906, Carnegie Institution of Washington.
19. Mayer AG: Rhythmical pulsation in scyphomedusae. II. In Papers from the Tortugas Laboratory of the Carnegie Institution of Washington, vol 1, Washington, DC, 1908, Carnegie Institution of Washington.
20. Mines GR: On dynamic equilibrium in the heart, *J Physiol (Lond)* 46:349, 1913.
21. Waldo AL, Wit AL: Mechanisms of cardiac arrhythmias: arrhythmia octet, *Lancet* 341:1189, 1993.

22. Lewis T: Observations upon flutter and fibrillation. IV. Impure flutter: theory of circus movement, *Heart* 7:293, 1920.

23. Allessie MA, Rensma W, Brugada J et al: Modes of atrial reentry. In Touboul P, Waldo AL, editors: *Atrial arrhythmias: current concepts and management,* St Louis, 1990, Mosby.

24. Moe GK, Pastelin G, Mendez R: Circus movement excitation of the atria. In Little RC, editor: *Physiology of atrial pacemakers and conductive tissue,* Mount Kisco, NY, 1980, Futura.

25. Allessie MA, Bonke FIM, Schopman FJG: Circus movement in rabbit atrial muscle as a mechanism of tachycardia. III. The "leading circle" concept: a new model of circus movement in cardiac tissue without the involvement of an anatomic obstacle, *Circ Res* 41:9, 1977.

26. Cranefield PF: *The conduction of the cardiac impulse: the slow response and cardiac arrhythmias,* Mount Kisco, NY, 1975, Futura.

27. Lesh MD, Spear JF, Moore EN: Myocardial anisotropy: basic electrophysiology and role in cardiac arrhythmias. In Zipes DP, Jalife J, editors: *Cardiac electrophysiology,* Philadelphia, 1990, WB Saunders.

28. Janse MJ, Opthof T: Mechanisms of ischemia-induced arrhythmias. In Zipes DP, Jalife J, editors: *Cardiac electrophysiology from cell to bedside,* ed 2, Philadelphia, 1995, WB Saunders.

29. Starmer CF, Biktashev VN, Romashko DN et al: Vulnerability in an excitable medium: analytical and numerical studies of initiating unidirectional propagation, *Biophys J* 65:1775, 1993.

30. Starobin J, Zilberter YI, Starmer CF: Vulnerability in one-dimensional excitable media, *Physica* 70:321, 1994.

31. Rosen MR: Fast-response action potential. In Podrid PJ, Kowey PR: *Cardiac arrhythmia mechanisms, diagnosis, and management,* Baltimore, 1995, Williams & Wilkins.

CHAPTER **6**

Concealed Conduction

Silent zones on the surface
  electrocardiogram 69
SA nodal electrogram 69
His bundle electrogram 70
The ECG related to
  activation of the
  conduction system 72
Concealed conduction 72

SILENT ZONES ON THE SURFACE ELECTROCARDIOGRAM

The discharge of the sinus (sinoatrial [SA]) node is a silent event because the magnitude of the electrical activity generated is too small to be picked up by the surface electrocardiogram (ECG). Indeed, it was not recorded directly at all until 1978.[1,2]

Like the SA nodal discharge, the electrical activity generated during depolarization of the atrioventricular (AV) node and His bundle is not strong enough to be recorded on the surface ECG. However, the PR interval offers a time frame for these events that is not available for the SA nodal discharge and conduction through the SA node to the atrial musculature. Initial activation of the AV node occurs only 0.03 or 0.04 seconds after the beginning of the P wave, with the His bundle and bundle branches activated during the PR segment.

Figure 6-1 illustrates electrical events in the heart and relates them to what is actually seen on the surface ECG. The discharge of the SA node occurs before the onset of the P wave. There also is a measurable conduction time between SA nodal discharge and depolarization of atrial myocardium as signaled by the P wave.

SA NODAL ELECTROGRAM

Direct recording of the electrical discharge of the human SA node was not available until the electrical potentials of the canine SA node were successfully recorded at Columbia University in 1978.[2] In 1979 and 1980, the same team developed a technique for direct recording of electrical potentials from the human SA node.[2,3]

Clinical Value

An understanding of SA conduction time illuminates the mechanism involved in type I and type II SA block and the difference between SA block and sinus arrest. These disorders are discussed in detail in Chapter 7. The SA node ECG may also prove useful in cardiac surgery as an aid to preventing damage to the SA node. It may also provide a better method for differentiating between normal and abnormal SA nodes.

SA Conduction Time

Conduction time between the SA node and the atrial myocardium (SA conduction time) is measured from the deflection on the SA nodal ECG, which is attributed to SA nodal electrical activity, to the beginning of the P wave (in bipolar records) or to the be-

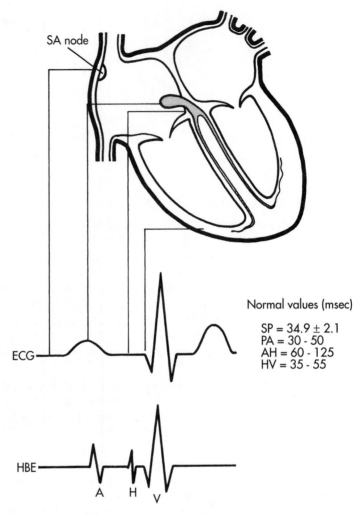

FIGURE 6-1 Electrical events in the heart as related to surface ECG and His bundle electrogram *(HBE)*. The approximate relationship of SA node discharge is also related to surface ECG. *SP,* SA conduction time; *PA,* intraatrial conduction time; *AH,* AV nodal conduction time; *HV,* His-Purkinje conduction time.

ginning of the high right atrial ECG (in unipolar records). In 15 patients without SA nodal dysfunction, SA conduction time was 34.9 ± 2.1 ms. Accurate measurement of SA conduction time permits differentiation between normal and abnormal SA nodal function.[2,3]

HIS BUNDLE ELECTROGRAM

The electrical activity in the His bundle was first recorded in 1960 in Europe[4] and in 1969 in the United States.[5]

TABLE 6-1   NONINVASIVE INTERVENTIONS TO DETERMINE SITE OF AV BLOCK; EFFECT ON AV CONDUCTION

INTERVENTION	AV NODAL CONDUCTION (TYPE I AV BLOCK)	SUBNODAL CONDUCTION (TYPE II AV BLOCK)
Atropine	Improves	Worsens
Exercise	Improves	Worsens
Catecholamines	Improves	Worsens
Carotid sinus massage	Worsens	Improves

Deflections

The deflections seen in the His bundle electrogram (HBE) are as follows (see Figure 6-1):

- **A wave.** The first deflection in the HBE represents atrial activation and is called the A wave. This deflection represents lower right atrial activation because the recording lead is either the bipolar His bundle lead or a low atrial lead.
- **H deflection.** The H deflection follows the A wave and represents His bundle electrical activity as recorded by a catheter lying at the base of the tricuspid valve and close to the His bundle.
- **V deflection.** The last deflection on the HBE represents ventricular activation and is concurrent with the QRS complex on the surface ECG.

Intervals and Normal Values

The HBE divides the PR interval into three components:

- **PA interval.** An approximate measurement of intraatrial conduction time from the area around the SA node to the lower right atrium. It is measured from the onset of the P wave on the standard ECG (or from the atrial deflection of a high right atrial electrogram) to the A wave on the HBE. The normal range for this interval is 30 to 50 ms.
- **AH interval.** Represents AV nodal conduction time. It is measured from the A wave on the HBE to the earliest onset of the His bundle potential. The normal range for this interval is 60 to 125 ms.
- **HV interval.** Conduction time through the His-Purkinje system (from the His bundle to the distal Purkinje fibers). The normal range for this interval is 35 to 55 ms.

Indications

The development of the catheter technique for recording HBEs has enabled the clinician to define the level of conduction delay within the AV junction and to establish the difference between type I and type II AV block. The extrapolation of data obtained from HBEs has actually lessened the clinical need to use the catheter technique. In most cases of AV block, the routine ECG, the clinical setting, and noninvasive interventions provide enough information to deduce correctly the site of block (Table 6-1). Even a diagnosis of concealed junctional extrasystoles, although not definitive, can generally be made from long continuous tracings.

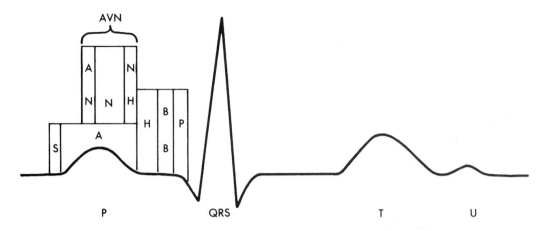

FIGURE 6-2 Sequence of activation through the conduction system as related to surface ECG. Note that the QRS complex begins only after most of the conduction system has already been activated. *S,* SA conduction; *A,* atria; *AVN,* AV node; *AN,* atrionodal; *N,* nodal (central); *NH,* nodal–His bundle; *H,* His bundle; *BB,* bundle branches; *P,* Purkinje fibers.

In the realm of research, HBEs will most certainly continue to contribute to the flow of information regarding reentrant phenomena, the mechanisms and actions of drugs, and the mechanisms of complex arrhythmias. The HBE will continue to be indispensable as a guide in the ablation of the AV node for control of ventricular rates in refractory atrial fibrillation or flutter, as well as in the ablation of atrial, AV, and ventricular arrhythmogenic substrates.

THE ECG RELATED TO ACTIVATION OF THE CONDUCTION SYSTEM

Figure 6-2 relates the ECG to the sequence of activation through the conduction system. Note that the SA node is activated before the P wave is inscribed and that the AV node is initially activated well before atrial depolarization is completed. An understanding of concealed conduction has proven to be most useful in interpreting arrhythmias that would otherwise be inexplicable in the surface ECG.

Activation of most of the His-Purkinje system naturally precedes activation of the working myocardium as represented by the QRS complex. The QRS complex therefore begins after most of the conduction system has already depolarized. An appreciation of this sequence helps with understanding the concept of concealed conduction in the bundle branches.

CONCEALED CONDUCTION

As long as the cardiac impulse is traveling in the specialized conduction system, it does not appear on the surface ECG tracing because of the small amount of tissue involved. However, if this impulse travels only a limited distance within the system, it can interfere with the formation or propagation of another impulse. When this interference can be recognized in the tracing because of an unexpected conduction delay or postponement of an

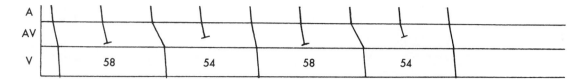

FIGURE 6-3 Diagram of atrial flutter with 2:1 AV conduction and alternation of the ventricular cycle length secondary to concealed deeper penetration of alternate blocked impulses (the first clinical invocation of concealed conduction). (From Kaufmann R, Rothberger CJ: *Z Ges Exp Med* 57:600, 1927.)

impulse, it is known as *concealed conduction*. It can be defined as the propagation of an impulse within the specialized conduction system of the heart that can be recognized only from its effect on the subsequent beat, interval (e.g., PR), or cycle.

Historical Background

The first indirect ECG evidence of concealed AV conduction appeared in 1925 when Lewis and Master[6] demonstrated in the canine heart the effect of blocked impulses on subsequent conduction. During this same period, Ashman[7] was performing similar experiments on the turtle heart. Twenty years before this time Erlanger[8] had noted concealed conduction in his studies on complete heart block and had postulated with Engelmann that delayed conduction was caused by incomplete penetration of the junctional tissues and the resultant partial refractoriness.

In 1927 Kaufmann and Rothberger[9] were the first to apply clinically the concept of concealed conduction. They proposed that the alternation of ventricular cycle length seen in a case of atrial flutter with 2:1 ventricular response was secondary to concealed deeper penetration into the AV junction by every other blocked flutter wave (Figure 6-3).

The term *concealed conduction* was not introduced until 1948, when Langendorf[10] succinctly defined it in the title of his published paper: *Concealed A-V Conduction: The Effect of Blocked Impulses on the Formation and Conduction of Subsequent Impulses.*

In 1950 Sodorstrom[11] and, later, Moe, Abildskov, and Mendez[12] showed that the irregular ventricular response in atrial fibrillation was a function of concealed conduction. The mechanism of concealed conduction was outlined in detail in 1956 by Katz and Pick[13] and in 1961 was demonstrated experimentally as a possibility in any part of the conduction system by Hoffman, Cranefield, and Stuckey.[14] Finally, in 1969, direct evidence of concealed AV conduction was obtained in His bundle recordings.[15]

Concealed Conduction in Atrial Fibrillation

The most common display of concealed conduction is seen in atrial fibrillation. In this arrhythmia literally hundreds of impulses are available each minute for conduction to the ventricles. Therefore it stands to reason that there can be little measurable variation in their spacing. The AV node would be expected to conduct whenever it became nonrefractory, which would be at regular intervals. This, however, is not what happens. The ventricular response to atrial fibrillation is chaotically irregular because

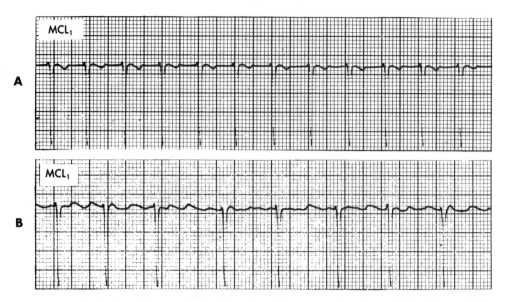

FIGURE 6-4 A, A regular supraventricular tachycardia at a rate of 148 beats/min. **B,** When atrial fibrillation develops, AV conduction to the ventricles is reduced to fewer than 100 beats/min.

numerous impulses are competing for pathways in the AV junction. Some penetrate incompletely, leaving the AV junction refractory yet not producing a QRS complex (concealed conduction); other impulses are blocked. A few do get through and result in (1) haphazard activation of the ventricles, and (2) a reduction in the number of impulses that pass the AV barrier. In fact, the more rapid the bombardment of the AV node by vagrant impulses from the fibrillating atria, the more frequent the concealed conduction and the slower the ventricular response.

Figure 6-4, *A,* illustrates a regular supraventricular tachycardia at a rate of 148 beats/min. In Figure 6-4, *B,* atrial fibrillation has developed in the same patient, with the ventricular rate reduced to fewer than 100 beats/min. In this patient it is evident that the AV junction is able to conduct 148 beats/min; however, when atrial fibrillation ensues, the AV junction can conduct only 100 beats/min because of concealed conduction.

Aberrant Ventricular Conduction Caused by Retrograde Concealed Conduction

Retrograde concealed conduction is a very common mechanism for aberrancy. The ECG shown in Figure 6-5 is from a patient with anteroseptal myocardial infarction. It illustrates a right bundle branch block (RBBB) aberration initiated and terminated by a left ventricular premature beat (VPB). The VPB retrogradely activates the right bundle branch (RBB) late so that the left bundle branch (LBB) can recover for the next sinus beat while the RBB remains refractory (phase 3 aberration). Conduction proceeds down the LBB. By this time the distal RBB has recovered and is again retrogradely activated late, leaving it again refractory for the next sinus beat, and so on. This scenario is

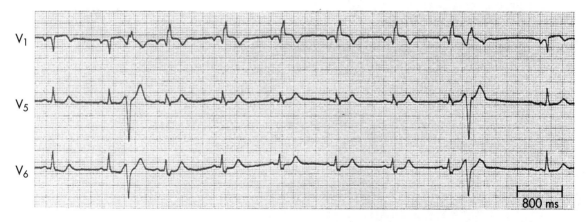

FIGURE 6-5 Phase 3 RBBB aberration caused by retrograde concealed conduction following a left ventricular VPB. The left ventricular VPB (fourth complex) penetrates the RBB late, leaving it refractory for the next sinus beat. Thus the next six sinus beats are conducted down the LBB and retrogradely up the RBB until another VPB breaks the pattern. (Courtesy Hein JJ Wellens, MD, The Netherlands.)

repeated for each ensuing sinus beat until another VPB breaks the cycle. The second VPB is followed by recovery of the refractory period of the RBB, which allows the next sinus beat to be conducted over both bundle branches. Note the retrograde P′ wave following the second VPB.

Interpolated Ventricular Extrasystoles with Concealed Retrograde Conduction

Ventricular extrasystoles often conduct retrogradely all the way to the atria. Kistin and Landowne[16] showed that this happened nearly half the time. It is therefore likely that a majority of ectopic ventricular impulses are conducted at least as far as the AV junction. This conduction is evident only if it has an effect on the next cycle; this effect is most likely if the next beat is due soon, such as the beat after an *interpolated* VPB. In such a case the VPB is sandwiched between two consecutive sinus beats. If the VPB penetrates retrogradely into the AV junction, the next sinus beat encounters refractory tissue and travels more slowly; thus the PR interval of the sinus beat following the VPB is prolonged.

In Figure 6-6 the PR interval after the VPB is so long that it creates the impression of supraventricular prematurity in the following beat. When the ventricular rhythm is irregular, the atrial rhythm often appears irregular also. The laddergram indicates the regularity of the sinus rhythm and the concealed retrograde conduction from the VPB. In Figure 6-7 there are three interpolated VPBs, all of which are followed by concealed retrograde conduction. In the laddergram the sinus P waves are right on time, which is not immediately perceived in the tracing. The PR prolongation after each VPB varies, depending on how soon the P wave follows the VPB. The closer it is, the longer the PR interval (a shorter RP results in a longer PR); the later the P, the shorter the PR.

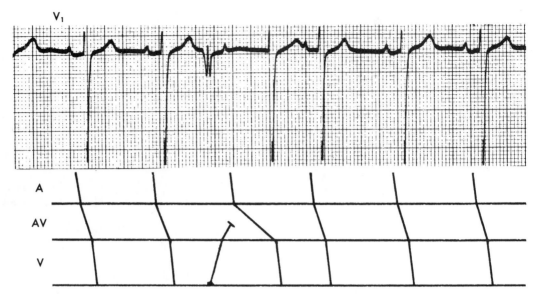

FIGURE 6-6 Third beat is an interpolated ventricular extrasystole which, thanks to retrograde concealed conduction, prolongs the next PR interval to approximately 0.50 second.

Figure 6-8 shows the progressive effect of interpolated ventricular bigeminy on the PR interval to produce a Wenckebach-like effect. Three of the P waves in this tracing are detectable only because of the way they distort the T waves, especially because this distortion occurs when a sinus P wave is expected (see the laddergram). The first VPB is interpolated, and its retrograde concealed conduction lengthens the following PR interval. Because the sinus rhythm is regular and the VPBs are precisely coupled, the next sinus P wave falls earlier on the downslope of the ectopic T wave, which results in an even longer PR interval. This sequence continues, with the sinus P waves falling progressively closer to the preceding ectopic beat. The fifth P wave of the series ends such a short RP interval that it is not conducted. The first three VPBs are interpolated; the fourth is not, and the Wenckebach-like cycle begins again.

Figure 6-9 is another example of ventricular bigeminy. However, because of the slower sinus rate in this example, the P waves are quite evident and the PR lengthening is easily appreciated. The sequence consists of two VPBs that are interpolated and a third that is not. The third VPB is followed by a ventricular escape beat.

Concealed Junctional Extrasystoles

Concealed junctional extrasystoles discharge the AV junction while both anterograde and retrograde conduction is blocked. Such an event is completely silent on the surface ECG. However, its diagnosis may be extremely important in patient management because concealed junctional beats can imitate type I (Wenckebach) and type II AV block and are themselves thought to indicate significant junctional disease.

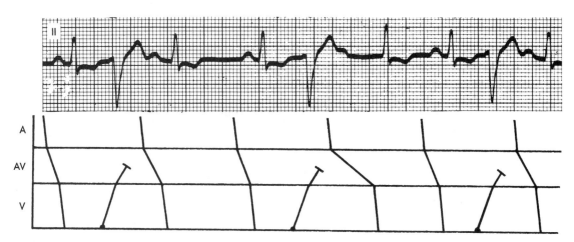

FIGURE 6-7 The second, fifth, and eighth beats are interpolated ventricular extrasystoles that prolong the ensuing PR intervals by concealed retrograde conduction.

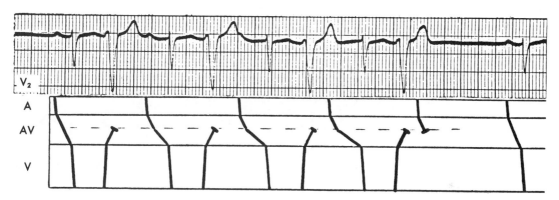

FIGURE 6-8 Interpolated ventricular bigeminy produces a Wenckebach-like effect because of retrograde concealed conduction. The first VPB lengthens the next PR, which automatically "pushes" the next couplet (sinus beat plus VPB) to the right and brings the ectopic beat nearer to the next P wave (shorter RP). Thus the next retrograde conduction is closer to the next descending impulse, and the PR is prolonged still further. This sequence is repeated until finally, after the fourth extrasystole, the descending impulse fails to get through.

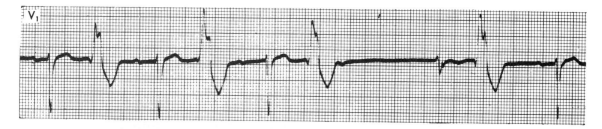

FIGURE 6-9 Ventricular bigeminy with concealed retrograde conduction that produces progressive lengthening of the PR interval until the fourth sinus impulse fails to get through. After the "dropped" beat, the cycle ends with a ventricular escape beat.

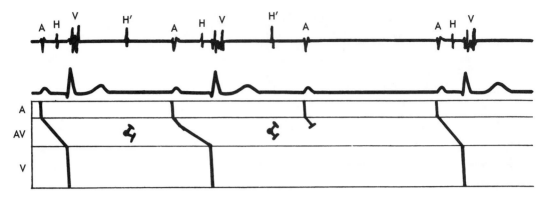

FIGURE 6-10 Diagrammatic representation of how concealed junctional extrasystoles can imitate Wenckebach conduction. The His bundle recording, ECG, and laddergram depict concealed junctional bigeminy that mimics the Wenckebach phenomenon. The first functional extrasystole lengthens the following AH and PR intervals; the next extrasystole prevents conduction altogether and simulates the dropped beat of a Wenckebach period.

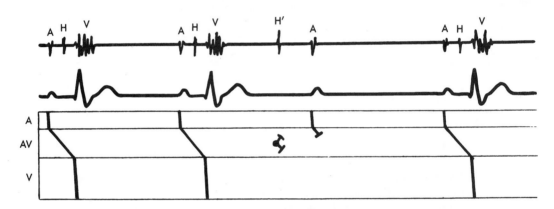

FIGURE 6-11 Diagrammatic representation of how concealed junctional extrasystoles can mimic type II AV block. Without prior lengthening of the PR interval, the junctional extrasystole prevents conduction of the next sinus impulse. *A*, Atrial activation; *H*, His bundle activation; *V*, ventricular activation; *H'*, junctional extrasystole.

Type I periodicity may be imitated in the presence of concealed junctional bigeminy because the PR may progressively lengthen until a beat is dropped (Figure 6-10). Type II AV block may be imitated if a single concealed junctional extrasystole suddenly prevents conduction of a sinus impulse (Figure 6-11) or if concealed penetration involves the proximal His-Purkinje system. Because the development of type II AV block is a widely accepted indication for a permanent implanted pacemaker, there is a serious responsibility to rule out concealed junctional extrasystoles.

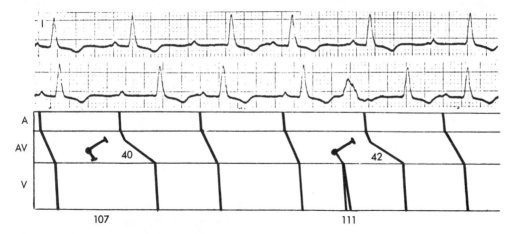

FIGURE 6-12 Strips are not continuous. In the top strip the two longer PR intervals and ventricular cycles are caused by concealed junctional extrasystoles (as diagrammed under the beginning of the bottom strip). Farther along in the bottom strip there is a junctional extrasystole conducted to the ventricles with LBBB aberration, producing the same effect on the next PR interval. (Courtesy Dr. Leo Schamroth, Johannesburg.)

ECG clues to concealed junctional extrasystoles

Although concealed junctional extrasystoles can be documented only with the aid of HBEs (which may indeed be necessary if there is a question of pacing the patient), they can be strongly suspected from the following clues:

1. Abrupt, unexplained lengthening of the PR interval
2. The presence of apparent types I and II AV block in the same tracing
3. Apparent type II block in the presence of a normal QRS complex
4. The presence of manifest junctional extrasystoles elsewhere in the tracing

In the top tracing of Figure 6-12 there is an abrupt and unexplained lengthening of the PR interval. This lengthening is not caused by the Wenckebach phenomenon because the next sinus impulse is conducted with a shorter PR interval and there are no non-conducted beats. In the bottom tracing there is the same abrupt and unexplained lengthening of the PR interval followed by two normally conducted beats and what looks like an interpolated VPB with concealed retrograde conduction to the atria, manifested by the long PR interval. Herein lies the clue to the abrupt and unexplained PR prolongations. As shown on the laddergram, if instead of a VPB the bizarre beat is a junctional extrasystole with aberration, the lengthening of the first three PR intervals becomes understandable—they are caused by the effect of concealed junctional extrasystoles.

In Figure 6-13 concealed junctional extrasystoles presumably cause PR lengthening and a dropped beat, simulating type II second-degree AV block. In Figure 6-14 concealed junctional extrasystoles are the most likely mechanism for the unexpected PR lengthening followed by PR shortening. The concealed junctional beats that occur after every second QRS complex leave the AV junction refractory and cause the next PR to lengthen. They also cause a bigeminal rhythm.

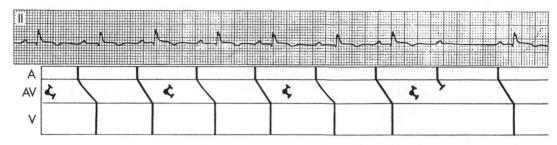

FIGURE 6-13 Concealed junctional extrasystoles every second beat are the most likely explanation for the alternating (shortened-lengthened-shortened-lengthened) PR intervals, the group beating, and the single dropped beat. The laddergram depicts this mechanism.

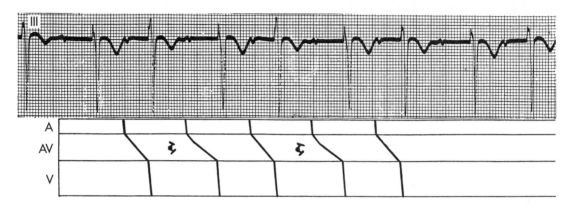

FIGURE 6-14 Concealed junctional extrasystoles again explain alternating PR intervals and group beating. The laddergram depicts this mechanism.

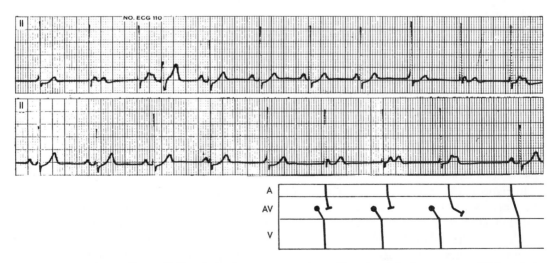

FIGURE 6-15 AV dissociation between an accelerated junctional rhythm at a rate of 74 beats/min and a slightly slower sinus rhythm. In the top strip the fourth beat is a ventricular capture conducted with aberration. At the end of the bottom strip there is another attempted capture, but the sinus impulse fails to reach the ventricle. However, as shown in the laddergram, it does reach and discharge the junctional pacemaker.

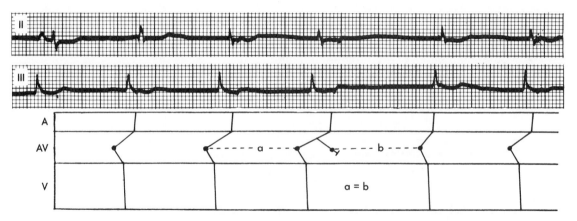

FIGURE 6-16 In lead II the first beat is a sinus beat. A mildly accelerated junctional rhythm takes over at a rate of 62 beats/min, with retrograde conduction to the atria. The RP lengthens progressively (potential retrograde Wenckebach), and a longer ventricular cycle develops after the fourth beat. The same sequence is repeated twice in lead III, for which the mechanism is diagrammed. A critical degree of retrograde conduction delay enables the retrograde impulse to reenter a downward path and discharge and reset the junctional pacemaker, although it fails to reach the ventricles.

Concealed Conduction Affecting Impulse Formation

In the bottom tracing of Figure 6-15 there is a sudden and unexpected interruption of an accelerated junctional rhythm (74 beats/min), which is dissociated from the slightly slower sinus rhythm. In the top tracing the junctional rhythm is interrupted when a sinus impulse (P wave in the T wave of the third junctional beat) is conducted to the ventricles (ventricular capture). After two normal sinus beats the accelerated junctional rhythm takes over again. Toward the end of the bottom tracing the same thing almost occurs a second time, but the sinus impulse fails to reach the ventricles. It does, however, discharge the AV pacemaker and interrupt the junctional rhythm. Thus concealed conduction is recognized because an expected beat fails to appear.

In Figure 6-16 another junctional rhythm has a sudden unexpected interruption. Each junctional beat is followed by a retrograde P′ wave, and the RP′ interval lengthens with each beat. Only when the RP′ interval has lengthened critically is the junctional rhythm abruptly interrupted. The readiest explanation is illustrated in the laddergram. Delayed retrograde conduction has permitted reentry with a resulting abortive reciprocal beat. The retrograde impulse with the longest RP′ interval turns down toward the ventricles but fails to reach its destination. However, it does succeed in discharging and thus resetting the junctional focus, leaving in its tracks an unexpected pause.

Figure 6-17 illustrates yet another form of concealed retrograde conduction. In this tracing a junctional escape rhythm of 36 beats/min results from an underlying sinus bradycardia and arrhythmia. Three VPBs can be seen in the two strips. In the top strip these VPBs do not disturb the basic junctional cycle length, which varies between 161

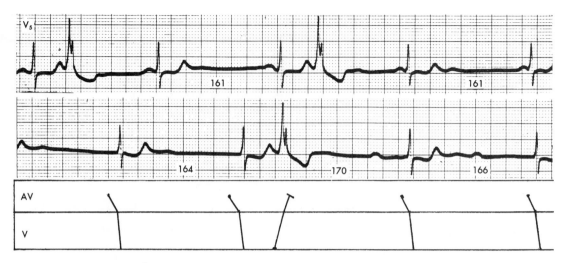

FIGURE 6-17 An idiojunctional pacemaker at a rate of 36 beats/min is dissociated from an irregular but even slower sinus rhythm. The two VPBs in the top strip do not interfere with the regularity of the junctional firing, but the VPB in the bottom strip does. This mechanism is diagrammed below the second strip. Through concealed retrograde conduction to the AV junction, this VPB resets the idiojunctional pacemaker.

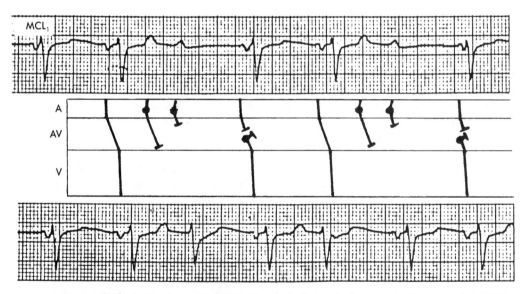

FIGURE 6-18 Strips are not continuous. On two occasions in the top strip there are pairs of APBs, neither of which is conducted. The first is not conducted because of refractoriness resulting from the preceding sinus conducted beat. The second is not conducted because of incomplete penetration of the junction by the preceding APB.

V_1

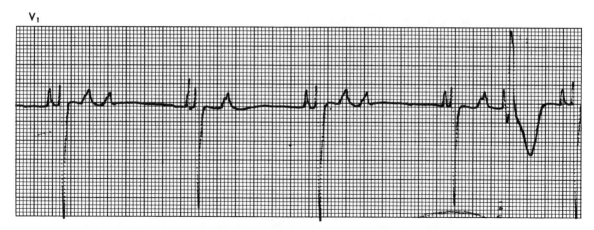

FIGURE 6-19 Bigeminal nonconducted APBs. After the first and third ventricular complexes there are two APBs in a row; the second of them is not conducted, probably because of incomplete penetration into the AV junction by the preceding APB. At the end of the strip an APB is conducted with RBBB aberration. There is an artifact in the second sinus P wave.

and 166 ms. However, the VPB in the second strip postpones the junctional beat, from which it can be inferred that the ventricular ectopic impulse has traveled retrogradely into the AV junction, discharged the junctional pacemaker, and reset its rhythm.

Figure 6-18 provides an interesting example of how consecutive atrial premature beats (APBs) can suggest some degree of AV block. In the top tracing there is an APB in the second and fourth T waves. Both APBs are immediately followed by a second APB late enough in the cycle to conduct normally to the ventricles. However, it is not conducted, suggesting AV block, and the pause ends with a junctional escape beat. In the bottom tracing (from the same patient), a single APB with the same coupling interval as in the top tracing is conducted on two occasions. If some APBs premature enough to land on the T wave can be conducted, it would stand to reason that the second of each pair of APBs in the top strip, which land well beyond the T wave, could be easily conducted. The explanation for this failure of conduction is that the first of each pair of APBs in the top strip has penetrated the AV junction and left it refractory so that the second APB of the pair is blocked.

In Figure 6-19 the same mechanism as described in the previous paragraph explains the failure of the second of a pair of APBs to be conducted when the first of the pair is conducted with RBBB aberration at the end of the tracing. The underlying rhythm is sinus with nonconducted atrial bigeminy.

SUMMARY

Conduction of the cardiac impulse through the heart is reflected on the surface ECG when the atrial or ventricular myocardium is activated. When the impulse is traveling within the SA node and perinodal fibers or within the AV node or His-Purkinje system, the amount of electrical current generated is too small to be seen on the surface ECG and is therefore "concealed." However, these currents can be recorded using invasive techniques such as SA nodal and His bundle electrograms. The existence of concealed conduction can be determined by its effects on what follows it. During atrial fibrillation, concealed conduction into the His-Purkinje system from the fibrillating atria is responsible for the irregular ventricular response in that not all impulses reach the ventricular myocardium but instead leave the conduction system refractory. Concealed conduction retrogradely into the fast pathway of the AV node is often observed after an interpolated ventricular extrasystole, which causes a long PR interval because the next sinus beat finds only the slow intranodal pathway available. Junctional extrasystoles that are blocked in both directions are concealed and affect the sinus impulse that follows.

REFERENCES

1. Cramer M, Hariman RJ, Hoffman BF: Electrograms from the canine sinoatrial pacemaker recorded in vitro and in situ, *Am J Cardiol* 42:939, 1978.
2. Hariman RJ, Krongrad E, Boxer RA, Weiss MB: Method for recording electrical activity of the sinoatrial node and automatic atrial foci during cardiac catheterization in human subjects, *Am J Cardiol* 45:775, 1980.
3. Hariman RJ, Krongrad E, Boxer RA, Bowman FO Jr: Methods for recording electrograms of the sinoatrial node during cardiac surgery in man, *Circulation* 61:10, 1980.
4. Giraud G: Variations de potentiel liées à l'activité du système de conduction auriculo-ventriculaire chez l'homme (enregistrement electrocardiographic endocavitairea), *Arch Mal Coeur* 53:757, 1960.
5. Scherlag BJ, Lau SH, Helfant RH et al: Catheter technique for recording His bundle activity in man, *Circulation* 39:13, 1969.
6. Lewis T, Master AM: Observations upon conduction in the mammalian heart: A-V conduction, *Heart* 12:209, 1925.
7. Ashman K: Conductivity in compressed cardiac muscle: supernormal phase in conductivity in compressed auricular muscle in the turtle heart, *Am J Physiol* 74:140, 1925.
8. Erlanger J: On the physiology of heart block in mammals, with special reference to the causation of Stokes-Adams disease, *J Exp Med* 7:676, 1905.
9. Kaufmann R, Rothberger CJ: Der-Uebergang von Kammerallorhythmien in Kammer-Arrhythmie in klinischen Fällen von Vorhofflattern, Alternans der Reisleitung, *Z Ges Exp Med* 57:600, 1927.
10. Langendorf R: Concealed A-V conduction: the effect of blocked impulses on the formation and conduction of subsequent impulses, *Am Heart J* 35:542, 1948.
11. Sodorstrom N: What is the reason for the ventricular arrhythmia in cases of atrial fibrillation? *Am Heart J* 40:212, 1970.
12. Moe GK, Abildskov JA, Mendez C: An experimental study of concealed conduction, *Am Heart J* 67:338, 1964.
13. Katz LN, Pick A: Clinical electrocardiography. I. *Arrhythmias,* Philadelphia, 1956, Lea & Febiger.
14. Hoffman BF, Cranefield PF, Stuckey JH: Concealed conduction, *Circ Res* 9:194, 1961.
15. Lau SH: A study of atrioventricular conduction in atrial fibrillation and flutter in man using His bundle recordings, *Circulation* 40:69, 1965.
16. Kistin AD, Landowne M: Retrograde conduction from premature ventricular contractions: a common occurrence in the human heart, *Circulation* 3:738, 1951.

CHAPTER 7

Sinoatrial Node Dysfunction

The SA node 85
24-hour heart rate
    variability 88
Increased heart rate 89
SA nodal reentrant
    tachycardia 89
SA exit block 92
Sick sinus syndrome 94

S INUS TACHYCARDIA AND SINUS BRADYCARDIA ARE WELL COVERED IN BASIC ELECTRO-
cardiography (ECG) books. This chapter deals with the anatomy and physiology of
the sinus (sinoatrial [SA]) node and the more advanced concepts of its arrhythmias.

THE SA NODE
Anatomy

The SA node is located superficially under the epicardium at the junction between
the superior vena cava and the right atrium (Figure 7-1). It is a spindle-shaped structure
of specialized cells with a central body and tapering ends. The head extends toward the
interatrial groove, and the tail extends toward the orifice of the inferior vena cava. In approximately 10% of individuals, the head extends across the crest of the atrial appendage
into the interatrial groove ("horseshoe" node) (see Figure 1-2).

The spread of electrical current between the SA and atrioventricular (AV) nodes is facilitated by isotropic conduction patterns within muscle bands composed of parallel
fibers that are located in the anterior limbus of the fossa ovalis, the crista terminalis,
and its continuation into the sinus septum. Broad wave fronts emanate from these bands
to activate adjacent atrial tissue. The preferential conduction between the two nodes
partly results from the isotropic construction of the muscle fibers in the bands as opposed to the anisotropic construction of the remainder of the right atrium.[1]

Physiology

The SA node is the dominant pacemaker of the heart. Its pacing function is determined by its low maximum diastolic membrane potential and steep phase 4. The means
by which SA nodal cells depolarize and reach threshold (-30 to -40 mV) is discussed
on p. 32.

Gomes and Winters[2] have found that the SA node has more than one pacing site
within it and that this large reserve capacity for automaticity casts more suspicion on the
failure of SA conduction as the culprit in so-called "sinus arrest." Their study involved
24 patients and the use of direct recordings of SA nodal potentials and suggests that
within the SA node itself are dominant and subsidiary pacing sites that produce sinus P
waves of different shapes and cycle lengths. The latent sinus pacemaker site has a longer
cycle length than does the dominant site.

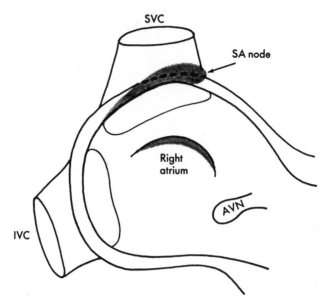

FIGURE 7-1 SA node. *SVC,* Superior vena cava; *IVC,* inferior vena cava; *AVN,* AV node.

Figure 7-2 is a gross representation of pacemaker shifts in the human SA node. Three shapes of sinus P waves result from shifts in pacing sites within the node. The primary site is in the upper portion of the SA node; two distal sites are illustrated. A shift to the subsidiary sites for one to six beats was noted after atrial stimulation at close coupling intervals in 56% of patients and during carotid sinus massage in 75% of patients. In Gomes and Winters' study,[2] spontaneous sinus pacemaker shifts were infrequent, suggesting that the so-called "wandering atrial pacemaker," a change in P wave morphology after overdrive pacing, or an early atrial premature beat may represent a shift to another site within the SA node rather than an atrial ectopic beat.

Another study used epicardial mapping on 14 patients at the time of surgery for Wolff-Parkinson-White (WPW) syndrome tachyarrhythmias and found multiple atrial pacemaker regions producing different patterns of global atrial activation and P waves of different shapes.[3] A typical sinus beat originated posteriorly and medial to the sulcus terminalis at the junction between the superior vena cava and the right atrium. Most of the patients in this study had more than one pacemaker site.

Conduction velocity in the SA node and the perinodal zone becomes slower and slower in response to more and more premature atrial extrasystoles, exhibiting behavior comparable to AV nodal tissue.[4] Thus an atrial extrasystole may enter the perinodal zone and conduct slowly through it or the body of the SA node, setting the scene for reentry. Rarely, it may also happen that the atrial extrasystole is early enough to arrive at the perinodal zone when the zone is in its absolute refractory period. In this case the rhythm of the SA node remains undisturbed and the next sinus beat appears on time, resulting in an interpolated atrial premature beat.

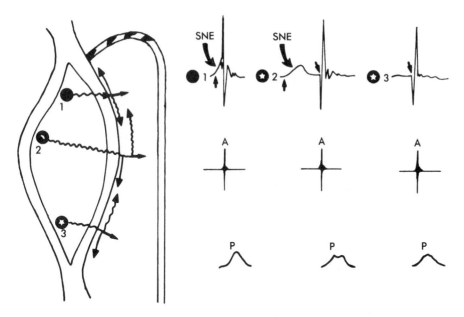

FIGURE 7-2 Pacemaker shift to alternate sites within the SA node results in different patterns to the SA node electrogram *(SNE)* and the sinus P wave. Dominant sinus pacemaker originates in the head end of the SA node *(1)*. *A*, Atrial potential; *P*, P wave. (From Gomes JA, Winters SL: The origins of the sinus node pacemaker complex in man: demonstration of dominant and subsidiary foci, *J Am Coll Cardiol* 9:45, 1987.)

Blood Supply

The SA node is supplied with blood by a large central artery with a rich supply of collateral vessels that are dense toward the center and thin toward the periphery of the node. The large central SA nodal artery originates from the initial portions of the right coronary artery in approximately 60% of cases and from the circumflex artery in 40% of cases. It passes through the interatrial groove and may be either epicardial or intramyocardial.[1] The disproportionately large size of the SA nodal artery is considered physiologically important in that its perfusion pressure may affect the sinus rate. Distention of the artery slows the sinus rate, whereas collapse causes an increase in rate.[4]

Nerve Supply

Parasympathetic and sympathetic influences modify both the rate of spontaneous depolarization in the SA node and the SA conduction time. Vagal stimulation prolongs SA conduction time and causes sinus slowing, an increase in intranodal conduction time, and lengthening of the effective and relative refractory periods of the SA node. Sympathetic stimulation shortens SA conduction time and causes an increase in the sinus rate because of steeper phase 4 depolarization.[3]

Temperature

Hypothermia inhibits the Na^+ pump, causing an accumulation of intracellular Na^+ and sinus slowing. Hyperthermia increases the sinus rate.

Diagnostic Evaluation of SA Node Function

The diagnostic approach for evaluating SA node function is individualized for each patient and depends on the patient's symptoms. The first step is usually ECG monitoring. Beyond this, the other diagnostic tools available for evaluation of suspected SA nodal dysfunction include the following:

- Ambulatory ECG recordings (24-hour, 48-hour tape recording)
- Ambulatory event recorders (intermittent, continuous loop)
- Exercise testing
- Tests for the autonomic nervous system (carotid sinus massage, Valsalva maneuver, upright tilt test, pharmacologic interventions)
- Clinical electrophysiologic testing (recovery times and secondary pauses after rapid atrial pacing, SA conduction time, SA node refractory period)

SA Conduction Time

SA conduction time is the interval between the exit of an impulse from the SA node to its arrival in atrial fibers. This measurement is made during electrophysiologic studies.[5,6]

24-HOUR HEART RATE VARIABILITY

Heart rate variability is the oscillation of the interval between consecutive heartbeats and between consecutive instantaneous heart rates. It is the *interval* between consecutive heartbeats that is being analyzed rather than the heart rate per se.

Clinical Value

Reduced heart rate variability is a powerful predictor of arrhythmia-related complications in patients who survive the acute phase of myocardial infarction.[7-10] Its predictive value is independent of left ventricular ejection fraction, the frequency of ventricular premature complexes, and the presence of late potentials on signal-averaged ECGs.[7,11]

History

The clinical value of heart rate variability for fetal distress was first reported by Hon and Lee.[12] The link between reduced heart rate variability and higher risk in postinfarction patients was first established in 1977.[13] After another decade heart rate variability was appreciated as a strong and independent predictor of mortality following acute myocardial infarction.[7-9]

Methods of Evaluation

In 1981 Akselrod, Gordon, and Ubel et al[15] introduced power spectral analysis of heart rate fluctuations as a quantitative probe of beat-to-beat cardiovascular control. Because of new digital, high-frequency, 24-hour multichannel ECG recorders available

TABLE 7-1 RISK STRATIFICATION FOR CARDIAC DEATH AFTER MYOCARDIAL INFARCTION

	SENSITIVITY (%)	SPECIFICITY (%)	POSITIVE PREDICTIVE ACCURACY (%)
Mean RR interval <700 ms	45	85	20
Heart rate variability <17 U	40	86	20
Left ventricular ejection fraction <35%	40	78	14

Sensitivity, The percentage of patients with a positive test result from all patients who died; *specificity,* the percentage of patients with a negative test result from all patients who did not die; *positive predictive accuracy,* the percentage of patients who died from all patients with a positive test result.

on the market today, heart rate variability has the potential to contribute significantly to risk stratification for postinfarction patients. The special report from the Task Force of the European Society of Cardiology and the North American Society of Pacing and Electrophysiology provides information regarding the measurement of heart rate interval, standards of measurement, physiologic interpretation, and clinical use of heart rate variability.[15]

INCREASED HEART RATE

Increased heart rate has been demonstrated to be a strong predictor of mortality after myocardial infarction.[16] A total of 579 patients surviving the acute phase of myocardial infarction were followed for at least 2 years, with evaluations of 24-hour mean RR interval (mean duration of all normal-to-normal RR intervals on the Holter recording), predischarge heart rate variability, and left ventricular ejection fraction. It was concluded that a predischarge 24-hour mean heart rate with an RR <700 ms is a strong predictor of mortality after myocardial infarction. This measurement competes with left ventricular ejection fraction and heart rate variability (Table 7-1).[10]

SA NODAL REENTRANT TACHYCARDIA

SA nodal reentrant tachycardia is thought to be a paroxysmal supraventricular tachycardia (PSVT) that uses the SA node as the slow arm of a reentry loop. In its sustained form it lasts more than 30 seconds and requires pacing, vagal maneuvers, or adenosine to terminate it.[17]

Not all investigators agree with the possibility of SA nodal reentry. Lesh and Kalman[18] classify tachycardias that might be called "SA nodal reentry" along with the group of "cristal tachycardias," which are named for their origin along the crista terminalis. They propose that sinus-like P waves can result from a focus on the crista terminalis, because the entire length of that structure can act as a substrate for atrial tachycardia. They also state that there is no clear evidence that SA node reentry acts differently from foci on the crista and that in vivo mapping of that structure has shown changes in the site of earliest SA node activation along with altered P wave axes under the influence of autonomic tone (see Chapter 4).

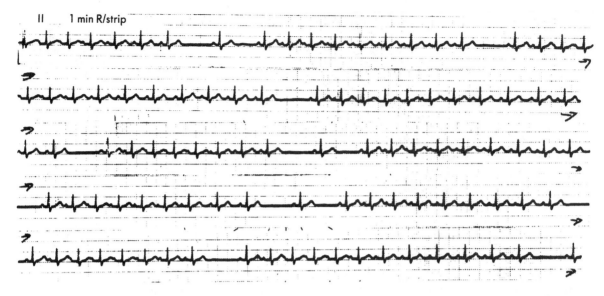

FIGURE 7-3 Repetitive paroxysmal supraventricular tachycardia. (From Curry PVL, Shenasa M: Atrial arrhythmias: clinical concepts. In Mandel WJ, editor: *Cardiac arrhythmias: their mechanisms, diagnosis and management,* Philadelphia, 1987, JB Lippincott.)

ECG Features

- **Heart rate.** Usually relatively slow (<150 beat/min), often with wide fluctuations
- **Rhythm.** PSVT; most attacks do not last longer than 10 to 20 beats[19]; however, they are repetitive and sensitive to changes in autonomic tone (including changes associated with normal breathing), which makes distinction from sinus arrhythmia sometimes difficult
- **QRS complex.** Narrow
- **P waves.** Look like sinus P waves but may not always be identical; precede rather than follow the QRS complexes, as is the case in the more common mechanisms of PSVT
  Figure 7-3 is an example of repetitive PSVT caused by SA nodal reentry.

ECG Documentation

The difficulty in ECG documentation of SA node disease lies in the fact that symptoms are relatively uncommon. For this reason, ECG event recorders may be more useful than the conventional magnetic tape recording systems.

Differential Diagnosis

SA nodal reentry can masquerade as sinus tachycardia, atrial tachycardia with block, and sinus arrhythmia. It is difficult to imagine SA nodal reentry tachycardia being mistaken for the two most common causes of PSVT (AV nodal reentry and circus movement tachycardia using an accessory pathway) because of the difference in P′ wave position, P′ wave polarity, and heart rate. The presence of 2:1 AV conduction excludes the possibility of an accessory pathway and is extremely rare (although theoretically possible) in AV nodal reentry.

History

The possibility of reentry through the SA node as a cause of PSVT was first suggested in 1943 and was conclusively documented by elaborate studies in the rabbit heart in 1968.[20,21] Until recently, SA nodal reentrant tachycardia was treated with drugs.[22] Surgical modification of the SA node offered a cure, but the morbidity of open heart surgery was significant.[23] With the refinement of the procedure for transvenous radiofrequency catheter ablation, the outlook for all patients with PSVTs has significantly improved.

Symptoms

Some bouts of SA nodal reentry tachycardia go unnoticed or are only slightly bothersome; more than half are associated with palpitations. In some cases the patient experiences angina, dyspnea, and syncope, especially when the tachycardia is associated with heart disease and sick sinus syndrome.

Mechanism

SA nodal reentry may develop without ectopic interference during a sinus rhythm or may be initiated by an atrial premature beat (APB) that arrives at the SA node before it has completely recovered excitability (during its relative refractory period).

There is slow conduction through the SA node itself or through atrial tissue adjacent to the SA node. This slow conduction provides the anatomic substrate for the leading circle type of reentry around a functionally refractory center.[6,24]

Atrial activation is a high-to-low sequence with a P wave configuration during the tachycardia similar to the sinus P waves.[17] The depolarization wave reenters the SA node or adjacent fibers and begins the loop again (Figure 7-4). The sequence of atrial activation is identical to that of sinus impulses.

Incidence

In 1978 Narula[25] demonstrated SA nodal reentry as the underlying mechanism in 8% of patients with PSVT. In 343 patients undergoing evaluation for PSVT and catheter ablation, 11 (3.2%) met stringent criteria for sustained SA nodal reentrant tachycardia.[17] This finding is similar to that observed by Josephson[26] (3%) and Wellens[27] (1.8%).

Treatment

In the acute symptomatic setting, SA nodal reentry should respond to vagal maneuvers and adenosine. The reentry circuit uses the SA node as the slow part of the reentry loop, just as AV nodal reentry and circus movement tachycardia of WPW use the AV node.

SA nodal modification with radiofrequency catheter ablation and preservation of normal SA nodal function is an effective and safe cure for SA nodal reentry tachycardia.[17,28,29] The radiofrequency energy is delivered in the high lateral right atrium at the sites of earliest atrial activation during the tachycardia.[17]

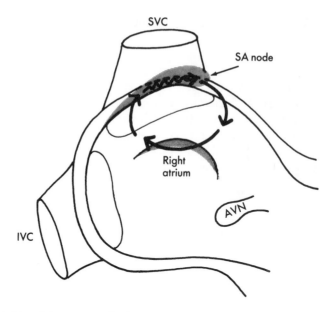

FIGURE 7-4 SA nodal reentry mechanism. *SVC,* Superior vena cava; *IVC,* inferior vena cava; *AVN,* AV node.

SA EXIT BLOCK

SA exit block occurs during the time between the actual discharge of the SA node and the arrival of the impulse in atrial tissue. It therefore does not result in atrial activation or a P wave. The conduction barrier is assumed to be in the SA node itself or in the perinodal zone. The block may be first, second, or third degree.

First-Degree SA Block

First-degree SA block is concealed because the actual firing of the SA node is not seen on the surface ECG and because all impulses are conducted at a fixed interval. Uncomplicated first-degree SA block in the ECG is indistinguishable from normal sinus rhythm. It can be identified by direct recording or indirect estimation of SA conduction time during electrophysiologic study.

Second-Degree SA Block

Second-degree SA block may be either type I or type II and is comparable to its second-degree AV block counterparts.

Type I

In type I second-degree SA block (sinus Wenckebach period) there is progressive lengthening of SA conduction time until finally a sinus beat is not conducted to the atria. Because the sinus discharge is a silent event, this arrhythmia can be inferred only because of a dropped P wave and the effect of the lengthening SA conduction times on

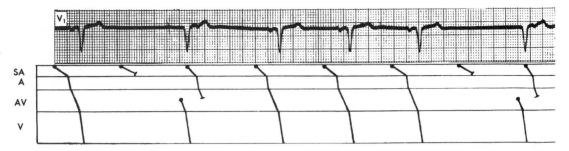

FIGURE 7-5 Sinus bradycardia, SA Wenckebach, and junctional escape beats. The second and last beats are junctional escape beats and are indicated by the two dots in the AV tier (see text).

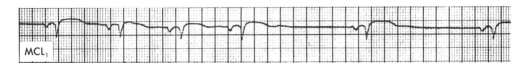

FIGURE 7-6 Type II second-degree SA block. The longer cycles equal exactly two of the basic sinus cycles.

the PP intervals. The signs of Wenckebach seen in this type of arrhythmia are (1) group beating, (2) shortening PP intervals, and (3) pauses that are less than twice the shortest cycle.

In Figure 7-5 the classical picture of SA Wenckebach is thwarted by underlying sinus bradycardia and junctional escape beats. The loss of every fifth P wave causes this mild sinus bradycardia to be more profound. The 4:3 SA Wenckebach period follows the first junctional escape beat. In the laddergram, the sinus rhythm is indicated by dots, and there is progressive conduction delay until a beat is not conducted, resulting in a dropped P wave. The long pause is interrupted by a junctional escape beat and is a reflection of the underlying sinus bradycardia. However, it is still less than twice the shortest sinus cycle.

Type II

In type II SA block there are dropped P waves without previous progressive prolongation of conduction times (and therefore without progressive shortening of PP intervals). The cycle of the dropped P wave is exactly equal to two of the basic sinus cycles (Figure 7-6). Sometimes two or more consecutive sinus impulses are blocked within the SA node, which creates considerably longer pauses.

Third-Degree SA Block

Third-degree SA block is usually compensated for by an atrial escape rhythm. With complete block in SA conduction there are no sinus P waves, but the SA node continues to discharge at regular intervals. This type of block cannot be differentiated clinically from sinus arrest, which is a total cessation of impulse formation within the SA node.

SICK SINUS SYNDROME

Sick sinus syndrome (SSS) encompasses a broad range of abnormalities, including disorders of impulse generation and conduction, failure of latent pacemakers, and susceptibility to paroxysmal or chronic atrial tachycardias.

History

As early as 1827, Adams[30] (and Stokes[31] two decades later) described syncopal attacks in patients with permanent bradycardia. In 1954 Short[32] presented the diverse clinical picture of SA nodal dysfunction in his classical paper on the syndrome of alternating bradycardia and tachycardia. The catchy alliterative title of *sick sinus syndrome* was coined by Lown[33] in 1967. This name was later popularized by Ferrer[34] and Rubenstein, Schulman, Yurchak, and DeSanctis[35] and was first used to characterize the situation following cardioversion for atrial fibrillation when there is unstable SA activity in the form of SA arrest or exit block.

ECG Features

Some of the ECG manifestations of SSS are as follows:
1. Sinus bradycardia that is persistent, severe, intermittent, or inappropriate
2. Sinus arrest with or without a new pacemaker arising
3. SA block
4. Failure of the sinus rhythm to follow termination of any supraventricular arrhythmia, whether the termination is spontaneous or electrically induced
5. Chronic atrial fibrillation with persistent slow ventricular rate in the absence of drugs
6. Alternating bradycardia and tachycardia (bradycardia-tachycardia syndrome)
7. Inappropriate SA node response to exercise or stress

Many patients with SSS may also have bundle branch block (BBB) and AV conduction abnormalities in the form of first-degree or second-degree AV block with prolonged AH interval (see Figure 6-1). Figure 7-7 illustrates SA nodal dysfunction in the form of the bradycardia-tachycardia syndrome. The first part of the tracing shows atrial fibrillation. When the paroxysm of atrial fibrillation ceases, a long pause ensues before the AV junction escapes.

Bradycardia-tachycardia syndrome is a common manifestation of SSS; atrial tachycardia and atrial fibrillation are more commonly observed than atrial flutter. Other rhythms seen are accelerated junctional rhythm and AV nodal reentry tachycardia. These tachycardias terminate spontaneously. The response of the SA node and subsidiary pacemakers to this overdrive suppression is exaggerated, leaving the patient with a long period of asystole or bradycardia that may result in syncope.

Pediatrics

SSS is seen in children during the postoperative period, usually following extensive intraatrial surgery (especially surgery for transposition of the great vessels). The rhythms seen are profound sinus bradycardia, periods of sinus arrest, atrial or junc-

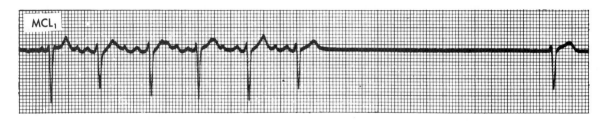

FIGURE 7-7 Sick sinus syndrome in the form of bradycardia-tachycardia syndrome.

tional rhythms, atrial flutter and, rarely, atrial fibrillation. The focus may switch from one to another, especially during the immediate postoperative period.

Mechanisms

A wide spectrum of abnormalities of both SA node automaticity and SA conduction causes the long sinus pauses of SSS. Complete SA block with an atrial escape rhythm can occur. It has also been shown that although the sinus impulse may not be able to conduct to the atria, conduction in the opposite direction (atriosinus) can occur and suppress the SA node. Following atrial tachyarrhythmias, the long pauses are the result of SA block and overdrive suppression of the SA node.

Causes

SSS is an acquired condition. It is usually encountered in the elderly but may be seen at any age, even in children and adolescents.[17,28-30] It is the result of a combination of abnormalities of the SA node itself (automaticity and SA conduction) and interdependence between these intrinsic properties and extrinsic factors such as the integrity of the autonomic nervous system, endocrine system, atrial muscle, and blood supply to the SA node.

SSS may be seen during the acute stage of inferior and lateral wall myocardial infarction, especially in the form of profound sinus bradycardia or even sinus arrest.[31-33] It is not known whether it is secondary to ischemia or local edema or is the result of autonomic neural influences.

Although SSS is most commonly idiopathic, it has been described as drug induced and is associated with infiltrative disorders such as coronary atherosclerosis, atrial amyloidosis, diffuse fibrosis, collagen vascular disease, infectious processes, and pericardial disease.

Drugs

The drugs most often implicated include cardiac glycosides, sympatholytic antihypertensive agents, β-blockers, calcium channel blockers, and membrane-active antiarrhythmic agents. Marked vagotonia, sometimes in combination with certain drugs, may be implicated in some cases of SSS.

Disease processes

There is still uncertainty regarding the disease processes that may cause intrinsic SA nodal dysfunction. In adult patients, coronary atherosclerosis is the most prominent disease linked to SSS. SSS is often intermittent and unpredictable and may occur in the absence of other cardiac diseases. The SA node itself may be partially or totally destroyed. There may be discontinuity between the SA node and atrial tissue; the nervous system surrounding the SA node or the atrial wall may be altered because of inflammatory or degenerative processes.[36]

Treatment

Treatment of SSS is determined by the patient's symptoms and ECG findings. The following are important therapeutic considerations[37]:

1. Thromboembolism (anticoagulation and preservation of organized atrial activation)
2. Symptoms of exertional intolerance (chronotropic support when indicated)
3. Survival (enhanced by physiologic pacing therapy and appropriate pharmacologic interventions)

Permanent cardiac pacemaker therapy is usually indicated when symptoms of dizziness and syncope are related to bradyarrhythmia in patients with SSS.[36] Data also support the beneficial use of oral theophylline in patients with SSS.[38,39]

SUMMARY

Physiologic arrhythmias originating in the SA node are sinus tachycardia, sinus bradycardia, and sinus arrhythmia. Other arrhythmias that originate in the SA node are SA nodal reentry, SA exit block, and the so-called sick sinus syndrome. SA nodal reentry is one of the mechanisms responsible for paroxysmal supraventricular tachycardia and accounts for approximately 8% of the symptomatic cases. It is recognized because of its abrupt beginnings that are unrelated to respirations, and it is difficult to differentiate from triggered activity in the vicinity of the SA node. SA block that can be noted on the surface ECG is second-degree. In type I second-degree SA block (SA Wenckebach) there are shortening PP intervals, pauses that are less than twice the shortest cycle, and group beating. In type II second-degree SA block there are dropped P waves without changes in PP intervals. Sick sinus syndrome, the term used with SA nodal dysfunction, is coupled with cerebral dysfunction. It usually involves not only the SA node but also includes a failure of adequate escape junctional beats.

REFERENCES

1. Ferguson TB Jr, Cox JL: Surgical treatment of arrhythmias. In Willerson JT, Cohn JN: *Cardiovascular medicine,* New York, 1995, Churchill Livingstone.
2. Gomes JA, Winters SL: The origins of the sinus node pacemaker complex in man: demonstration of dominant and subsidiary foci, *J Am Coll Cardiol* 9:45, 1987.
3. Boineau JP, Canavan TE, Schuessler RB et al: Demonstration of a widely distributed atrial pacemaker complex in the human heart, *Circulation* 77:1221, 1988.
4. Jordan JL, Mandel WJ: Disorders of sinus function. In Mandel WJ, editor: *Cardiac arrhythmias: their mechanisms, diagnosis, and management,* Philadelphia, 1980, JB Lippincott.
5. Gomes JAC, Kang PS, El-Sherif N: The sinus node electrogram in patients with and without sick sinus syndrome: techniques and correlation between directly measured and indirectly estimated sino-atrial conduction time, *Circulation* 66:864, 1982.

6. Allessie MA, Bonke FIM: Re-entry within the sino-atrial node as demonstrated by multiple micro-electrode recordings in the isolated rabbit heart. In Bonke FIM, editor: *The sinus node: structure, function, and clinical relevance,* The Hague, 1978, Martinus Nijoff.

7. Kleiger RE, Miller JP, Bigger JT, Moss AJ, and the Multicenter Post-Infarction Research Group: Decreased heart rate variability and its association with increased mortality after acute myocardial infarction, *Am J Cardiol* 59:256, 1987.

8. Malik M, Farrell T, Cripps T, Camm AJ: Heart rate variability in relation to prognosis after myocardial infarction: selection of optimal processing techniques, *Eur Heart J* 10:1060, 1989.

9. Bigger JT, Fleiss JL, Steinman RC et al: Frequency domain measures of heart period variability and mortality after myocardial infarction, *Circulation* 85:164, 1992.

10. Copie X, Hnatkova K, Staunton A et al: Predictive power of increased heart rate versus depressed left ventricular ejection fraction and heart rate variability for risk stratification after myocardial infarction: results of a two-year follow-up study, *J Am Coll Cardiol* 27:270, 1996.

11. Farell TG, Bashir Y, Cripps T et al: Risk stratification for arrhythmic events in postinfarction patients based on heart rate variability, ambulatory electrocardiographic variables and the signal-averaged electrocardiogram, *J Am Coll Cardiol* 18:687, 1991.

12. Hon EH, Lee ST: Electronic evaluations of the fetal heart rate patterns preceding fetal death: further observations, *Am J Obstet Gynecol,* 87:814, 1965.

13. Wolf MM, Varigos GA, Hunt D, Sloman JG: Sinus arrhythmia in acute myocardial infarction, *Med J Aust* 2:52, 1978.

14. Akselrod S, Gordon D, Ubel FA et al: Power spectrum analysis of heart rate fluctuation: a quantitative probe of beat-to-beat cardiovascular control, *Science* 213:220, 1981.

15. Task Force of the European Society of Cardiology and the North American Society of Pacing and Electrophysiology: Heart rate variability: standards of measurement, physiological interpretation and clinical use, *Circulation* 93:1043, 1996.

16. Wannamethee G, Shaper AG, MacFarlane PW, Walker M: Risk factors for sudden cardiac death in middle-aged British men, *Circulation* 91:1749, 1995.

17. Sanders WE, Sorrentino RA, Greenfield RA et al: Catheter ablation of sinoatrial node reentrant tachycardia, *J Am Coll Cardiol* 23:926, 1994.

18. Lesh MD, Kalman JM: To fumble flutter or tackle "tach"? Toward updated classifiers for atrial tachyarrhythmias, *J Cardiovasc Electrophysiol* 7:460, 1996.

19. Curry PVL, Shenasa M: Atrial arrhythmias: clinical concepts. In Mandel WJ, editor: *Cardiac arrhythmias, their mechanisms, diagnosis, and management,* Philadelphia, 1980, JB Lippincott.

20. Barker PS, Wilson FN, Johnson FD: The mechanism of auricular paroxysmal tachycardia, *Am Heart J* 26:435, 1943.

21. Han J, Malozzi AN, Moe GK: Sinoatrial reciprocation in the isolated rabbit heart, *Circ Res* 22:355, 1968.

22. Gomes JA, Hariman RJ, Kang PS, Chowdry IH: Sustained symptomatic sinus node reentrant tachycardia: incidence, clinical significance, electrophysiologic observations and the effects of antiarrhythmic agents, *J Am Coll Cardiol* 5:45, 1985.

23. Kerr CR, Klein GG, Guiraudon GM, Webb JG: Surgical therapy for sinoatrial reentrant tachycardia, *Pacing Clin Electrophysiol* 11:776, 1988.

24. Benditt DG: Sinus node dysfunction. In Willerson JT, Cohn JN, editors: *Cardiovascular medicine,* New York, 1995, Churchill Livingstone.

25. Narula OS: Sinus node reentry: a mechanism for supraventricular tachycardia, *Circulation* 50:1114, 1974.

26. Josephson ME: *Clinical cardiac electrophysiology: techniques and interpretations,* Philadelphia, 1993, Lea & Febiger.

27. Wellens HJJ: Role of sinus node reentry in the genesis of sustained cardiac arrhythmias. In Bonke FKM, editor: *The sinus node: structure, function and clinical relevance,* The Hague, 1978, Martinus Nijhoff.

28. Gomes JA, Mehta D, Langan MN: Sinus node reentrant tachycardia, *Pacing Clin Electrophysiol* 18:1045, 1995.

29. Kay GN, Chong F, Epstein AE et al: Radiofrequency ablation for treatment of primary atrial tachycardias, *J Am Coll Cardiol* 21. 1, 1993.

30. Adams R: Cases of disease of the heart, *Dublin Hosp Rep* 4:353, 1827.

31. Stokes W: Observations on some cases of permanent slow pulse, *Dublin J Med Sci* 2:73, 1846.

32. Short DS: The syndrome of alternating bradycardia and tachycardia, *Br Heart J* 16:208, 1954.

33. Lown B: Electrical reversion of cardiac arrhythmias, *Br Heart J* 29:469, 1967.

34. Ferrer MI: The sick sinus syndrome, *Circulation* 47:635, 1973.

35. Rubenstein JJ, Schulman CL, Yurchak PM, DeSanctis RW: Clinical spectrum of the sick sinus syndrome, *Circulation* 46:5, 1972.

36. Zipes DP: Specific arrhythmias: diagnosis and treatment. In Braunwald E, editor: *Heart disease,* Philadelphia, 1992, WB Saunders.

37. Benditt DG, Sakaguchi S, Goldstein MA et al: Sinus node dysfunction: pathophysiology, clinical features, evaluation, and treatment. In Zipes DP, Jalife J, editors: *Cardiac electrophysiology from cell to bedside,* ed 2, Philadelphia, 1995, WB Saunders.

38. Saito D, Matsubara K, Yamanari H et al: Effects of oral theophylline on sick sinus syndrome, *J Am Coll Cardiol* 21:1199, 1993.

39. Alboni P, Ratto B, Cappato R et al: Clinical effects of oral theophylline in sick sinus syndrome, *Am Heart J* 122:1361, 1991.

CHAPTER 8

Atrial Fibrillation

Classification 99
Descriptive designations 99
Electrocardiogram recognition 99
Mechanism 102
Tachycardia-induced cardiomyopathy and electrical remodeling 104
Symptoms 104
Physical findings 104
Incidence 105
Pediatrics 106
Thromboembolism 106
Treatment 106

T HE ATRIA ARE QUIVERING CHAMBERS THAT CONNECT THE GREAT VESSELS WITH THE ventricles. Atrial fibrillation is disorganized electrical activity of the atria that results in an irregular heartbeat, hemodynamic compromise, and a risk of thromboembolism.

CLASSIFICATION

Acute atrial fibrillation has an onset within 24 to 48 hours and usually converts spontaneously or in response to an antiarrhythmic agent. If cardioversion is necessary, anticoagulation is not first required. *Chronic atrial fibrillation* may be paroxysmal, persistent, or permanent.

Lone atrial fibrillation occurs in the absence of any other clinical evidence that would suggest a primary cardiac disorder.[1] Patients with lone atrial fibrillation have no history of transient ischemic attacks (TIAs), stroke, hypertension, diabetes, angina, myocardial infarction (MI), or heart failure.

DESCRIPTIVE DESIGNATIONS

Paroxysmal atrial fibrillation converts to sinus rhythm spontaneously at least once and may consistently be triggered by atrial ectopic beats (Figure 8-1), predominant vagal tone, sympathetic activity, or paroxysmal supraventricular tachycardia (PSVT). The paroxysmal form of atrial fibrillation may be accompanied by severe dyspnea and be the most debilitating because of its abrupt onset.

Vagally-mediated atrial fibrillation is an uncommon form of fibrillation and was first described by Coumel, Attuel, and Leclercq.[2] It is found in middle-aged men; episodes occur postprandially or during sleep or rest. The *catecholamine-sensitive* form of atrial fibrillation is found in young women; episodes are provoked by stress, exercise, caffeine, or alcohol.

Persistent atrial fibrillation requires intervention for conversion to sinus rhythm. Atrial fibrillation that has been persistent for many years is often assumed to be permanent. *Permanent atrial fibrillation* resists attempts at cardioversion and the maintenance of sinus rhythm.

ELECTROCARDIOGRAM RECOGNITION
Heart Rate

In uncontrolled atrial fibrillation, the heart rate is 100 to 180 beats/min. Slower rates suggest disease of atrioventricular (AV) conduction; faster rates suggest an accessory AV pathway (broad QRS complex, irregular rhythm) or enhanced AV nodal conduction (narrow QRS complex). The ventricular rate during atrial fibrillation is governed

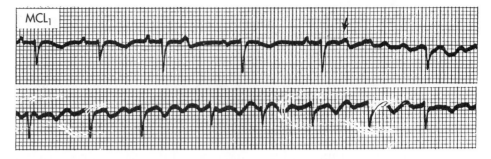

FIGURE 8-1　An atrial premature beat *(arrow)* initiates atrial fibrillation.

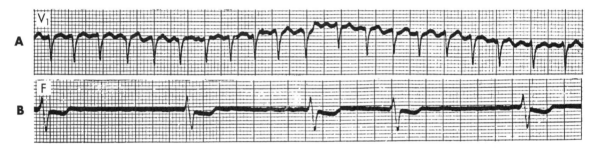

FIGURE 8-2　The extremes of ventricular response in atrial fibrillation. **A,** The ventricular response is approximately 190 beats/min. **B,** A slow ventricular response of approximately 40 beats/min.

by the effective refractory period in the AV node and, in the case of Wolff-Parkinson-White syndrome, by the refractory period in the accessory pathway, which varies among patients. The rate is slower when a rate-control drug such as verapamil, a β-blocker, or digitalis is being taken.

The ventricular response to atrial fibrillation is either *controlled* or *uncontrolled,* a designation that is related to the slope of the ratio of cardiac output to ventricular rate. For example, by decreasing the ventricular response, there is an increase in cardiac output.

Figure 8-2 shows wide swings in the heart rate; Figure 8-2, *A,* illustrates an uncontrolled atrial fibrillation with an unusually rapid ventricular response of approximately 190 beats/min. The usual uncontrolled response to atrial fibrillation is approximately 140 to 150 beats/min. However, that rate can be increased by the presence of sympathetic stimulation (exercise, fear, anger), even in patients taking digitalis for rate control. Figure 8-2, *B,* illustrates atrial fibrillation with a slow ventricular response of approximately 40 beats/min because of high-grade AV block. AV conduction is evident because of the irregular rhythm.

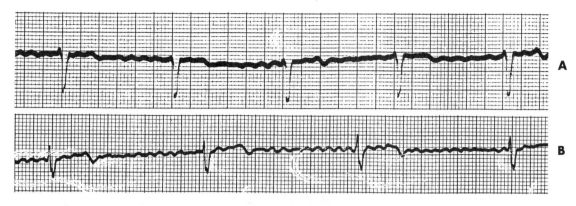

FIGURE 8-3 Both strips are from lead III in different patients. **A,** Atrial fibrillation with an independent junctional or fascicular rhythm (the patient had right bundle branch block and left axis deviation). The ventricular rate is 51 beats/min. **B,** Atrial fibrillation with complete AV block and a junctional escape rhythm at a rate of 36 beats/min.

Rhythm

The heart rhythm is irregular in atrial fibrillation unless complete AV block is present or AV conduction has been compromised either by pathologic or drug-induced complete AV block or by drug-induced junctional or fascicular ventricular tachycardia.

In Figure 8-3 the absolute regularity and the bradycardia seen in the two tracings (51 beats/min in Figure 8-3, *A*; 36 beats/min in Figure 8-3, *B*) are indications of complete AV block. The narrow QRS complex indicates a junctional escape rhythm. In patients who are taking digitalis, regularization of the rhythm or group beating is an indication of possible digitalis toxicity.

Fibrillatory Line

The coarse and fine fibrillatory lines that characterize atrial fibrillation represent the unorganized electrical activity of the atria. Figure 8-4 shows examples of coarse, medium, and fine atrial fibrillation. As is evident in Figure 8-4, *A*, the coarseness is so marked that the undulations all but obscure the QRS complexes.

Figure 8-5 illustrates a "straight line" atrial fibrillation. The diagnosis is made because of the absence of evident atrial activity and the irregular ventricular response. In the case of AV block (regular ventricular response), the diagnosis is made on the basis of the patient's history and past ECGs.

QRS Complexes

With atrial fibrillation, the QRS complexes are narrow unless bundle branch block is also present or the patient has an accessory pathway.

Warning Arrhythmias

- **Postoperative.** Numerous supraventricular ectopic beats, PSVT, and episodes of nonsustained atrial fibrillation and flutter[3]

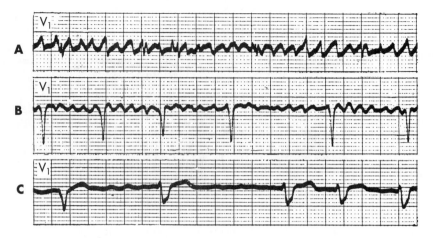

FIGURE 8-4 Coarse (**A**), medium (**B**), and fine (**C**) atrial fibrillatory lines.

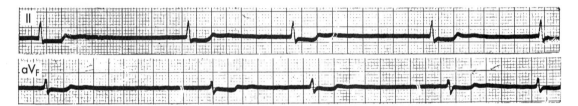

FIGURE 8-5 "Straight-line" atrial fibrillation.

- **Post-myocardial infarction.** Rapid atrial tachycardia (340 beats/min) that lasts up to 30 seconds before the fibrillatory pattern takes over[4]

Distinguishing Features

Uncomplicated atrial fibrillation is recognized on the electrocardiogram (ECG) because of the absence of P waves and an irregular ventricular response. Nevertheless, this explanation is an oversimplification. Clinically, atrial fibrillation has many faces. The fibrillatory line can be anything from very coarse (and confused with atrial flutter) to a straight line (and confused with a junctional rhythm). Atrial fibrillation can be associated with the ECG pattern of left ventricular hypertrophy, AV block, junctional tachycardia, fascicular ventricular tachycardia, ventricular ectopic beats, and MI. Figure 8-6 is an example of an ECG that is strongly suggestive of mitral stenosis: atrial fibrillation with right axis deviation.

MECHANISM

Figure 8-7 diagrammatically illustrates the atrial activity of atrial fibrillation. There is a pattern of large macroreentry with transition to multiple wavelets of reentry. These

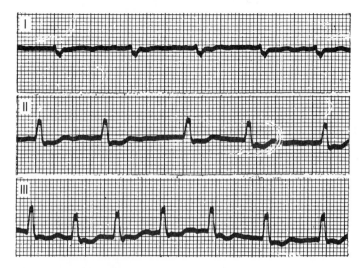

FIGURE 8-6 Atrial fibrillation with right axis deviation in a patient with mitral stenosis.

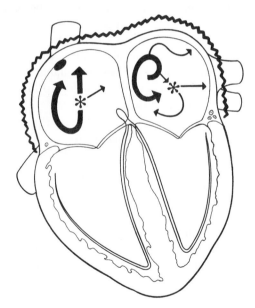

FIGURE 8-7 Diagrammatic representation of the mechanism of atrial fibrillation. Large macroreentry patterns give off multiple wavelets of reentry. These wavelets contribute to the propagation of atrial fibrillation.

wavelets contribute to the propagation of atrial fibrillation. The anatomic course of the spiraling wave fronts change from beat to beat.[5,6]

Concealed Conduction

Concealed conduction is electrical activity not seen on the surface ECG. The erratic and rapid atrial activity that occurs during atrial fibrillation results in incomplete penetration of the AV node so that not all impulses are propagated to the ventricular myocardium. Such impulses are not seen on the surface ECG and are thus "concealed." However, such impulses do leave the AV conduction tissue refractory, resulting in irregular RR intervals (see p. 73).

TACHYCARDIA-INDUCED CARDIOMYOPATHY AND ELECTRICAL REMODELING
Cardiomyopathy

Atrial fibrillation has been shown to be associated with left and right atrial enlargement, which is both a cause and a consequence of the arrhythmia and is thought to be its mechanism in acute MI.[7,8] For decades it was assumed that patients experienced atrial fibrillation because of cardiomyopathy when actually the cardiomyopathy was the result of the tachycardia. The ejection fraction markedly improves after the heart rate is controlled.

Electrical Remodeling

Daoud, Bogun, and Goyal et al[9] have demonstrated that even a few minutes of pacing-induced atrial fibrillation significantly shortens the right atrial effective refractory period, with recovery over 5 to 8 minutes. Goette, Honeycutt, and Langberg[10] have shown that even brief exposure to rapid atrial rates may cause mitochondrial swelling and disorganization and possible lysis of the cristae—changes that occurred in animals treated with verapamil. Such changes in atrial physiology promote the perpetuation of atrial fibrillation and facilitate reinduction.

SYMPTOMS
- Palpitations
- Hemodynamic compromise
- Polyuria (may be profound enough to cause hypovolemic hypotension)

PHYSICAL FINDINGS
- Varying intensity of the first heart sound
- Absence of "a" waves in the jugular pulse (no atrial contractions). (Note in the jugular pulse tracing in Figure 8-8 that because there is no atrial relaxation there is no "x" descent. Even in the presence of a regular independent ventricular rhythm, atrial fibrillation is easily diagnosed with an eye on the jugular and a finger on the carotid artery.)
- Irregular arterial pulse
- Pulse deficit (radial pulse less than the apical pulse)
- Possible thromboembolism (peripheral, coronary, pulmonary, or cerebral)
- Possible signs of decreased cardiac output, heart failure, and decreased cerebral oxygen supply

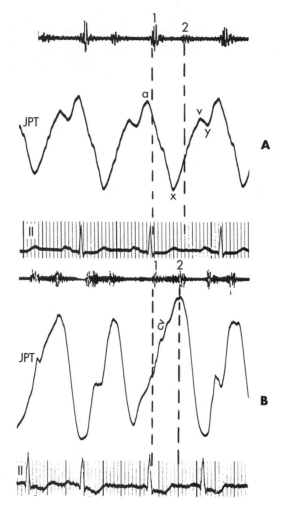

FIGURE 8-8 Two records of a phonocardiogram, jugular pulse tracing *(JPT)*, and ECG from the same patient. **A,** During sinus rhythm, systole is mainly occupied by a collapsing venous pulse ("x" descent). **B,** During atrial fibrillation, systole is entirely occupied by a progressively positive "cv" wave.

INCIDENCE

Atrial fibrillation is one of the most common symptomatic sustained arrhythmias seen in clinical practice.[11] It affects 2.2 million Americans and accounts for up to 15% of all stroke syndromes. Its prevalence doubles in successive decades of life above 50 years of age, reaching 8% to 10% per year at 80 to 89 years of age.[12] Nearly 10% of persons older than 80 years of age have a history of atrial fibrillation.[13]

Postoperative atrial fibrillation is seen in at least 25% to 30% of patients after coronary artery bypass grafting and in 60% of patients after valvular surgery. It usually appears on the second or third postoperative day.[14]

PEDIATRICS

Atrial fibrillation is rare in the pediatric age group. When present, it is characterized by rapid and chaotic atrial depolarization and a rapid ventricular response that sometimes exceeds 300 beats/min. On the surface ECG there may be grossly irregular atrial fibrillatory waves, or they may not be seen at all.

THROMBOEMBOLISM

With atrial fibrillation, thrombi can form inside the left atrium because of a stasis of blood. When a thrombus embolizes, it may lodge in the brain and cause a stroke, which results in death or severe neurologic deficit in 50% to 70% of episodes.[15] Each year approximately 70,000 strokes are caused by emboli from the fibrillating left atrium, and it is estimated that approximately one third of all persons in atrial fibrillation will experience a peripheral vascular event.[16]

TREATMENT

Treatment of atrial fibrillation has three main goals and three treatment categories. Treatment goals are rate control, anticoagulation, and conversion to sinus rhythm. Treatment categories are acute, paroxysmal, and persistent or permanent. The initial approach to therapy may change once the response to simple treatment has been observed.

DC Cardioversion
Risk of embolism

The risk of embolism following pharmacologic or electrical cardioversion is 1% to 5%. This risk is decreased by several weeks of anticoagulation with warfarin before and immediately following cardioversion.[17]

Mechanism of thromboembolism

There are two mechanisms for thromboembolism following cardioversion:
1. Because blood is not being propelled through the atria during fibrillation, a thrombus may form in the left atrial appendage and embolize following cardioversion.
2. Cardioversion itself may cause thrombogenesis and thromboembolism because of atrial stunning.

Atrial stunning

Following DC cardioversion, the atrial A-wave velocity is immediately depressed, creating an environment for thrombus formation. The atria begin to show recovery only between 4 and 7 days; recovery is not complete until weeks or months after the procedure. Recovery time appears to be related to the duration of atrial fibrillation preceding cardioversion. With atrial fibrillation of short duration, the left atrium recovers within 1 week; with atrial fibrillation of long duration, recovery occurs much later.

Surgery

A surgical cure for atrial fibrillation is based on the fact that the mechanism for this condition is reentry. Reentry may be prevented if the atrium is segmented into smaller geographic regions by linear ablation. The disadvantages of surgery are thoracotomy, cardiopulmonary bypass, and significant surgical morbidity.

The corridor operation designed by Guiraudon[18] in 1985 uses scalpel incisions and cryosurgery to isolate a band of atrial tissue between the high right atrium and the AV node from the rest of the fibrillating atrium. This procedure eliminates the critical mass necessary to support fibrillation. Both atrial appendages are amputated, and the pulmonary veins are isolated from the left atrium. Sinus rhythm proceeds in the corridor, but the rest of the atria may fibrillate. Besides the surgical disadvantages already mentioned there is a high incidence of atrial arrhythmias, a need for permanent pacing, and a loss of atrial function.[19]

The maze operation was developed by Cox, Schuessler, and D'Agostino et al[20] in 1991. Lesions are made within the atria to increase the total length and number of anatomic boundaries in the atria and thus interrupt potential reentry circuits.[21] Left and right atrial appendages are removed, and a large part of the left atrium is excluded around the pulmonary veins. This procedure has reported success rates between 84% and 98%. Atrial fibrillation may occur early following surgery and disappears after a few weeks.[22-24] This procedure not only prevents atrial fibrillation from occurring but also preserves sinus rhythm and AV conduction and prevents thromboembolism.

A simplified approach to the idea of segmenting the atrium is presented with the compartment operation, in which two vertical incisions are made to divide the atrium into three separate compartments more easily and quickly than in the maze operation. In long-term follow-up the success rates are 64%, with very low complication rates.

Cure by Catheter?

Because of the surgical successes, investigators are working on several catheter techniques using radiofrequency energy in an effort to emulate the surgical procedure. The drag technique places a conventional radiofrequency ablation catheter in the atrium; during ongoing electrical energy it is dragged along the atrial wall, hopefully leaving a lesion in its wake. Ring electrode or coil electrode catheters may also be used to create long linear lesions.

SUMMARY

Atrial fibrillation is recognized on the ECG because of the absence of P waves and an irregular ventricular response, which results in a drop in cardiac output up to 20%, a tendency to develop thromboembolism, and an increased mortality. This condition may be either acute with a rapid uncontrolled ventricular response or chronic with a paroxysmal and persistent or permanent form. Treatment involves rate control, antithrombotic therapy, and attempts to convert to normal sinus rhythm.

REFERENCES

1. Evans W, Swann P: Lone auricular fibrillation, *Br Heart J* 16:189,1954.
2. Coumel P, Attuel P, Leclercq JF: Arrhythmias auriculaires d'origine vagale ou catécholergique. Effects comparés du traitment béta-bloqueur et phénomènes d'échappement, *Arch Mal Coeur* 75:373, 1982.

3. Frost L, Molgaard H, Christiansen EH et al: Atrial ectopic activity and atrial fibrillation/flutter after coronary artery bypass surgery: a case-base study controlling for confounding from age, beta-blocker treatment, and time distance from operation, *Int J Cardiol* 50:153, 1995.

4. Bennett MA, Pentacost BL: The pattern of onset and spontaneous cessation of atrial fibrillation in man, *Circulation* 41:981, 1970.

5. Allessie MA, Lammers WJEP, Bonke FIM, Hollen J: Experimental evaluation of Moe's multiple wavelet hypothesis of atrial fibrillation. In Zipes DP, Jalife J, editors: *Cardiac arrhythmias,* New York, 1985, Grune & Stratton.

6. Falk RH, Podrid PJ: *Atrial fibrillation: mechanism and management,* New York, 1991, Raven Press.

7. Gosselink ATM, Crijns HJGM, Hamer HPM et al: Changes in left and right atrial size after cardioversion of atrial fibrillation: role of mitral valve disease, *J Am Coll Cardiol* 22:1666,1993.

8. Sanfilippo AJ, Abascal VM, Sheenan M et al: Atrial enlargement as a consequence of atrial fibrillation, *Circulation* 82:792, 1990.

9. Daoud EG, Bogun F, Goyal R et al: Effect of atrial fibrillation on atrial refractoriness in humans, *Circulation* 94:1600, 1996.

10. Goette A, Honeycutt C, Langberg JJ: Electrical remodeling in atrial fibrillation: time course and mechanisms, *Circulation* 94:2968, 1996.

11. The National Heart, Lung and Blood Institute Working Group on Atrial Fibrillation: Atrial fibrillation: current understandings and research imperatives, *J Am Coll Cardiol* 22:1830, 1993.

12. Benjamin EJ, Levy D, D'Agostino RB et al: Impact of atrial fibrillation of the risk of death: the Framingham Study [abstract], *J Am Coll Cardiol* Feb (special issue), 230A, 1995.

13. Wolf PA, Benjamin EJ, Belanger AJ et al: Secular trends in the prevalence of atrial fibrillation: the Framingham study, *Am Heart J* 131:790, 1996.

14. Antman EM: Medical management of the patient undergoing cardiac surgery. In Braunwald E, editor: *Heart disease,* Philadelphia, 1992, WB Saunders.

15. Cairns JA, Connolly SJ: Nonrheumatic atrial fibrillation: risk of stroke and role of antithrombotic therapy, *Circulation* 84:469, 1991.

16. Halperin JL, Hart RG: Atrial fibrillation and stroke: new ideas, persisting dilemmas, *Stroke* 19:937, 1988.

17. Bjerkelund CJ, Ornigh OM: The efficacy of anticoagulant therapy in preventing embolism related to DC electrical conversion of atrial fibrillation, *Am J Cardiol* 23:208, 1969.

18. Guiraudon GM, Campbell CS, Jones DL et al: Combined sinoatrial nodel–atrioventricular node isolation: a surgical alternative to His bundle ablation in patients with atrial fibrillation [abstract], *Circulation* 72:III, 1985.

19. Doevendans PA, Wellens HJJ: Atrial dissection for atrial fibrillation: when, how much and where? *J Am Coll Cardiol* 28:991, 1996.

20. Cox JL, Schuessler RB, D'Agostino JH Jr et al: The surgical treatment of atrial fibrillation. III. Development of a definitive surgical procedure, *J Thorac Cardiovasc Surg* 101:569, 1991.

21. Ong JJC, Lee JJ, Tseng-Ong LSY et al: Anatomic boundaries as a mechanism for termination of meandering reentrant wave fronts during atrial fibrillation, *Circulation* 94(8 suppl):2045, 1996.

22. Cox JL, Boineau JP, Scheussler RB et al: Operations for atrial fibrillation, *Clin Cardiol* 14:827, 1991.

23. Ferguson TB Jr, Cox JL: Successful surgical treatment for atrial fibrillation, *Prim Cardiol* 18:15, 1992.

24. Cheng TO: Atrial fibrillation, stroke, and antithrombotic treatment, *Am Heart J* 127:961, 1994.

CHAPTER 9

Atrial Flutter

Historical perspective in humans 109
Electrophysiologic classification 110
Pertinent atrial structures 110
ECG findings common to all forms of atrial flutter 112
Pediatrics 113
Typical atrial flutter 115
True atypical atrial flutter 122
Incisional reentrant atrial tachycardia 124
Differential diagnosis 124
Physical signs 124
Clinical setting and incidence 125
Ablation of automatic and reentrant atrial tachycardia 126
Chemical ablation in the future? 126
Anticoagulation 126

ATRIAL FLUTTER IS A RAPID AND REMARKABLY REGULAR FORM OF ATRIAL TACHYCARDIA that is sustained by a macroreentrant circuit. It is usually paroxysmal and lasts for periods that vary from seconds to hours or, occasionally, days. Chronic atrial flutter is unusual.[1] It is estimated that there are 200,000 cases of new onset atrial flutter in the United States each year and that within the first 30 months of diagnosis, fewer than 60% of deaths are a result of cardiovascular disease.[2]

Atrial flutter involves macroreentry around fixed or functional, anatomic or surgical barriers (conduction blocks). It is possible to record electrical activity that spans the length of the cycle and to reset and entrain the circuit from multiple atrial sites.[3] Within this reentry circuit there is a 30- to 50-ms gap of excitable tissue *(excitable gap),* which has been demonstrated by *transient entrainment* of the tachycardia (i.e., the ability to capture the reentry circuit with atrial pacing).[4]

Flutter fibrillation appears as a coarse atrial fibrillation on surface leads and is commonly seen as a transitional stage from fibrillation to flutter in patients taking class I antiarrhythmic drugs. In such cases flutterlike atrial activity coexists with zones of desynchronized depolarizations.[5,6]

HISTORICAL PERSPECTIVE IN HUMANS

- **1906.** The first electrocardiogram (ECG) of atrial flutter in humans was published by Einthoven. In 1911 Jolly and Ritchie drew a clear distinction between atrial fibrillation and flutter in the ECG.
- **1951.** Prinzmetal, Corday, and Brill et al[7] offered evidence that the main difference between atrial tachycardia and atrial flutter is that flutter represents a faster discharge from the ectopic focus in the atrium. They also described the negative P′ and the development of the positive atrial repolarization wave (Ta) as the atrial rate accelerated.
- **1950 to 1960.** Atrial flutter was thought to be an intraatrial reentrant rhythm that used the left atrium with a current traveling in a caudocranial direction and the right atrium with a current in a craniocaudal direction.[8]
- **1956 to 1970.** Mapping studies suggested that the reentry circuit of atrial flutter was confined to the right atrium.[9,10]
- **1977 to 1984.** Demonstrations that the reentry circuit of atrial flutter could be transiently entrained and interrupted with atrial pacing in humans following open heart surgery provided strong evidence that atrial flutter is an intraatrial reentrant rhythm with an excitable gap.[11-14]
- **1986 to 1993.** Mapping studies concluded the following[14a-c]:
  1. The reentrant circuit is confined to the right atrium.

2. The reentrant current travels counterclockwise—caudocranial in the interatrial septum and craniocaudal in the right atrial free wall.

3. An area of slow conduction is present in the posteroinferior part of the circuit.

4. The wave front circulates around anatomic obstacles (central areas that do not conduct), including the inferior vena cava and a functional barrier in the atrial septum.

- **1994 to 1997.** Activation and entrainment mapping better define the protected pathway and conduction barriers during type I atrial flutter. Atrial flutter is reclassified according to electrophysiologic guidelines.[3] The use of intracardiac echocardiography is used to visualize structures that cannot be seen with fluoroscopy (fossa ovalis, crista terminalis, eustachian ridge, coronary sinus os, venae cavae).[15-18] The critical elements of the reentrant circuits of type I atrial flutter are established using concealed entrainment techniques and techniques for precise placement of ablative lesions.[19] The mechanism of initiation of counterclockwise and clockwise rotation of the reentrant circuit and the site of unidirectional block is defined using standardized induction protocol.[19a]

ELECTROPHYSIOLOGIC CLASSIFICATION

Atrial flutter has received its name because of its unique "sawtooth" appearance on the surface ECG. A classification on the basis of features directly assessed from activation mapping and entrainment techniques offers a better understanding of the mechanisms of atrial flutter and is presented in this chapter for that reason and because of its future potential. A more precise classification from the surface ECG may eventually be possible as more data are accumulated from activation mapping, entrainment techniques, and comparisons with surface ECGs.

Currently, however, the subclassification of atrial flutter is not very accurate when patients are evaluated solely on the basis of their surface ECG because of the wide rate range and the crossover in rates and P′ wave patterns. Perhaps the clinical classification of atrial flutter should wait until electrophysiologic studies have been performed, because atrial flutter is potentially curable. Even if an atypical (possibly nonablatable) form of atrial flutter is noted, electrophysiologic studies are still performed to see if the substrate of the mechanism can be ablated.[20]

If mapping data are available, atrial flutter is classified according to the boundaries and rotation of the reentrant loop. Three major categories are offered[3]:

1. Typical atrial flutter (Type I)
   a. Counterclockwise rotation of the reentrant circuit
   b. Clockwise rotation of the reentrant circuit
2. True atypical atrial flutter (Type II)
3. Incisional reentrant atrial tachycardia

PERTINENT ATRIAL STRUCTURES

Figure 9-1 illustrates the atrial structures that help to form a protected pathway for the macroreentrant circuit of atrial flutter.

The **crista terminalis** is the terminal crest of the right atrium; it is a ridge on the internal surface of the right atrium and is located laterally to the orifices of the superior

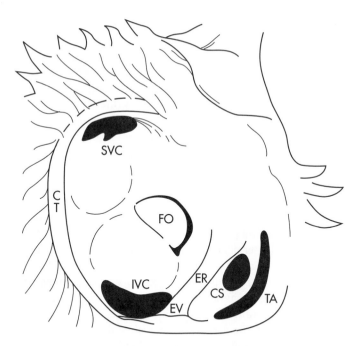

FIGURE 9-1 Pertinent anatomic landmarks in the right atrium. The eustachian ridge *(ER)* lies between the inferior vena cava *(IVC)* and the tricuspid annulus *(TA)*. (See text.) *CS*, Coronary sinus; *CT*, crista terminalis; *EV*, eustachian valve; *FO*, fossa ovalis; *SVC*, superior vena cava.

and inferior venae cavae. It corresponds to a groove on the external surface called the *sulcus terminalis.* The portion of the atrium behind the crista terminalis is smooth; it develops from the sinus venosus, an embryonic structure. The portion of the atrium in front of the crista terminalis develops from the primitive atrium and is trabeculated.

The **eustachian valve** is the valve of the inferior vena cava and forms the inferior lip of the inferior vena cava. Together with the eustachian valve, the **eustachian ridge** forms a barrier to conduction between the inferior vena cava and coronary sinus.

The **coronary sinus** is the terminal portion of the great cardiac vein, which empties into the right atrium. The orifice of the coronary sinus opens between the orifice of the inferior vena cava and the tricuspid annulus. It is guarded by a fold that is often perforated like a piece of lace and is known as the *valve of the coronary sinus.*

The **fossa ovalis** is a depression on the right interatrial septum that represents the remains of the fetal *foramen ovale.* The fossa ovalis does not participate in the macroreentrant circuit of atrial flutter but is included in Figure 9-1 for its landmark value.[21] A forceps passed up the inferior vena cava in a cadaver heart is usually blocked by the crescentic upper margin of the fossa ovalis. However, in approximately 25% of cases it passes onward through a valvelike slit in the septum (foramen ovale) and into the left atrium. This is the course much of the blood follows until birth.

The **tricuspid annulus** is a fibrous ring that surrounds the orifice of the tricuspid valve. This type of ring surrounds each of the four orifices guarded by a valve. The aortic ring is the strongest and is like a cuff. Without the rings, the orifices would stretch and the valves would be rendered incompetent.

ECG FINDINGS COMMON TO ALL FORMS OF ATRIAL FLUTTER

- **Ventricular rate.** The rate depends on AV conduction ratio; it is usually 140 to 160 beats/min because of a 2:1 AV conduction ratio. In this range flutter should be considered. However, all other tachycardias may also have a rate in this range.
- **Ventricular rhythm.** The rhythm is regular if there is a fixed AV conduction ratio. Group beating occurs if there is Wenckebach conduction. The rhythm is irregular if there is variable AV conduction.
- **Effect of carotid sinus massage.** This procedure may temporarily slow the ventricular rate because of AV block (Figure 9-2), or it may have no effect.
- **AV conduction ratio.** Conduction ratios are usually even (e.g., 2:1, 4:1, 6:1). With a normal AV node there is usually a physiologic AV block with 2:1 conduction, but the ratio may be 4:1 or variable. Higher degrees of AV block can occur in patients with AV nodal disease or increased vagal tone or can occur with drugs that cause AV block. A 1:1 conduction ratio may be seen in patients with an accessory pathway, in patients with a short PR interval (Lown-Ganong-Levine syndrome), during exertion, or in patients taking catecholamines or sympathomimetic amines. In patients taking class I antiarrhythmic agents (especially class Ic), the atrial rate may slow down to as little as 180 to 200 beats/min. With the slower atrial rate, 1:1 AV conduction is more likely (Figure 9-3).

In a patient with an accessory pathway, atrial flutter is indistinguishable from ventricular tachycardia, even with 2:1 conduction (see Chapter 17). In this situation, the patient is usually seriously compromised hemodynamically and requires immediate electrical cardioversion.

Wenckebach conduction often causes group beating (Figures 9-4 to 9-6). Atrial impulses that appear to be completely blocked actually penetrate into different levels of the AV junction (concealed conduction), with 2:1 conduction at the level of the proximal AV node and Wenckebach conduction of the beats that reach the distal level of the AV node.[22]

In 1996 Page, Wharton, and Prystowsky[23] presented data supporting a mechanism (other than two levels of AV nodal block) to explain the 2:1 and 4:1 conduction in atrial flutter. These investigators demonstrated that heightened vagal tone could substantially

CSM

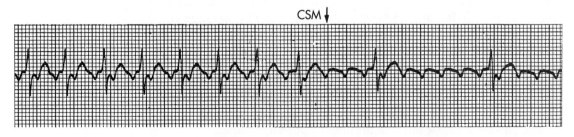

FIGURE 9-2 Counterclockwise typical atrial flutter with a 2:1 AV conduction ratio that changes to 4:1 and 6:1 in response to carotid sinus massage *(CSM)*.

prolong the effective refractory period of the AV node and block two consecutive atrial impulses. The second blocked beat would increase the AV nodal effective refractory period enough to prevent the next beat from conducting, thus producing 4:1 conduction.

PEDIATRICS

Atrial flutter is a common mechanism in the neonate; atrial rates usually approach 400 beats/min with 2:1 conduction.[24] In the neonate this arrhythmia is usually associated with normal cardiac structure. It can be treated by transesophageal overdrive pacing or external synchronized cardioversion. In some cases the condition never returns once treated. Most infants outgrow this arrhythmia by 12 to 18 months of age.[25,26]

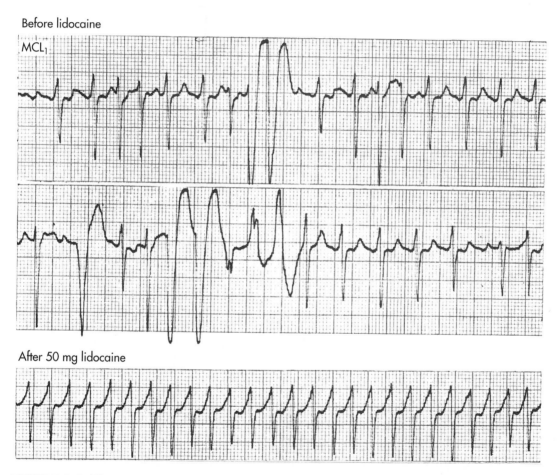

FIGURE 9-3 The upper two strips are continuous and show typical atrial flutter (rate = 285 beats/min), with varying AV conduction interrupted by multiform anomalous beats. The bottom strip was recorded after the administration of 50 mg of lidocaine. The atrial rate has decreased to 265 beats/min, with an alarming acceleration of the ventricular rate because of 1:1 conduction.

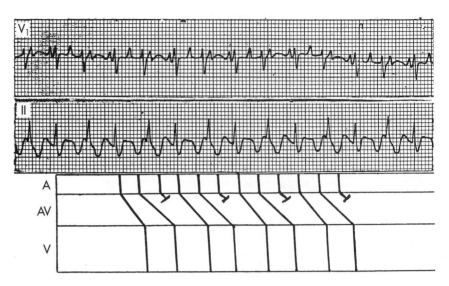

FIGURE 9-4 Counterclockwise typical atrial flutter at a rate of 268 beats/min with 3:2 Wenckebach periods.

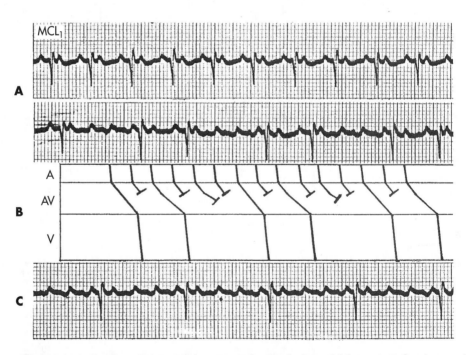

FIGURE 9-5 The effect of propranolol on AV conduction during atrial flutter. **A,** Before therapy, the atrial rate is 262 beats/min with 2:1 conduction. **B,** The atrial rate is unchanged less than 1 minute after intravenous administration of 2 mg propranolol. However, the drug has produced 2:1 conduction at the proximal AV node and 3:2 Wenckebach conduction at the distal AV node, resulting in a bigeminal rhythm. **C,** Later the atrial rate slowed slightly to 252 beats/min, and propranolol has now produced 2:1 block of the alternate impulses so that the net AV ratio is now 4:1.

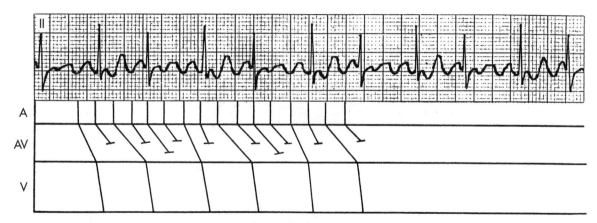

FIGURE 9-6 The laddergram demonstrates the mechanism of atrial flutter with Wenckebach conduction. The atrial tier *(A)* shows a regular atrial rhythm. In the upper level of the atrioventricular *(AV)* tier there is 2:1 conduction. In the lower level of the AV node there is 3:2 Wenckebach conduction. These two mechanisms result in group beating.

TYPICAL ATRIAL FLUTTER (TYPE I)

Typical atrial flutter, sometimes called "type I atrial flutter,"* is found in two forms according to the direction of rotation of its macroreentrant circuit. A counterclockwise rotation is common; a clockwise rotation is rare. Both forms are seen in patients with or without heart disease and do not require a scar from prior atriotomy.[3] Both forms can be cured by radiofrequency ablation.[20] During sinus rhythm, both forms share similar right atrial conduction disturbances and normal left atrial conduction times.[27]

Counterclockwise Typical Atrial Flutter
Mechanism

Barriers to conduction play an important role in the maintenance of the macroreentrant circuit of atrial flutter. They provide a protected pathway for the wave front and prevent stray currents from traversing the smooth-walled posterior right atrium and terminating the mechanism by introducing refractory tissue.[21]

Figure 9-7 demonstrates the pathway thought to sustain this most common form of atrial flutter as constructed from activation and entrainment mapping during electrophysiologic studies. Confirmation of this complex circuit currently awaits high-density mapping.[21]

Counterclockwise typical atrial flutter travels the following pathway (see Figure 9-7):
1. Note the line drawn in the superior and lateral aspect of the right atrium. This broad, inferiorly directed wave front is confined by a *posterior barrier* (line of fixed conduction block) formed by the *crista terminalis* and the *eustachian valve* and *eustachian ridge,* which together form a line of conduction block between the inferior vena cava and coronary sinus.

---

*To add confusion, other terms used to identify the typical macroreentrant form of atrial flutter are "classic," "common," "usual," "type A," and orthodromic."

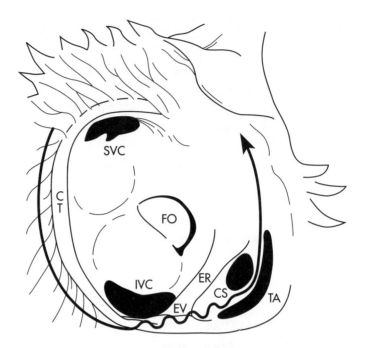

FIGURE 9-7 The macroreentrant path taken by counterclockwise typical atrial flutter. (See text.) *CS*, Coronary sinus; *CT*, crista terminalis; *EV*, eustachian valve; *ER*, eustachian ridge; *FO*, fossa ovalis; *IVC*, inferior vena cava; *SVC*, superior vena cava; *TA*, tricuspid annulus.

2. The wave front proceeds along a continuous *anterior barrier* formed by the *tricuspid annulus*.[21] Together the posterior and anterior barriers form a continuous protected pathway.[28]
3. The wave front continues its loop, ascending the septum between the coronary sinus ostium and the septal tricuspid annulus.
4. The upper link in the circuit is above the superior vena cava, from which point it completes its clockwise circle anterior to the superomedial portion of the crista terminalis.[21,29]

Note that in Figure 9-7 the macroreentrant wave front does not bridge the barrier of the crista terminalis at any point. The cycle length of this circuit is 200 to 400 ms (300 to 150 beats/min) and depends on atrial size, underlying disease, and the presence of antiarrhythmic drugs.[21]

The isthmus of slow conduction

It is now well established that one critical element of both forms of the typical atrial flutter reentrant circuit is a narrow isthmus of slow conduction. This isthmus can be interrupted by a lesion created by radiofrequency energy. Such a lesion eliminates the possibility of such a reentrant circuit being initiated or sustained and thus provides a cure.

Both the posterior isthmus and the septal isthmus can be interrupted. The posterior isthmus lies in the low posterior right atrium between the inferior vena cava and the tri-

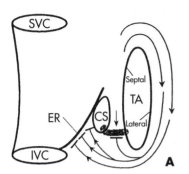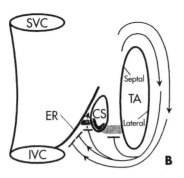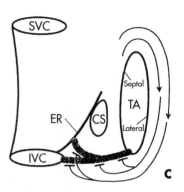

FIGURE 9-8 Schematics of the right atrium in the right anterior oblique projection illustrate the three approaches used for ablation of counterclockwise typical atrial flutter. **A,** Ablation *(arrow)* across the septal isthmus from the tricuspid annulus *(TA)* to the posteroapical margin of the coronary sinus *(CS)* ostium. **B,** The ablation line can be extended along the posterior margin of the coronary sinus ostium to the eustachian ridge *(ER)* in patients who have conduction through this space *(dashed arrow)*. **C,** Ablation line across the posterior isthmus from the tricuspid annulus to the inferior vena cava *(IVC)* or the eustachian valve and ridge. *SVC,* Superior vena cava. (From Nakagawa H, Lazzara R, Khastgir T et al: Role of the tricuspid annulus and the eustachian valve/ridge on atrial flutter: relevance to catheter ablation of the septal isthmus and a new technique for rapid identification of ablation success, *Circulation* 94:407, 1996.)

cuspid annulus.[30,31] The septal isthmus, from the tricuspid annulus to the posteroapical margin of the coronary sinus ostium, is the narrower of the two possible ablation sites (Figure 9-8, *A*). In patients who do not have conduction in the narrow space between the coronary sinus ostium and the eustachian ridge, this ablation line should produce a complete arc of conduction block that extends from the tricuspid annulus to the coronary sinus ostium and the inferior vena cava and eliminates both forms of typical atrial flutter.

In patients who do have conduction in the narrow space between the coronary sinus ostium and the eustachian ridge, the ablation line is extended along the posterior margin of the coronary sinus ostium and to the eustachian ridge (Figure 9-8, *B*).

Figure 9-8, *C* shows the longer ablation line across the posterior isthmus from the tricuspid annulus to the inferior vena cava or eustachian ridge.[32] One study has demonstrated that successful ablation can be verified by a change in the polarity of the P wave with low lateral right atrial pacing (negative before ablation; positive after successful ablation).[33]

The genesis of flutter waves

Although atrial flutter is generated by a reentry circuit in the right atrium, the P′ wave polarity on the ECG is determined primarily by the sequence of activation in the left atrium, activating it in an inferior/superior direction.

In counterclockwise typical atrial flutter (type I), the F waves in the inferior leads are composed of a negative component (the P′ wave) and a positive component (the Ta wave), producing a very distinctive sawtooth pattern that varies slightly among patients.

This pattern is easier to spot when the AV conduction ratio is 4:1. Figures 9-9 to 9-12 illustrate 2:1 and 4:1 AV conduction ratios. In both forms of typical atrial flutter (counterclockwise and clockwise right atrial rotation), the ECG pattern of the F waves is similar in the inferior leads (i.e., "sawtooth"). However, the P′ wave pattern may be opposite (negative in counterclockwise rotation and positive in clockwise rotation).

ECG recognition

- **Atrial rate.** Ranges from 240 to 340 beats/min (long excitable gap); rate may be slower (e.g., in right atrial enlargement); overlap in rate between the typical and true atypical atrial flutter.
- **Atrial rhythm.** Regular.
- **P′ wave axis.** Superior.
- **Flutter wave.** Familiar sawtooth appearance. The P′ wave is the negative component of the flutter wave in lead aV_F. The Ta wave (atrial repolarization) is positive.

In Figure 9-10 note that no atrial activity is seen in lead I. Because the amplitude of the flutter waves is approximately the same in leads II and III, there will be no sign of them in lead I. This demonstrates Einthoven's equation (II = I + III). In lead V_1 there is a positive P′ wave with a correspondingly negative P′ wave in leads V_5 and V_6.

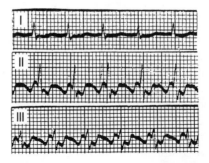

FIGURE 9-9 Typical atrial flutter with 2:1 AV conduction. The F waves in leads II and III are of approximately equal amplitude. Because I + III = II, there is no sign of atrial activity in lead I.

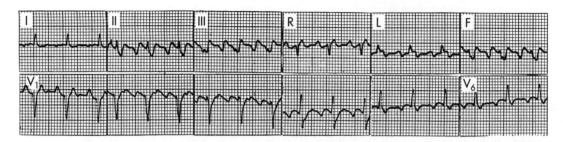

FIGURE 9-10 Typical atrial flutter in a 12-lead tracing. Note the sawtooth pattern in leads II, III, and aV_F, the positive P′ waves in V_1, and the negative ones in V_5 and V_6. Evidence of atrial activity, as usual, is minimal in lead I.

Acute treatment

Acute treatment of typical atrial flutter depends on the clinical setting.[1] DC cardioversion (<50 joules) or rapid atrial pacing are preferred choices; antiarrhythmic drug therapy may be initiated before either.

The goals of drug therapy are to[34]:

1. Slow the ventricular rate.
2. Restore sinus rhythm. An Na^+ channel blocker may be combined with a Ca^{2+} channel–blocking drug or digitalis to prevent 1:1 conduction. This combination is advisable because if the class Ia drug does not restore sinus rhythm it may slow the flutter rate, with the undesirable effect of an AV conduction ratio of 1:1. Feld

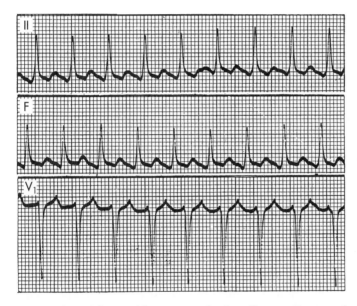

FIGURE 9-11 Typical atrial flutter with 2:1 AV conduction. Alternate F waves coincide with the ventricular complex, and the diagnosis could easily be missed. The positive P′ waves in lead V_1 coincide with the T wave.

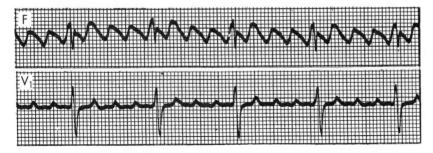

FIGURE 9-12 Typical atrial flutter with 4:1 AV conduction. With this conduction ratio the flutter waves are easily seen. Note the positive little P′ waves in V_1.

and colleagues have observed this phenomenon in 10% of patients treated with type I drugs—particularly in patients with structural heart disease. Sotalol may be more effective in interrupting this type of reentry because of its ability to prolong the refractory period in atrial flutter.[20]

3. Enhance the effect of rapid atrial pacing.
4. Maintain sinus rhythm once converted.

For cases of chronic obstructive pulmonary disease or for cases in which the patient has recently eaten, rapid atrial pacing or antiarrhythmic drugs to slow the ventricular response are preferred to DC cardioversion, which requires an anesthetic. In postoperative patients who have an epicardial wire, rapid atrial pacing is performed to convert the atrial flutter.

Long-term treatment—a cure

There has been a recent and dramatic change in the therapeutic approach to atrial flutter.[20] This change has evolved because of the understanding of the mechanism of atrial flutter and because of the rapid expansion of applications for transvenous radiofrequency energy. In the past, many drug studies considered atrial flutter and atrial fibrillation as a unit when they are in fact separate entities.

Over the last decade radiofrequency ablation has been successful in eliminating typical atrial flutter.[31,35] The ability to terminate or ablate type I atrial flutter is identical for the more common counterclockwise and the less common clockwise types. A lesion is created with radiofrequency energy to interrupt conduction through the isthmus formed by the eustachian ridge (the slow arm of the reentry circuit).[36] Others have been successful in ablating the septal isthmus, which lies between the coronary sinus ostium and the tricuspid annulus.[32] With the introduction of improved catheter technology, other sites that are easier to ablate may eventually be identified. This procedure has the same success rate in both forms of typical atrial flutter.

In most patients, the mechanism of success of this procedure is the creation of a persistent bidirectional conduction block in the inferior vena cava–tricuspid annulus isthmus. The procedure has been shown to be successful in patients both with and without associated atrial fibrillation.[31,35,37-40]

Recurrences of atrial flutter are associated with failure to achieve a permanent block in the isthmus. Coumel's group demonstrated that right atrial activation was a fusion of different wave fronts before ablation, whereas following ablation of the isthmus the caudocranial wave front was eliminated and right atrial activation appeared to be dependent on a single superior/inferior wave front.[41]

Radiofrequency catheter ablation has become a very effective method in the treatment of AV nodal reentry tachycardia and accessory pathway ablation, where there is a high success rate and low risk. Experienced physicians are achieving a 90% success rate with the initial attempt to cure atrial flutter. The recurrence rate is 10% or less.[31,42] Patients with typical atrial flutter, a normal right atrial size, and no history of atrial fibrillation have been shown to have the best short- and long-term results from radiofrequency ablation.[43] Verification of a complete line of block between the tricuspid annulus and the eustachian valve and ridge is a reliable criterion for long-term ablation success.[32] Chu, Kalman, and Kwasman et al[44] report that intracardiac echocardiography augments fluoroscopy during catheter ablation by visualizing anatomic landmarks, ensuring stable endocardial contact, and assisting in transseptal puncture (for ablation of left atrial foci and left-sided accessory pathways). In more than 50 consecutive cases of radiofrequency catheter ablation by Feld and colleagues,[20] pericardial effusion developed late after the procedure in only one patient.

Clockwise Typical Atrial Flutter
Mechanism

Figure 9-13 demonstrates the pathway of clockwise typical atrial flutter—the less common form of typical atrial flutter. Its circuit is anatomically identical to that of the counterclockwise rotation but travels in the clockwise direction with similar cycle lengths.

Genesis of flutter waves

In clockwise typical atrial flutter, the F wave in the inferior leads is usually composed of a positive component (the P′ wave) and a negative component (the Ta wave). The path of the macroreentrant circuit is the same as for the counterclockwise form. However, its direction is reversed and descends the interatrial septum and left posterior paraseptal portion of the atria and crosses the inferior right atrium.[6]

ECG recognition

- **Atrial rate.** Same as counterclockwise.
- **Atrial rhythm.** Regular.

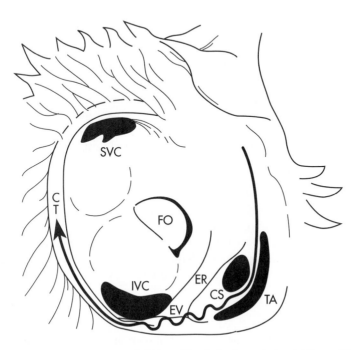

FIGURE 9-13 The macroreentrant path followed by clockwise typical atrial flutter. The route is the same as that of counterclockwise atrial flutter but in the opposite direction.

- **P′ wave axis.** Usually inferior but may be superior.
- **Flutter wave.** The sawtooth flutter waves in the inferior leads may have a positive P′ wave (and negative Ta wave) caused by the inferior P′ axis. However, some cases of clockwise typical atrial flutter have a superior P′ wave axis so that the sawtooth flutter waves are identical to those of the more common counterclockwise form of atrial flutter.[45] The P′ waves in V_1 may have an undulating diphasic pattern or may mimic the positive P′ wave of the more common counterclockwise mechanism.[20]

Acute and long-term treatment

The treatment for clockwise typical atrial flutter is the same as for counterclockwise typical atrial flutter.

TRUE ATYPICAL ATRIAL FLUTTER (TYPE II)

A rare form of rapid macroreentrant atrial tachycardia is called "true atypical atrial flutter" by some electrophysiologists and is sometimes clinically known as "type II atrial flutter."[3] Unfortunately, it appears necessary to use the qualifying adjective true because the term *atypical* is also used to identify the clockwise form of typical atrial flutter.* With a standard classification, it would seem that eventually the "true" could be dropped from this term.

Mechanism

The path of the reentry loop in true atypical atrial flutter has not been as thoroughly studied as that of typical atrial flutter. Using esophageal leads and His bundle electrocardiography, Puech and colleagues[6,10] have shown that activation of the upper part of the right atrium precedes that of the low atrial septum, with the depolarization wave descending along the interatrial septum and the left posterior paraseptal aspect of the atria. The conduction barriers and activation sequence of either type of typical atrial flutter are not present. The mechanism of true atypical atrial flutter is said to be a leading circle–type of reentry with a very small excitable gap that is difficult to penetrate and ablate and probably represents a heterogenous group of arrhythmias.[46-48] New evidence suggests that not all cases of true atypical atrial flutter are functional reentry. Further classification awaits more detailed mapping.[45]

Genesis of Flutter Waves

In true atypical atrial flutter (type II), the F waves differ from those of typical atrial flutter in that the P′ wave is positive in both the frontal plane and precordial leads. The positive component of the F wave (the P′ wave) reflects the descending limb of the reentry circuit in the intraatrial septum and left atrium—the chamber that determines the shape of the P′ wave. The ascending limb of the reentry circuit is not reflected on the surface ECG.

---

*True atypical atrial flutter is also sometimes called "uncommon," "rare," "antidromic," "type B," "unusual," "fast," and "left atrial."

ECG Recognition

- **Atrial rate.** Ranges from 340 to 433 beats/min (short excitable gap), with overlap with the typical form of atrial flutter.[1,49]
- **Atrial rhythm.** Regular, although a shortening of the atrial interval may be seen following the QRS complex.[49]
- **P′ wave axis.** Inferior.
- **Flutter wave.** The P′ component of the flutter wave is positive in the inferior leads (similar to the clockwise form of typical atrial flutter). The P′ component in the precordial leads is also positive (Figure 9-14). An atrial rate of more than 340 beats/min clinically distinguishes true atypical atrial flutter (Type II) from typical atrial flutter (Type I).

Acute Treatment

True atypical atrial flutter is difficult to terminate.

Long-Term Treatment

Radiofrequency ablation of true atypical atrial flutter is difficult to achieve. Nevertheless, most patients remain candidates for electrophysiologic studies.[50, 51] Therefore

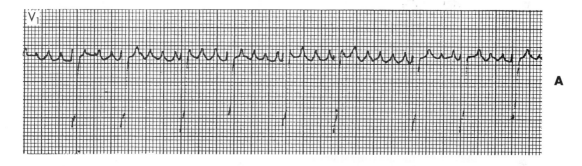

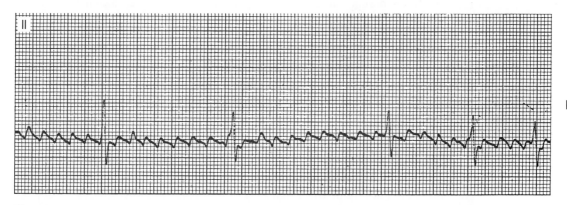

FIGURE 9-14   True atypical (type II) atrial flutter. **A,** The atrial rate is 428 beats/min with variable conduction. **B,** The atrial rate is 345 beats/min with high-grade AV block.

even if the P′ component of the flutter waves is positive in the inferior leads (as they are in true atypical atrial flutter), electrophysiologic studies are still performed to determine if the substrate of the mechanism can be ablated.[20] In one study of 75 consecutive patients undergoing catheter ablation of typical atrial flutter, additional atypical types were found in 11 patients. In three of these patients, the circuit was confined to the right atrial free wall and was successfully ablated with a linear lesion directed at the lateral right atrium.[52]

INCISIONAL REENTRANT ATRIAL TACHYCARDIA

Intraatrial reentrant atrial tachycardia is a well described complication in as many as 25% of patients following repair of complex congenital heart disease. Although this type of tachycardia is often classified as atrial flutter, it differs significantly from typical atrial flutter.[53-55] In order to be more specific, Lesh and Kalman[3] have called these tachycardias "incisional reentrant atrial tachycardias" rather than simply "atrial flutter." The studies by Baker, Lindsay, and Bromberg et al[53] suggest that the incidence of incisional reentrant atrial tachycardia may be substantially reduced if atriotomy incisions are altered slightly to coincide with nonconductive atrial borders such as the inferior or superior vena cava, pulmonary veins, and valve annuli. (For more information, see p. 132.)

DIFFERENTIAL DIAGNOSIS

With a less rapid atrial rate (e.g., 200 beats/min), chronic monomorphic atrial tachycardia may be difficult to distinguish from atrial flutter. In other cases of atrial flutter (especially true atypical atrial flutter), the typical sawtooth pattern may not be seen because concealment of part of the atrial depolarization on the surface ECG produces an isoelectric line between F waves. The atrial rhythm can help distinguish between these two supraventricular tachycardias on the surface ECG. In atrial flutter the rhythm is regular; in chronic atrial tachycardia the atrial rate changes in response to variations of the autonomic nervous system.[6]

Even when the typical sawtooth pattern is present, atrial flutter can be missed when the flutter waves are superimposed on the QRS complex or T wave. Vagal maneuvers are valuable in providing temporary AV block to reveal the underlying flutter waves.

PHYSICAL SIGNS

- **Neck veins.** Rapid, rippling flutter waves may be seen in the jugular venous pulse if the conduction ratio is 4:1; with a 2:1 ratio there is little chance of seeing this phenomenon. Figure 9-15 is a jugular pulse tracing of the flutter (f) waves that can be seen in the neck veins.
- **Heart sounds.** The first heart sound has a constant intensity if the AV relationship remains constant. It is sometimes possible to hear the rapid sounds of the atrial contractions at the 4:1 ratio, but there is little chance of hearing them at the 2:1 ratio.
- **Pulse.** In atrial flutter with a fixed conduction ratio the pulse is regular. If there is a variable conduction ratio, the irregularity of the ventricular rhythm exactly mimics that of atrial fibrillation.

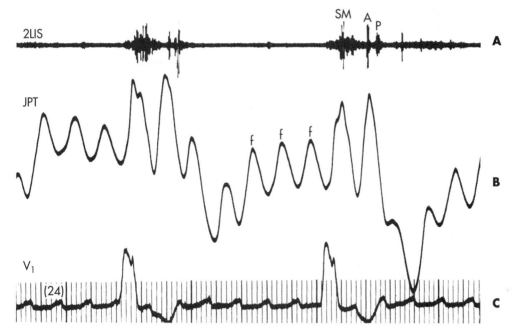

FIGURE 9-15 A demonstration of the flutter waves *(f)* that may be seen in the neck veins during atrial flutter with more than a 4:1 conduction ratio. The tracings are from a 70-year-old man with atrial flutter, complete heart block, and an idioventricular rhythm from the left ventricle. **A,** A phonocardiogram showing an ejection systolic murmur *(SM)* and wide splitting of the second heart sound *(A, P).* **B,** A jugular pulse tracing *(JPT)* showing prominent venous flutter waves related to atrial activation in the ECG **(C).**

CLINICAL SETTING AND INCIDENCE

Acute or transient atrial flutter is one of the atrial tachyarrhythmias that is a typical complication following open heart surgery. Supraventricular tachycardia (SVT) occurs in 30% of patients, one third of whom have atrial flutter that may convert to atrial fibrillation and back again, especially immediately after surgery.[56] In this clinical setting, atrial flutter is probably caused by the diffuse sterile pericarditis and atrial inflammation associated with the surgical procedure.[57] Atrial flutter may also be seen during the acute phase of myocardial infarction and in patients with pulmonary embolism with or without preexisting cardiac disease.[58]

Chronic atrial flutter is rare and is most often seen in persons over 40 years of age. It is commonly associated with organic heart disease, which makes termination and prevention of the arrhythmia important.[59]

Patients with accessory pathways who develop atrial flutter are particularly at risk for sudden death because of the high rate of ventricular response, which sometimes can be 1:1.

ABLATION OF AUTOMATIC AND REENTRANT ATRIAL TACHYCARDIA

It is possible to ablate the focus for automatic and reentrant atrial tachycardias, the majority of which arise in the crista terminalis. Some occur in the left atrium and can be approached with a transseptal technique. Atrial tachycardias after surgery for congenital heart disease and reentry around a surgical scar, anatomic defect, or atriotomy incision have also been successfully ablated.[39,60]

CHEMICAL ABLATION IN THE FUTURE?

An interesting experimental technique has emerged in the form of chemical ablation for atrial flutter. Goette, Honeycutt, and Fleischman et al[61] report success and safety in using transcatheter ethanol infusion in five dogs to produce transmural lesions that ablate the entire isthmus between the lip of the inferior vena cava and the tricuspid annulus.

ANTICOAGULATION

There is no clear consensus regarding the use of anticoagulants in patients with atrial flutter. Some investigators do not anticoagulate or look for clots with transesophageal echo unless there is severe heart disease with a history of transient ischemic attacks or stroke. However, in one study of nine consecutive patients with chronic atrial flutter, transesophageal echocardiogram revealed several minutes of atrial stunning after cardioversion, which suggests that short-term anticoagulation may be appropriate for cardioversion.[62] Data from 85 consecutive patients undergoing cardioversion for atrial flutter suggest that clinically apparent thromboemboli may occur in chronic atrial flutter and that anticoagulation is recommended awaiting further studies.[63] Waldo suggests that aspirin therapy should be considered in patients less than 75 years of age and that warfarin therapy should be considered on an individual basis.[1] In one study of 12 patients, three were found to have left atrial thrombus warranting postponement of radiofrequency ablation.[64]

TABLE 9-1   TYPES AND FEATURES OF ATRIAL FLUTTER

TYPE	MECHANISM	P′ WAVE AXIS	ATRIAL RATE (BEATS/MIN)
Counterclockwise typical	Counterclockwise macroreentry	Superior	240-340 beats/min
Clockwise typical	Clockwise macroreentry	Usually inferior; may be superior	240-340 beats/min
True atypical	Macroreentry	Inferior	340-433 beats/min
Incisional	Macroreentry	May vary with scar location	Varies

Note: A superior P′ wave axis has negative P′ waves and positive Ta waves that form the sawtooth pattern in leads II, III, and aV$_F$. An inferior P′ wave axis has positive P′ waves and negative Ta waves in those leads.

SUMMARY

Atrial flutter is a rapid, regular atrial rhythm with a rate of approximately 300 beats/min and a unique ECG pattern. There are four major types of atrial flutter (Table 9-1). Typical atrial flutter (type I) has a rate of 240 to 340 beats/min and can be interrupted with rapid atrial pacing; it can be further broken down into counterclockwise and clockwise rotation of the reentry circuit. True atypical atrial flutter (type II) has a rate of greater than 340 beats/min with a short excitable gap. With true atypical atrial flutter, it is difficult to cardiovert, ablate, or even slow the rapid ventricular rate pharmacologically. A cure is available for typical atrial flutter in the form of radiofrequency ablation of the slow arm of the intraatrial reentry circuit. Incisional reentrant atrial flutter is a complication in 25% of cases of repair of complex congenital heart disease.

REFERENCES

1. Waldo A: Atrial flutter: mechanisms, clinical features, and management. In Zipes DP, Jalife J, editors: *Cardiac electrophysiology from cell to bedside,* ed 2, Philadelphia, 1995, WB Saunders.
2. Uribe W, Vidaillet H, Granada J et al: Incidence and cause of death among patients with atrial flutter in the general population, *Circulation* 94 (8;suppl):2269, 1996.
3. Lesh MD, Kalman JM: To fumble flutter or tackle "tach"? Toward updated classifiers for atrial tachyarrhythmias, *J Cardiovasc Electrophysiol* 7:460, 1996.
4. Waldo AL, Carlson MD, Biblo LA, Henthorn RW: The role of transient entrainment in atrial flutter. In Touboul P, Waldo AL, editors: *Atrial arrhythmias: current concepts and management,* St Louis, 1990, Mosby.
5. Puech P, Grolleau R, Rebuffat G: Intraatrial mapping of atrial fibrillation in man. In Kulbertus H, Olsson JB, Schlepper M, editors: *Atrial fibrillation,* Mölndal, Sweden, 1982, AB Hassle.
6. Puech P, Gallay P, Grolleau R: Mechanism of atrial flutter in humans. In Touboul P, Waldo AL: *Atrial arrhythmias; current concepts and management,* St Louis, 1990, Mosby.
7. Prinzmetal M, Corday E, Brill IC et al: *The auricular arrhythmias,* Springfield, Ill, 1951, Charles C Thomas.
8. Rytand DA: The circus movement (entrapped circuit wave) hypothesis of atrial flutter, *Arch Intern Med* 65:125, 1966.
9. Puech P: *L'Activité electrique auriculaire normale et pathologique,* Paris, 1956, Masson & Cie.
10. Puech P, Latour H, Grolleau R: Le flutter et ses limites, *Arch Mal Coeur* 63:116, 1970.
11. Waldo AL, MacLean WAH, Karp RB et al: Entrainment and interruption of atrial flutter with atrial pacing: studies in man following open heart surgery, *Circulation* 56:737, 1977.
12. Inour H, Matsuo H, Takayanagi K, Murao S: Clinical and experimental studies of the effects of extrastimulation and rapid pacing on atrial flutter: evidence of macroreentry with an excitable gap, *Am J Cardiol* 48:623, 1981.
13. Waldo AL: Cardiac pacing: role in diagnosis and treatment of disorders of cardiac rhythm and conduction. In Rosen MR, Hoffman BF, editors: *Cardiac therapy,* Boston, 1983, Martinus Nijhoff.
14. Waldo AL, Plumb VJ, Henthorn RW: Observations on the mechanism of atrial flutter. In Surawicz B, Reddy CP, Prystowsky EN, editors: *Tachycardias,* The Hague, 1984, Martinus Nijhoff.
14a. Cosio FG, Arribas F, Palacios J et al: Fragmented electrograms and continuous electrical activity in atrial flutter, *Am J Cardiol* 57:1309, 1986.
14b. Olshansky B, Okumura K, Henthorn RW, Waldo AL: Characterization of double potentials in human atrial flutter: studies during transient entrainment, *J Am Coll Cardiol* 15:833, 1990.

14c. Klein GJ, Guiraudon GM, Sharma AD, Milstein S: Demonstration of macroreentry and feasibility of operative therapy in the common type of atrial flutter, *Am J Cardiol* 57:587, 1986.

15. Chu E, Fitzpatrick AP, Chin MC et al: Radiofrequency catheter ablation guided by intracardiac echocardiography, *Circulation* 89:1301, 1994.

16. Chu E, Kalman JM, Kwasman MA et al: Intracardiac echocardiography during radiofrequency catheter ablation of cardiac arrhythmias in man, *J Am Coll Cardiol* 24:1351, 1994.

17. Kalman JM, Lee RJ, Fisher WG et al: Radiofrequency catheter modification of sinus node function guided by intracardiac echocardiography, *Circulation* 90(4; pt 2):207:I-41, 1994 (abstract).

18. Kalman JM, Fitzpatrick AP, Chin MC et al: Efficiency of heating with radiofrequency energy is related to stability of tissue contact evaluation by intracardiac echocardiography, *Circulation* 90(4; pt 2):1454:I-270, 1994 (abstract).

19. Van Hare GF, Waldo AL: The atrial flutter reentrant circuit: additional pieces of the puzzle, *Circulation* 94:244, 1996.

19a. Olgin JE, Kalman JM, Saxon LA et al: Mechanism of initiation of atrial flutter in humans: site of unidirectional block and direction of rotation, *J Am Coll Cardiol* 29:376, 1997.

20. Feld G: Catheter ablation for atrial flutter (Session ACC96-327). From Morady F, Borggrefe M, Epstein L et al: *Changing concepts in treatment of supraventricular tachycardia,* American College of Cardiology 45th Annual Scientific Sessions, Orlando, March 24-27, 1996.

21. Kalman JM, Olgin JE, Saxon LA et al: Activation and entrainment mapping defines the tricuspid annulus as the anterior barrier in typical atrial flutter, *Circulation* 94:398, 1996.

22. Langendorf R: Concealed A-V conduction: the effect of blocked impulses on the formation and conduction of subsequent impulses, *Am Heart J* 35:542, 1948.

23. Page RL, Wharton JM, Prystowsky EN: Effect of continuous vagal enhancement on concealed conduction and refractoriness within the atrioventricular node, *Am J Cardiol* 77:260, 1996.

24. Porter CJ: Premature atrial contractions and atrial tachyarrhythmias. In Gillette PC, Garson A Jr, editors: *Pediatric arrhythmias: electrophysiology and pacing,* Philadelphia, 1990, WB Saunders.

25. Dunnigan A, Benson DW Jr, Benditt DG: Atrial flutter in infancy: diagnosis, clinical features, and treatment, *Pediatrics* 75:725, 1985.

26. Gillette PC, Zeigler VL, Case CL: Pediatric arrhythmias: are they different? In Zipes DP, Jalife J: *Cardiac electrophysiology from cell to bedside,* ed 2, Philadelphia, 1995, WB Saunders.

27. Aziz AA, Saoudi N, Nair M et al: Intra- and interatrial conduction abnormalities in atrial flutter: a comparison between clockwise and counterclockwise right atrial rotation, *J Am Coll Cardiol* 27(suppl A):189-A,1996.

28. Olgin JE, Kalman JM, Fitzpatrick AP, Lesh MD: Role of right atrial endocardial structures as barriers to conduction during human type I atrial flutter: activation and entrainment mapping guided by intracardiac echocardiography, *Circulation* 92:1839, 1995.

29. Arribas F, Lopez-Gil M, Nunez A et al: The upper link of the common atrial flutter circuit, *Circulation* 90(suppl I):I, 1994.

30. Olshansky B, Okumura K, Hess PG, Waldo AL: Demonstration of an area of slow conduction in human atrial flutter, *J Am Coll Cardiol* 16:1639, 1990.

31. Feld GK, Fleck P, Chen PS et al: Radiofrequency catheter ablation for the treatment of human type I atrial flutter: identification of a critical zone in the reentrant circuit by endocardial mapping techniques, *Circulation* 86:1233, 1992.

32. Nakagawa H, Lazzara R, Khastgir T et al: Role of the tricuspid annulus and the eustachian valve/ridge on atrial flutter: relevance to catheter ablation of the septal isthmus and a new technique for rapid identification of ablation success, *Circulation* 94:407, 1996.

33. Mackall JA, Ozin MB, Carlson MD et al: A simple predictor of successful radiofrequency ablation of atrial flutter, *Circulation* 94(8; suppl):3950, 1996.
34. Rosen MR, Strauss HC, Janse MJ: The classification of antiarrhythmic drugs. In Zipes D, Jalife J, editors: *Cardiac electrophysiology from cell to bedside*, ed 2, St Louis, 1995, WB Saunders.
35. Cosio FG, Lopeq-Gil M, Goicolea A et al: Radiofrequency ablation of the inferior vena cava–tricuspid valve isthmus in common atrial flutter, *Am J Cardiol* 71:705, 1993.
36. Lesh MD, Van Hare GF: Status of ablation in patients with atrial tachycardia and flutter, *Pacing Clin Electrophysiol* 17:1026, 1994.
37. Movsowitz C, Callans DJ, Schwartzman D et al: The results of atrial flutter ablation in patients with and without a history of atrial fibrillation, *Am J Cardiol* 78:93, 1996.
38. Calkins H, Leon AR, Deam G et al: Catheter ablation of atrial flutter using radiofrequency energy, *Am J Cardiol* 73:353, 1994.
39. Lesh MD, Van Hare GF, Epstein LM et al: Radiofrequency catheter ablation of atrial arrhythmias, *Circulation* 89:1074, 1994.
40. Kirkorian G, Moncada E, Chevalier P et al: Radiofrequency ablation of atrial flutter: efficacy of an anatomically guided approach, *Circulation* 90:2804, 1994.
41. Cauchemez B, Haissaguerre M, Fischer B et al: Electrophysiological effects of catheter ablation of inferior vena cava–tricuspid annulus isthmus in common atrial flutter, *Circulation* 93:284, 1996.
42. Saoudi N, Atallah G, Deschamps D et al: The role of transient entrainment in atrial flutter. In Touboul P, Waldo AL, editors: *Atrial arrhythmias: current concepts and management*, St Louis, 1990, Mosby.
43. Nath S, Mounsey JP, Haines DE, DiMarco JP: Predictors of acute and long-term success after radiofrequency catheter ablation of type I atrial flutter, *Am J Cardiol* 76:604, 1995.
44. Chu E, Kalman JM, Kwasman MA, Jue JC et al: Intracardiac echocardiography during radiofrequency catheter ablation of cardiac arrhythmias in humans, *J Am Coll Cardiol* 24:1351,1994.
45. Lesh MD: Personal communication, August 13, 1996.
46. Allessie MA, Lammers WJEP, Bonke FIM, Hollen J: Intraatrial reentry as a mechanism for atrial flutter induced by acetylcholine in rapid pacing in the dog, *Circulation* 70:123, 1984.
47. Ravelli F, Disertori M, Cozzi F et al: Ventricular beats induce variations in cycle length of rapid (type II) atrial flutter in humans: evidence of leading circle reentry, *Circulation* 89:2107, 1994.
48. Aziz AA, Saoudi N, Nair M et al: Intra- and interatrial abnormalities in atrial flutter: a comparison between clockwise and counterclockwise right atrial rotation, *J Am Coll Cardiol* 27(suppl A):768-5:189A, 1996.
49. Wells JL Jr, MacLean WAH, James TN, Waldo AL: Characterization of atrial flutter: studies in man after open heart surgery using fixed atrial electrodes, *Circulation* 60:665, 1979.
50. Kirkorian G, Moncada E, Defeo M et al: Radiofrequency ablation of atrial tissue is also effective in atypical atrial flutter, *Circulation* 90:1802, 1994 (abstract).
51. Satake S, Okishiga K, Azegami K et al: Radiofrequency catheter ablation of uncommon type atrial flutter, *Circulation* 90:3201, 1994 (abstract).
52. Kall J, Rubenstein D, Kopp D et al: Characterization and catheter ablation of right atrial free wall atypical atrial flutter, *Circulation* 94 (8; suppl):3949, 1996.
53. Baker BM, Lindsay BD, Bromberg BI et al: Catheter ablation of clinical intraatrial reentrant tachycardias resulting from previous atrial surgery: localizing and transecting the critical isthmus, *J Am Coll Cardiol* 28:411, 1996.

54. Triedman JK, Jenkins KJ, Colan SD et al: Intra-atrial reentrant tachycardia after palliation of congenital heart disease: characterization of multiple macroreentrant circuits using fluoroscopically based three-dimensional endocardial mapping, *J Cardiovasc Electrophysiol* 8:259, 1997.

55. Muller GI, Deal BJ, Strasburger JF et al: Electrocardiographic features of atrial tachycardias after operation for congenital heart disease, *Am J Cardiol* 71:122, 1993.

56. Waldo AL, MacLean WAH: *Diagnosis and treatment of arrhythmias following open heart surgery: emphasis on the use of epicardial wire electrodes,* Mt Kisco, NY, 1980, Futura.

57. Pagé PL, Plumb VJ, Okumura K, Waldo AL: A new animal model of atrial flutter, *J Am Coll Cardiol* 8:872, 1986.

58. Brugada P, Gorgels AP, Wellens HJJ: The electrocardiogram in pulmonary embolism. In Wellens HJJ, Kulbertus HE, editors: *What's new in electrocardiography,* The Hague, 1981, Martinus Nijhoff.

59. Wellens HJJ: Atrial flutter: progress but no final answer, *J Am Coll Cardiol* 17:1235, 1991.

60. Morady F, Borggrefe M, Epstein L et al: *Changing concepts in treatment of supraventricular tachycardia.* American College of Cardiology 45th Annual Scientific Sessions, Orlando, Florida, March 24-27, 1996 (ACC96-327).

61. Goette A, Honeycutt C, Fleischman S et al: Transcatheter subendocardial infusion: a novel technique for ablation of atrial flutter, *J Am Coll Cardiol* 27(suppl A):401A, 1996.

62. Weiss R, Marcovitz P, Knight BP et al: Evaluation of atrial stunning after cardioversion of chronic atrial flutter, *Circulation* 94 (8; suppl):409:I-71, 1996 (abstract).

63. Pagadala P, Gummadi SS, Olshansky B: Thromboembolic risk of chronic atrial flutter: is the risk underestimated? *Circulation* (90; pt 4):2141:I-398, 1994 (abstract).

64. Prater S, Wadas M, Reynertson S et al: Incidence of atrial thrombus in patients with type I atrial flutter undergoing catheter ablation, *Circulation* 94 (8; suppl):4257, 1996.

CHAPTER 10

Atrial Tachycardia

Classification and
  mechanisms 131
Clinical implications 131
Incisional reentrant atrial
  tachycardia 132
Focal atrial tachycardia 134
Chaotic or multifocal atrial
  tachycardia 135
Nonparoxysmal atrial
  tachycardia 135
Nonsustained paroxysmal
  atrial tachycardia 138
Differential diagnosis 138
Location of focal atrial
  tachycardias 139
P' wave configuration as a
  guide to locations of
  atrial foci 139
Pediatrics 140
Postoperative atrial
  warning arrhythmias 140
Incidence 142
Medical treatment 142
Radiofrequency catheter
  ablation for a cure 142

A TRIAL TACHYCARDIA IS AN UNCOMMON CAUSE OF SYMPTOMATIC SUPRAVENTRICULAR tachycardia that may result in the development of dilated cardiomyopathy, particularly in children.[1] In all of its forms, the mechanism of atrial tachycardia does not require either the sinus (sinoatrial [SA]) node or the atrioventricular (AV) node for sustenance. Therefore the paroxysmal supraventricular tachycardias of SA nodal reentry (see Chapter 7), AV nodal reentry, and AV reentry using an accessory pathway (see Chapter 11) are excluded from this definition. Atrial tachycardia is also distinguished from atrial fibrillation (see Chapter 8) and atrial flutter (see Chapter 9).

The recognition of the mechanism of the arrhythmia is essential because radiofrequency ablation of automatic and reentrant atrial tachycardia, atrial flutter, AV nodal reentry tachycardia, and accessory pathways has a high success rate. In experienced hands there are no complications related to energy application.[2-4] Management strategies are not well defined because of the paucity of data on the long-term effectiveness of pharmacologic and nonpharmacologic therapies.[5]

CLASSIFICATION AND MECHANISMS

- Incisional reentrant atrial tachycardia (intraatrial microreentry)
- Focal atrial tachycardia (abnormal automaticity)
- Incessant* atrial tachycardia (intraatrial reentry)
- Nonparoxysmal (focal) atrial tachycardia (triggered activity)
- Chaotic atrial tachycardia (multifocal abnormal automaticity)
- Nonsustained paroxysmal atrial tachycardia

The mechanisms of atrial tachycardia have already been covered in Chapter 5. Although the designation "ectopic atrial tachycardia" is often used in the literature, the term is unequivocally redundant.[1,5,6] An atrial tachycardia is certainly ectopic because it is not a sinus rhythm.

CLINICAL IMPLICATIONS

In its incessant form, atrial tachycardia often causes tachycardiomyopathy, which is reversible after the tachycardia has been cured by surgery or radiofrequency ablation.[7]

---

*The term *incessant* is incorrectly used in the literature (as it is also in *incessant* junctional tachycardia). These two arrhythmias do in fact cease from time to time. "Frequently recurring" or "persistent" would have been better had the other term not gained popular usage before the characteristics of the arrhythmia were fully evaluated.

It is possible for a patient to have more than one mechanism causing the supraventricular tachycardia.[8-10]

INCISIONAL REENTRANT ATRIAL TACHYCARDIA

Incisional reentrant atrial tachycardia is a sustained supraventricular tachycardia caused by a microreentry circuit, usually around an intraatrial scar. This type of tachycardia is characterized by its sudden onset and termination and may or may not be associated with AV block. Reentry may be confirmed in the electrophysiology laboratory by entrainment and by demonstrating initiation and termination of the tachycardia with programmed electrical stimulation. Following surgery for complex congenital heart disease (e.g., Mustard, Senning, or Fontan procedure; atrial septal defect repair), incisional reentrant atrial tachycardia may develop in as many as 25% of patients and is difficult to manage with antiarrhythmic drug therapy.[11,12]

Mechanism

High density atrial activation sequence maps demonstrate that incisional reentrant atrial tachycardia uses diverse circuits different from those of typical atrial flutter.[13] In the absence of atrial hypertension or stretch in an acute canine model, the Fontan suture lines alone were found to permit the induction of atrial flutter. An essential electrophysiologic substrate is an isthmus of myocardium between the atriotomy and the atriopulmonary connection. Interruption of conduction through this isthmus terminates the atrial flutter in this model and suggests a technique for the ablation of atrial flutter in patients who have undergone a classic Fontan procedure.[14]

Figure 10-1, *A,* is a 12-lead electrocardiogram (ECG) that illustrates reentrant atrial tachycardia of 240 beats/min with alternating 3:1 and 2:1 AV conduction. This ECG is from a 36-year-old woman with an intraatrial scar (from a past atrial septal defect repair) extending obliquely from the right atrial appendage to the low right atrium. Figure 10-1, *B,* shows the scar, the reentrant circuit with its slow arm, and the position of the catheter at the site of successful ablation. The tachycardia terminated promptly after ablation and could not be reinduced.

Long-Term Treatment

Incisional atrial reentrant tachycardia circuits can be ablated with radiofrequency energy with a high success rate.[2] Until recently, successful ablation involved mapping and entrainment techniques that identify a protected isthmus.[2,15] However, Baker, Lindsay, and Bromberg et al[11] suggest that the region of slow conduction does not need to be identified to achieve long-term success and that detailed entrainment studies are not required to identify the critical isthmus. They have demonstrated that incisional atrial reentrant tachycardia can be successfully ablated by using focused activation mapping in the immediate vicinity of atriotomy scars and by performing radiofrequency ablation to transect a critical isthmus of conductive tissue between two nonconductive regions. They also suggest that the incidence of postoperative intraatrial reentrant tachycardia may be diminished by slightly altering the surgical procedures so that the atriotomy incision is made along the natural nonconductive borders of the atria (e.g., inferior vena cava, superior vena cava, pulmonary veins, and valve annuli).

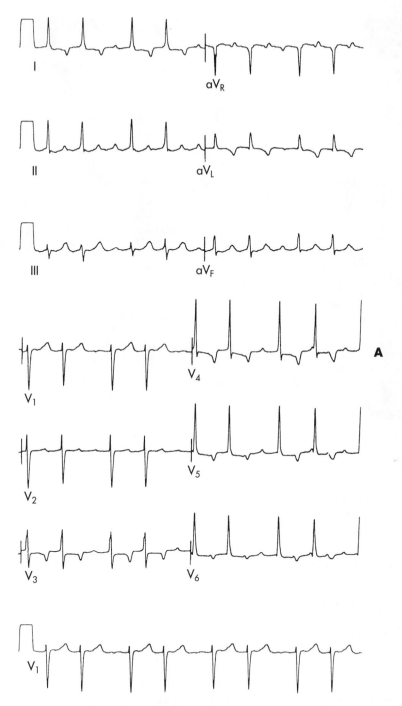

FIGURE 10-1 A, Reentrant atrial tachycardia of 240 beats/min with alternating 3:1 and 2:1 AV conduction (note the group beating). P waves are positive in lead I and in the inferior leads. The P waves are negative in aV_R and negative or isoelectric in leads V_1 and aV_L.   *Continued*

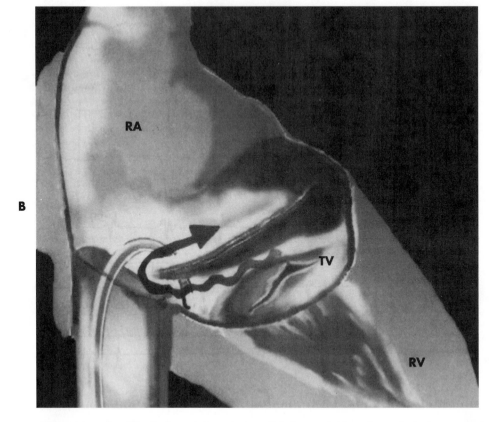

FIGURE 10-1, Cont'd. B, An artist's rendering of the heart of this patient, which shows an atriotomy scar from an old surgery for atrial septal defect. Also shown are the presumed reentry circuit (note its slow arm inferior to the scar) and the radiofrequency catheter poised for successful ablation of the circuit. *RA,* Right atrium; *RV,* right ventricle; *TV,* tricuspid valve. (From Lesh MD, Van Hare GF, Epstein LM et al: Radiofrequency catheter ablation of atrial arrhythmias: results and mechanisms, *Circulation* 89:1074, 1994.)

FOCAL ATRIAL TACHYCARDIA

Focal atrial tachycardia is a supraventricular tachycardia that is initiated and sustained by abnormal automaticity from a nonsinus atrial focus. Figure 10-2 shows atrial tachycardia sites that were successfully ablated in 30 patients.[16]

Focal atrial tachycardia is characterized by the following:
- Prolonged episodes of atrial tachycardia that commonly show a "warm-up" heart rate at initiation and a "cool-down" at termination
- Distinctly visible P′ waves with an abnormal axis and configuration during the tachycardia
- Failure to be initiated or terminated with programmed atrial stimulation[16,17]

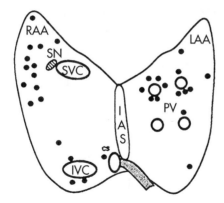

FIGURE 10-2   The dots in this figure indicate 31 sites for atrial tachycardia that were successfully ablated in 30 patients. *CS,* Coronary sinus; *IAS,* interatrial septum; *IVC,* inferior vena cava; *LAA,* left atrial appendage; *PV,* pulmonary veins; *RAA,* right atrial appendage; *SN,* SA node; *SVC,* superior vena cava. (From Tang CW, Scheinman MM, Van Hare GF et al: Use of P wave configuration during atrial tachycardia to predict site of origin, *J Am Coll Cardiol* 26:1315, 1995.)

P′ waves at the onset of the tachycardia are similar in shape to the subsequent P′ waves. The presence of second-degree AV block does not interrupt the automatic atrial tachycardia.

Incessant atrial tachycardia is characterized by its presence more than half the day. Figure 10-3 is a 12-lead ECG that demonstrates incessant atrial tachycardia with a focus in the right atrial appendage. Figure 10-4 is from a patient with a left atrial focus near the right superior pulmonary vein.

CHAOTIC OR MULTIFOCAL ATRIAL TACHYCARDIA

Chaotic or multifocal atrial tachycardia is a supraventricular tachycardia with more than two P′ wave shapes (Figure 10-5). It is initiated and sustained by abnormal automaticity and is often associated with chronic obstructive pulmonary disease. There are at least three P′ wave patterns in each tracing in Figure 10-5. In Figure 10-5, *B,* note that the P′ waves bear the pointed, prominent stamp of P-pulmonale. The beats ending the longest cycles may be junctional or ventricular escapes. The negative QRS complex in lead II indicates left axis deviation, which is an occurrence in a minority of patients with chronic cor pulmonale.

NONPAROXYSMAL ATRIAL TACHYCARDIA

Nonparoxysmal atrial tachycardia is a focal supraventricular tachycardia that is initiated and sustained by triggered activity and is usually but not exclusively associated with digitalis toxicity (Figure 10-6). Because of the rate and the drug, there is often 2:1 AV block. This condition is exacerbated by catecholamines and a shortening of the cycle length.

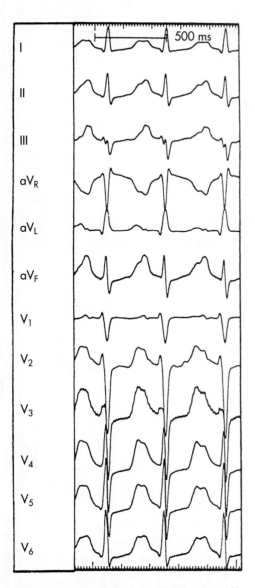

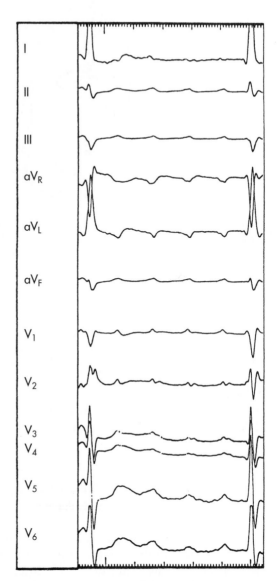

FIGURE 10-3 An incessant atrial tachycardia with the focus in the right atrial appendage. (From Tang CW, Scheinman MM, Van Hare GF et al: Use of P wave configuration during atrial tachycardia to predict site of origin, *J Am Coll Cardiol* 26:1315, 1995.)

FIGURE 10-4 An incessant atrial tachycardia with the focus in the left atrium at the right superior pulmonary vein. (From Tang CW, Scheinman MM, Van Hare GF et al: Use of P wave configuration during atrial tachycardia to predict site of origin, *J Am Coll Cardiol* 26:1315, 1995.)

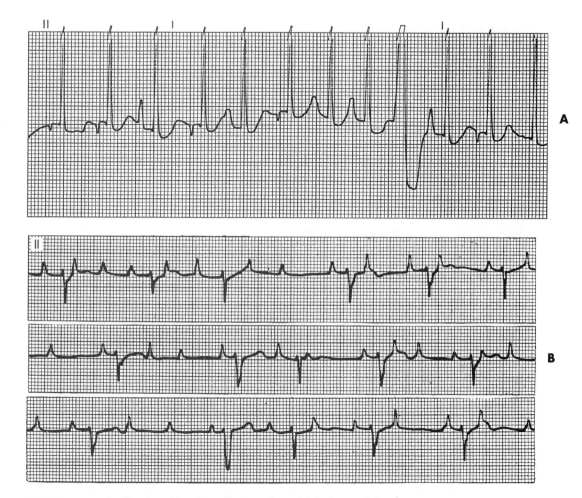

FIGURE 10-5 A, Chaotic atrial tachycardia. Note the multiple shapes of the P′ waves. There is also one ventricular premature beat in the center of the tracing. **B,** Chaotic atrial tachycardia with varying AV block from a patient with severe emphysema.

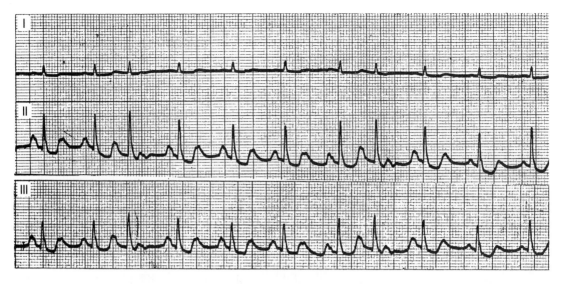

FIGURE 10-6 Nonparoxysmal atrial tachycardia caused by digitalis toxicity in a 68-year-old man suffering from chronic obstructive pulmonary disease and pulmonary cancer and taking digoxin 0.25 mg/day. (Courtesy William P Nelson, MD.)

NONSUSTAINED PAROXYSMAL ATRIAL TACHYCARDIA

Nonsustained paroxysms of atrial tachycardia consist of four to six beats with P′ waves that are different in shape from the sinus P wave and identical to each other (Figure 10-7). They usually go unnoticed by the patient and probably have the same clinical significance and mechanism as atrial premature beats.

DIFFERENTIAL DIAGNOSIS

On the surface ECG, atrial tachycardia is easily distinguished from atrial flutter, atrial fibrillation, AV nodal reentry tachycardia, and AV reentry tachycardia using an accessory pathway simply by the location and shape of the P′ waves:

- **Atrial tachycardia.** P′ waves are usually all the same shape and at a conductible interval in front of the QRS complex. There may or may not be AV block.
- **Atrial flutter.** P′ waves are usually negative in the inferior leads with a positive Ta wave, producing a characteristic sawtooth pattern. There is usually 2:1 or 4:1 AV conduction (see Chapter 9).
- **Atrial fibrillation.** Absent P waves (see Chapter 8).
- **AV nodal reentry tachycardia.** P′ waves are usually buried within the QRS complex (see Chapter 12).
- **AV reentry with an accessory pathway.** P′ waves always separate from the QRS complex and usually immediately follow it; AV block would preclude this mechanism and therefore is never seen (see Chapter 12).

There are, of course, other clues from the ECG, history, and physical examination that help in the differential diagnosis. These clues are discussed in the chapters that discuss each arrhythmia.

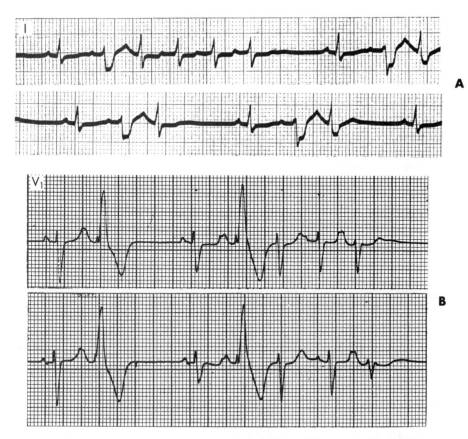

FIGURE 10-7 A, The strips are continuous. Sinus rhythm interrupted by pairs of atrial premature beats and a five-beat salvo of atrial tachycardia with right bundle branch block (RBBB) and probably left posterior hemiblock aberration (negative complex in lead I). The ninth and fifteenth beats show RBBB aberration without the hemiblock. **B,** Sinus rhythm interrupted by atrial premature beats and a four-beat salvo of atrial tachycardia. The first beat in each salvo is conducted with RBBB aberration. Note that the last beat in the bottom strip ends a shorter cycle than the preceding beats and shows the earliest signs of RBBB aberration (shrinkage of the S wave and a rudimentary r′ wave).

LOCATION OF FOCAL ATRIAL TACHYCARDIAS

Lesh and Kalman[12] have classified focal atrial tachycardias according to their location:
- Cristal tachycardias (distributed along the long axis of the *crista terminalis*)[18]
- Atrial tachycardia of pulmonary venous origin *(pulmonary venous ostia* location)
- Septal atrial tachycardia (arise from the septum and do not involve AV nodal tissue)

The term *focal atrial tachycardia* was used when the tachycardia did not qualify for the locations along the crista terminalis, pulmonary venous ostia, or atrial septum.

P′ WAVE CONFIGURATION AS A GUIDE TO LOCATIONS OF ATRIAL FOCI

In a study of 31 consecutive patients with atrial tachycardia resulting from either abnormal automaticity or triggered activity, Tang et al[16] used detailed atrial endocardial mapping to successfully ablate a single atrial focus with radiofrequency energy. P' wave configuration was analyzed from 12-lead ECGs during the tachycardia with spontaneous or pharmacologically induced atrioventricular block. Their findings indicate that analysis of P' wave configuration in leads aV_L and V_1 was most helpful in distinguishing right atrial from left atrial foci:

- **Lead aV_L.** A positive or biphasic P' wave indicates a right atrial focus (sensitivity 88%; specificity 79%).
- **Lead V_1.** A positive P' wave in lead V_1 indicates a left atrial focus (sensitivity 93%; specificity 88%).
- **Leads II, III and aV_F.** These leads provide clues for differentiating superior from inferior foci.[16] For example, a negative P' wave indicates an inferior focus; a positive P' wave indicates a superior focus.

In Figure 10-8, leads aV_L and V_1 are taken from patients with right and left atrial foci. Note the positive or biphasic P' waves in lead aV_L in the patients with right atrial foci. Note the positive P' waves in lead V_1 in the patients with left atrial foci.

Figure 10-9 is an example of an inferior atrial focus. Note the negative P' waves in lead II and the varying AV conduction. The fact that all atrial impulses are not conducted differentiates this type of tachycardia from AV nodal reentry tachycardia (usually 1:1 conduction) and a circus movement tachycardia using an accessory pathway in the retrograde direction (always 1:1 conduction).

PEDIATRICS

Congenital defects such as atrial septal defect and Wolff-Parkinson-White syndrome are commonly associated with the mechanisms in pediatric arrhythmias.

AV reciprocating tachycardia using an accessory pathway is the most common arrhythmia in the neonate, with 50% of infants demonstrating overt Wolff-Parkinson-White syndrome during sinus rhythm.[19]

Chaotic atrial tachycardia in neonates and infants may be associated with atrial septal defect. It is often mistaken for atrial flutter but is more difficult to control and may be more persistent, requiring up to three or four drugs. If the ventricular rate is controlled with drugs but the atrial rate continues unabated, atrial dilatation will result and the arrhythmia will worsen and lead to congestive heart failure.[20]

Unlike reentrant supraventricular arrhythmias, automatic rhythm disturbances *(focal atrial tachycardia)* in children are rare and more resistant to standard pharmacologic therapy. Two of the more common pediatric automatic rhythms are atrial and junctional tachycardia.[21,22]

Radiofrequency ablation is reserved for those rare infants who fail aggressive medical regimens or for situations complicated by ventricular dysfunction, severe symptoms, or complex congenital heart disease.[23,24]

POSTOPERATIVE ATRIAL WARNING ARRHYTHMIAS

In a study of 128 consecutive patients undergoing elective coronary artery bypass grafting, Frost, Molgaard, and Christiansen et al[25] found that the number of supraventricular ectopic beats per hour increased during each of the last 7 hours before the on-

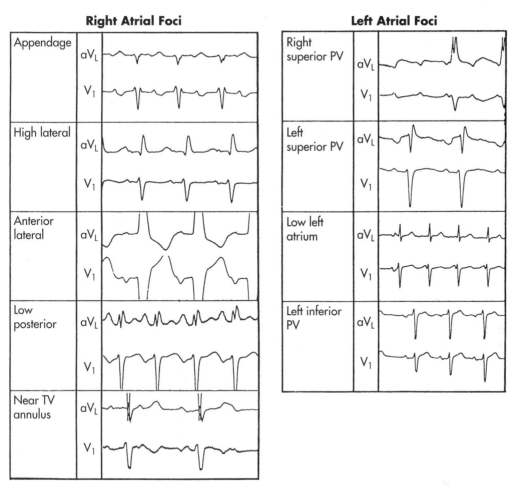

FIGURE 10-8 Leads aV_L and V_1 from nine patients with atrial tachycardia. The P' wave configuration, especially in these two leads, helps to separate right from left atrial foci. A positive P' wave in lead V_1 supports a left atrial focus. A positive P' wave in lead aV_L supports a right atrial focus. (From Tang CW, Scheinman MM, Van Hare GF et al: Use of P wave configuration during atrial tachycardia to predict site of origin, *J Am Coll Cardiol* 26:1315, 1995.)

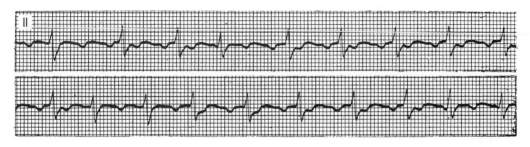

FIGURE 10-9 Atrial tachycardia at a rate of 202 beats/min with varying AV conduction, mostly 2:1. The negative P' wave identifies an inferior atrial focus, and the AV block eliminates the possibility of AV nodal reentry tachycardia or circus movement tachycardia using an accessory pathway. The mechanism may be automatic or reentry.

set of atrial fibrillation or flutter. Episodes of paroxysmal supraventricular tachycardia and nonsustained atrial fibrillation and flutter increased in a similar manner.

INCIDENCE

In 17 years of experience in the clinical electrophysiology laboratory, Wellens, Rodriquez, and Smeets et al studied 1834 patients with supraventricular tachycardia. Atrial tachycardia was diagnosed in 130 patients (7%), 25% of whom had the "incessant" form. In this group of patients, 40% presented with dilated cardiomyopathy.[7]

MEDICAL TREATMENT

Paroxysmal atrial tachycardia is sometimes treated medically with verapamil or a β-blocker. However, because drug therapy usually fails for incessant atrial tachycardia, ablation or surgical isolation of the focus is necessary. In patients with tachycardiomyopathy, the decision to ablate is clear-cut.[7]

RADIOFREQUENCY CATHETER ABLATION FOR A CURE

Ablation of automatic and reentrant atrial tachycardia and atrial flutter have had a high success rate and have caused no complications from energy application. However, repeat procedures may be required for long-term success, especially in patients with atrial flutter. The mechanism by which ablation is successful for intraatrial reentry involves severing a critical isthmus of slow conduction bounded by anatomic or structural obstacles. Automatic arrhythmias are abolished by causing lesions at the focus of abnormal impulse formation. Radiofrequency ablation of drug refractory atrial tachycardias avoids the need for His bundle ablation and permanent pacing.[1-3,5,6]

REFERENCES

1. Tracy CM, Swartz JF, Fletcher RD et al: Radiofrequency catheter ablation of ectopic atrial tachycardia using paced activation sequence mapping, *J Am Coll Cardiol* 21:910, 1993.
2. Lesh MD, Van Hare GF, Epstein LM et al: Radiofrequency catheter ablation of atrial arrhythmias: results and mechanisms, *Circulation* 89:1074, 1994.
3. Lesh MD, Van Hare GF: Status of ablation in patients with atrial tachycardia and flutter, *Pacing Clin Electrophysiol* 17(5; pt 2):1026, 1994.
4. Wellens HJJ: Atrial tachycardia: how important is the mechanism? *Circulation* 90:1576, 1994.
5. Prager NA, Cox JL, Lindsay BD et al: Long-term effectiveness of surgical treatment of ectopic atrial tachycardia, *J Am Coll Cardiol* 22:85, 1993.
6. Walsh EP, Saul JP, Hulse JE et al: Transcatheter ablation of ectopic atrial tachycardia in young patients using radiofrequency current, *Circulation* 86:1138, 1992.
7. Wellens HJJ, Rodriquez LM, Smeets JLRM et al: Tachycardiomyopathy in patients with supraventricular tachycardia with emphasis on atrial fibrillation. In Olsson SB, Allessie MA, Campbell RWF, editors: *Atrial fibrillation: mechanisms and therapeutic strategies,* Armonk, NY, 1994, Futura.
8. Triedman JK, Jenkins KJ, Colan SD et al: Intra-atrial reentrant tachycardia after palliation of congenital heart disease: characterization of multiple macroreentrant circuits using fluoroscopically based three-dimensional endocardial mapping, *J Cardiovasc Electrophysiol* 8:259, 1997.

9. Tritto M, Calabrese P, Massari V, Tricarico G: Intra-atrial and atrioventricular nodal reentrant tachycardia in the same subject diagnosed at transesophageal electrophysiologic study, *Cardiologia* 39:137, 1994.

10. Haissaguerre M, Saoudi N: Role of catheter ablation for supraventricular tachyarrhythmias, with emphasis on atrial flutter and atrial tachycardia, *Curr Opin Cardiol* 9:40, 1994.

11. Baker BR, Lindsay BD, Bromberg BI et al: Catheter ablation of clinical intraatrial reentrant tachycardias resulting from previous atrial surgery: localizing and transecting the critical isthmus, *J Am Coll Cardiol* 28:411, 1996.

12. Lesh MD, Kalman JM: To fumble flutter or tackle "tach"? Toward updated classifiers for atrial tachyarrhythmias, *J Cardiovasc Electrophysiol* 7:460, 1996.

13. Triedman JK, Jenkins KJ, Colan SD et al: High-density transcatheter mapping shows diverse mechanisms for atrial reentrant tachycardia after congenital heart surgery, *J Am Coll Cardiol* 27(suppl A):768-6:189A,1996.

14. Gandhi SK, Bromberg BI, Schuessler RB et al: Characterization and surgical ablation of atrial flutter after the classic Fontan repair, *Ann Thorac Surg* 61:1666, 1996.

15. Triedman JK, Saul JP, Weindling SN, Walsh EP: Radiofrequency ablation of intra-atrial reentrant tachycardia after surgical palliation of congenital heart disease, *Circulation* 91:707, 1995.

16. Tang CW, Scheinman MM, Van Hare GF et al: Use of P wave configuration during atrial tachycardia to predict site of origin, *J Am Coll Cardiol* 26:1315, 1995.

17. Naheed ZJ, Strasburger JF, Benson DW Jr, Deal BJ: Natural history and management strategies of automatic atrial tachycardia in children, *Am J Cardiol* 15:405, 1995.

18. Kalman J, Olgin J, Fitzpatrick A et al: "Cristal tachycardia": relationship of atrial tachycardias to the crista terminalis identified using intracardiac echocardiography, *PACE* 18:261, 1995.

19. Ludomirsky A, Garson A Jr: Supraventricular tachycardia. In Gillette PC, Garson A Jr, editors: *Pediatric arrhythmias: electrophysiology and pacing,* Philadelphia, 1990, WB Saunders.

20. Gillette PC, Zeigler VL, Case CL: Pediatric arrhythmias: are they different? In Zipes DP, Jalife J, editors: *Cardiac electrophysiology from cell to bedside,* ed 2, Philadelphia, 1995, WB Saunders.

21. Case CL, Gillette PC: Automatic atrial and junctional tachycardias in the pediatric patient: strategies for diagnosis and management, *Pacing Clin Electrophysiol* 16:1323, 1993.

22. Douglas DE, Case CL, Shuler CO, Gillette PC: Successful radiofrequency catheter ablation of atrial muscle reentry tachycardia in a young adult, *Clin Cardiol* 18:51, 1995.

23. Weindling SN, Saul JP, Walsh EP: Efficacy and risks of medical therapy for supraventricular tachycardia in neonates and infants, *Am Heart J* 131:66, 1996.

24. Bauersfeld U, Gow RM, Hamilton RM, Izukawa T: Treatment of atrial ectopic tachycardia in infants <6 months old, *Am Heart J* 129:1145, 1995.

25. Frost L, Molgaard H, Christiansen EH et al: Atrial ectopic activity and atrial fibrillation/flutter after coronary artery bypass surgery: a case-base study controlling for confounding from age, beta-blocker treatment, and time distance from operation, *Int J Cardiol* 30:153, 1995.

CHAPTER 11

Reciprocal (Echo) Beats

AV junction (V-A-V
    sequence) 145
Ventricles (V-A-V sequence)
    145
RP′ interval in V-A-V
    sequences 147
Atria (A-V-A sequence) 147

REENTRY USING THE ATRIOVENTRICULAR (AV) NODE MAY BE AN ISOLATED OCCURRENCE and produce a single reciprocal or echo beat. A single impulse, having activated either the atria or the ventricles, returns to activate them for a second time. Reciprocal beats were called "return extrasystoles" by Scherf and Shookhoff[1] in 1926. The term *reciprocal* was introduced in 1913 by Mines.[2]

Figure 11-1 diagrammatically illustrates the three main forms of reciprocal beats, which depend on their site of origin: the AV junction, the ventricles, and the atria.

AV JUNCTION (V-A-V SEQUENCE)

In general, a reciprocal beat occurs when the retrograde conduction to the atria from an ectopic junctional beat is long enough to permit reactivation of the ventricles.

Reciprocal beating is one of the mechanisms that produce allorhythmia (i.e., a repeated arrhythmic sequence). Figure 11-2 is an example of reciprocal beats producing an allorhythmia of three beats. Each trio consists of two junctional beats followed by a reciprocal beat.

VENTRICLES (V-A-V SEQUENCE)

Half of all ventricular premature beats travel retrogradely to the atria via the His bundle and AV node and may return to reactivate the ventricles (V-A-V sequence). Virtually all ventricular premature beats activate the atria retrogradely in the presence of an accessory pathway (Wolff-Parkinson-White syndrome) because of the easy access to the atrium via this accessory pathway.

Figure 11-3 is an example of a ventricular ectopic rhythm with retrograde Wenckebach conduction and ventricular echoes. The tracing begins with a run of ventricular tachycardia. Retrograde conduction from the first two beats lengthens until the third finally blocks (3:2 retrograde Wenckebach period). There are two sinus beats before the beginning of the next run of ventricular rhythm, which is interrupted after only two beats by a ventricular echo. Reciprocal beats do not change the management of ventricular arrhythmias. They merely provide an alert to the possibility that a paroxysmal supraventricular tachycardia *(PSVT)* may develop.

In the top strip of Figure 11-4 there is ventricular tachycardia with a 4:3 retrograde Wenckebach period. Note that the RP′ intervals get longer until the impulse fails to reach the atria. In the bottom strip of Figure 11-4, a laddergram is provided to illustrate a reciprocal beat with fusion. The second retrograde impulse spawns an anterograde impulse to the ventricles; this impulse fuses with the next beat of the ventricular tachycardia.

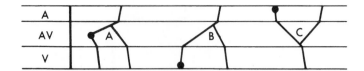

FIGURE 11-1 Three forms of reciprocal beating. **A,** Junctional rhythm with reciprocal beat. **B,** Ventricular ectopic beat with reciprocal beat. **C,** Reversed reciprocal beat.

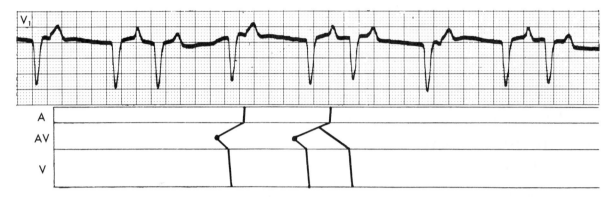

FIGURE 11-2 AV rhythm with left bundle branch block and reciprocal beating. The allorhythmia consists of two junctional beats with lengthening retrograde conduction, the second of which is followed by a reciprocal beat. The three-beat sequence then repeats itself.

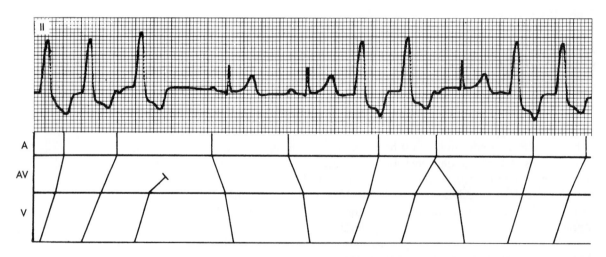

FIGURE 11-3 Ventricular ectopic beats manifest retrograde Wenckebach conduction to the atria. The first group of ventricular ectopic beats has lengthening RP′ intervals until, after the third complex, retrograde conduction is blocked. The next group of ventricular ectopic beats also has retrograde Wenckebach conduction. However, after the second complex the impulse returns to the ventricles to produce a ventricular echo. (From Conover MH: *Cardiac arrhythmias*, ed 2, St Louis, 1978, Mosby.)

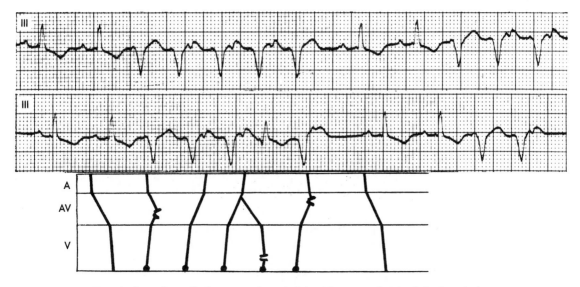

FIGURE 11-4 Ventricular tachycardia (rate = 145 beats/min), with retrograde Wenckebach period in the top strip and a reciprocal beat in the bottom strip.

RP′ INTERVAL IN V-A-V SEQUENCES

In Figure 11-4, which illustrates V-A-V sequences, the retrograde P′ that was followed by the ventricular reciprocal beat ended a long RP′ interval. This interval is usually 0.24 seconds or longer and may be as long as 0.60 seconds or more. Occasionally the RP′ is shorter than 0.24 seconds; reciprocal beating may be possible even with an RP′ interval of only 0.12 seconds. The shorter RP′s are more often seen with junctional than with ectopic ventricular rhythms.

At first it seems surprising that reentry can occur after a short RP′ interval because delayed conduction, although not absolutely essential for reentry, is a common component of the circuit. The short RP′ appears to indicate relatively rapid retrograde conduction. However, it is important to remember that in AV junctional rhythms the RP′ interval is not a measure of retrograde conduction alone but instead represents the *difference* between anterograde and retrograde conduction times. Therefore very slow retrograde conduction, which is conducive to reentry, can be masked by correspondingly slow anterograde conduction (Figure 11-5). Impulse *b* has considerable slowing of retrograde conduction, yet the masking effect of correspondingly slow anterograde conduction produces the same RP′ interval as that of the faster-conducted impulse *(a)*. This masquerade is possible because the junctional discharge is a silent event and is not seen on the surface ECG.

ATRIA (A-V-A SEQUENCE)

When an atrial impulse is conducted with some delay (prolonged PR) through the AV junction (e.g., at the end of a Wenckebach cycle), it may return to the atria through another pathway to produce an atrial echo.[3,4]

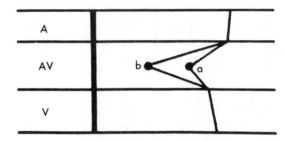

FIGURE 11-5 The RP' interval of junctional beats remains unchanged provided the difference between retrograde and anterograde conduction remains the same.

At times it is impossible to differentiate an atrial echo beat from a nonconducted atrial premature beat. Sometimes the fact that an atrial echo beat appears only after a lengthening of the PR interval affords the necessary differential clue. There is no reason for an atrial extrasystole to be dependent on lengthening AV conduction, whereas a measure of conduction delay is clearly a promoter of reentry (Figure 11-6). In the top strip of Figure 11-6, none of the beats with the shorter PR intervals are followed by an inverted P wave. The one beat with a lengthened PR interval is followed by an inverted P wave, which establishes it as an echo rather than as a nonconducted extrasystole. In each of the lower strips the third and last P wave of a 3:2 Wenckebach period is followed by a retrograde P wave without an intervening QRS complex. This pattern undoubtedly represents an atrial echo and is shown in the laddergram below the bottom strip. Just as the anterogradely reciprocal beat (ventricular echo) can complete its circuit without activating the atria, so the reversed reciprocal beat (atrial echo) can complete its return journey without involving the ventricles.[4-6]

In patients with Wolff-Parkinson-White syndrome, an atrial premature beat (APB) depolarizes the ventricles and can easily gain access to the atria via the accessory pathway to produce an atrial echo beat. Figure 11-7, *A*, is an example of an APB that activates the ventricles in the normal way but then returns to the atria through an accessory pathway located in the posterior septum. Note the retrograde P' wave in the T wave of the premature beat. Figure 11-7, *B*, is taken from the same patient, a 12-year-old girl who presented in the emergency room with PSVT. The sequence that produced the single atrial echo beat in Figure 11-7, *A*, now sees the depolarization wave repeatedly returning to the ventricles via the AV node and back up the accessory pathway to the atria to support PSVT (see Chapter 12).

SUMMARY

Because of normally slow conduction through the AV node, it is possible for this structure to produce a reciprocal beat or to support a reentry circuit in the absence of an AV nodal pathologic condition. This is especially true because of the presence of pathways approaching the AV node, one with a faster conduction velocity and longer refractory period than the other. Because of the longer refractory period of the faster con-

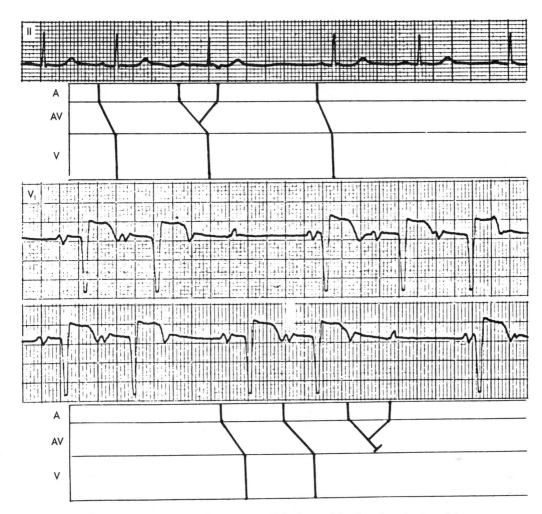

FIGURE 11-6   Atrial echoes. Lead II illustrates an atrial echo resulting from lengthening of the preceding PR interval. The strips of V_1 are not continuous; each shows a 3:2 AV Wenckebach period in which the third and last sinus impulse of the group, which fails to reach the ventricles, returns to the atria to produce an echo.

ducting pathway, an early atrial premature beat may be conducted only down the slow pathway, resulting in a long P′R interval and giving the fast pathway time to complete its refractory period. The impulse may then return to the atria via the fast pathway to produce a single reciprocal beat or to begin the sustained circuit that supports AV nodal reentry tachycardia. Such a scenario is also possible following ventricular premature beats with retrograde conduction to the atria either through the His bundle and AV node or via an accessory pathway.

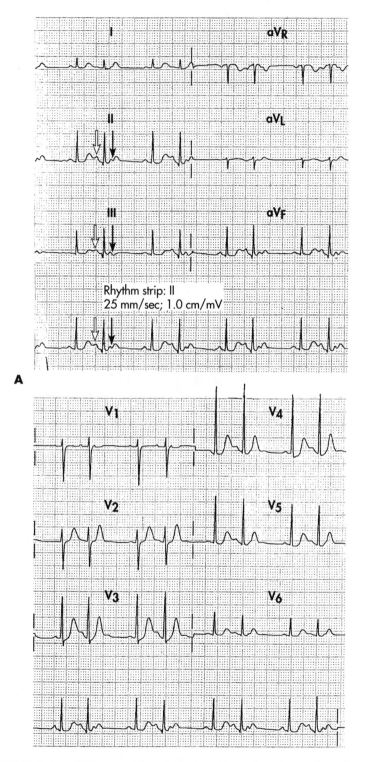

FIGURE 11-7 **A,** An atrial premature beat *(open arrow)* is conducted normally to the ventricles and returns to the atria via a posterior septal accessory pathway to produce a retrograde P′ wave in the inferior leads *(solid arrow)*. This repeated sequence produces a bigeminal rhythm.

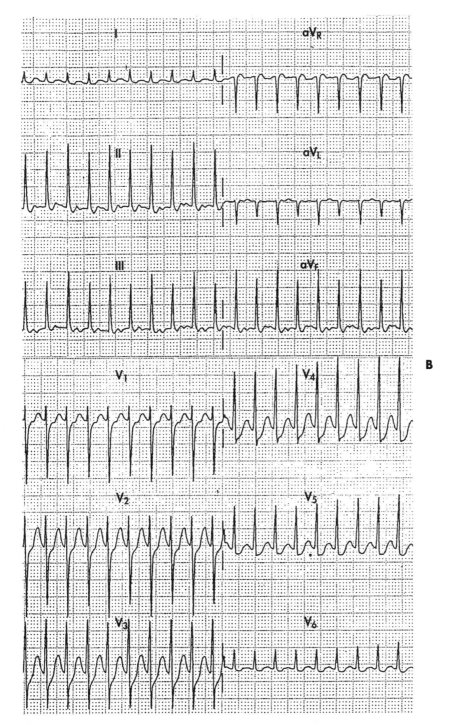

FIGURE 11-7, CONT'D B, Lead II from the same patient. In this case the sequence perpetuates itself. Once retrograde conduction up the accessory pathway is initially completed, the impulse returns repeatedly in a circus movement to the ventricles, through the AV node, and to the atria through the accessory pathway.

REFERENCES

1. Scherf D and Shookhoff C: Experimentelle Untersuchungen über die "Umkehr-Extrasystole," *Wien Arch Inn Med* 12:501, 1926.
2. Mines GR: On dynamic equilibrium in the heart, *J Physiol (Lond)* 46:349, 1913.
3. Kistin AD: Atrial reciprocal rhythm, *Circulation* 32:687, 1965.
4. Pick A: Mechanisms of cardiac arrhythmias: from hypothesis to physiologic fact, *Am Heart J* 86:249, 1973.
5. Pick A, Langendorf R: *Interpretation of complex arrhythmias*, Philadelphia, 1979, Lea & Febiger.
6. Bix HH, Marriott HJL: Reciprocal beats masquerading as ventricular captures, *Am J Cardiol* 4:128, 1959.

CHAPTER 12

Narrow QRS Paroxysmal Supraventricular Tachycardia

Terminology 153
Classification 153
Relative incidence 154
Maintenance and interruption of a reentry circuit 154
Emergency response 155
Importance of recording multiple leads during tachycardia 155
Methods of vagal stimulation 156
Carotid sinus massage 156
Bedside diagnosis 157
AV nodal reentrant tachycardia 157
Orthodromic circus movement tachycardia 160
Atypical AV nodal reentrant tachycardia 171
Incessant junctional tachycardia (atypical orthodromic circus movement tachycardia) 173
Differentiating the reciprocating supraventricular tachycardias 174
Pediatrics 176

TERMINOLOGY

- **Orthodromic** [*ortho-* running in the right direction + *dromic* conduction]. Normal (anterograde) conduction through the AV node.
- **Antidromic.** In the opposite direction of the normal current through the atrioventricular (AV) node.
- **Reciprocating.** The return of an impulse to its place of origin.
- **Circus movement.** Any reentry circuit, but commonly used to refer to the AV reentry circuit that uses an accessory pathway and the AV node.
- **Paroxysmal.** Beginning and ending abruptly.

CLASSIFICATION (NARROW AND BROAD QRS TYPES OF PAROXYSMAL SUPRAVENTRICULAR TACHYCARDIA)
Common Forms (Narrow QRS)

- AV nodal reentrant tachycardia (50%)
- Orthodromic circus movement tachycardia (40%)[1]

Uncommon Forms (Narrow QRS)

- AV nodal reentrant tachycardia (atypical)
- Incessant junctional reciprocating tachycardia (circus movement tachycardia using a slow accessory pathway)
- Sinoatrial (SA) nodal reentrant tachycardia (see Chapter 7)
- Intraatrial reentrant tachycardia (see Chapter 10)

Uncommon Forms (Broad QRS)

- Antidromic circus movement tachycardia (see Chapter 17)
- Circus movement tachycardia using a nodoventricular or fasciculoventricular fiber
- Circus movement tachycardia using two accessory pathways (see Chapter 17)

153

RELATIVE INCIDENCE (NARROW QRS PAROXYSMAL SUPRAVENTRICULAR TACHYCARDIA)

Out of a total of 708 patients with symptomatic paroxysmal supraventricular tachycardia (PSVT) seen at the Hospital of the University of Pennsylvania (280 patients) and at the University of Limburg in Maastricht, The Netherlands (428 patients), 50% had AV nodal reentrant tachycardia (AVNRT) in both institutions. The second most common mechanism was circus movement tachycardia (CMT) (that is, atrioventricular reentry using a concealed, retrogradely conducting bypass tract (39% in Pennsylvania and 27% in Maastricht), 10% of whom had CMT using a slowly conducting accessory pathway. Atrial tachycardia was the mechanism in 19% of the Maastricht series (versus 11%).[1] (See Table 12-1.)

MAINTENANCE AND INTERRUPTION OF A REENTRY CIRCUIT

In 1908 Mayer[2] accurately described the conditions for reentry in the following words:

> This wave will maintain itself indefinitely, provided the circuit be long enough to permit each and every point of the wave to remain at rest for a certain period of time before the return of the wave through the circuit. This single wave going constantly in one direction around the circuit may maintain itself for days traveling at a uniform rate. The circuit must, however, be long enough to allow each point to rest for an appreciable interval of time before the return of the wave. The wave is actually "trapped" in the circuit and must constantly drive onward through the tissue. The point from which the wave first arises is of no more importance in maintaining the rhythmical movement than is any other point on the ring.

A circus movement is interrupted if a temporary block is created within the circuit (e.g., vagal maneuver, adenosine, or a calcium channel blocker) or if a well-timed impulse, nat-

---

TABLE 12-1 TYPES OF NARROW QRS SUPRAVENTRICULAR TACHYCARDIA

	HOSPITAL OF THE UNIVERSITY OF PENNSYLVANIA (280 PATIENTS)	UNIVERSITY OF LIMBURG, MAASTRICHT, THE NETHERLANDS (428 PATIENTS)
AVNRT	141	216
AV reentry	108	131
Rapidly conducting accessory pathway	97	116
Slowly conducting accessory pathway	11	15
Atrial tachycardia	31	77

From Josephson ME, Wellens HJJ: Differential diagnosis of supraventricular tachycardia, *Cardiol Clin* 8:411, 1990.
AVNRT, Atrioventricular nodal reentrant tachycardia.

ural or artificial, finds the nonrefractory gap between the head and the tail of the circulating wave and produces refractoriness. Further discussion of reentry can be found on p. 56.

EMERGENCY RESPONSE

Emergency treatment for the two most common mechanisms of PSVT (AVNRT and CMT) is exactly the same, which relieves the emergency team of the need to make a hurried diagnosis. Once the tachycardia is recorded and terminated, there is time to carefully evaluate the tracings obtained during the tachycardia and compare them with the postconversion sinus rhythm.

Hemodynamically Stable Patient

- **Record** the tachycardia in at least five leads (I, II, III, V_1, V_6).
- **Terminate** the tachycardia.[3]
    1. Vagal maneuver, if unsuccessful, then:
    2. Adenosine 6 mg IV rapidly. If unsuccessful, the dosage is increased to 12 mg; this may be repeated once. If not adenosine, verapamil may be given (10 mg IV over 3 minutes; reduce to 5 mg if the patient is taking a β-blocker or is hypotensive). If unsuccessful, then:
    3. Procainamide 10 mg/kg body weight IV over 5 minutes. If unsuccessful, then:
    4. Electrical cardioversion
- **Record** the sinus rhythm in the same leads.
- **Stabilize** the patient and obtain a history.
- **Diagnose** by close examination of the tracings with and without the tachycardia.
- **Refer** for radiofrequency ablation if CMT or refractory AVNRT is diagnosed.

Hemodynamically Unstable Patient

- **Record** the rhythm in at least five leads.
- **Terminate** with synchronized DC cardioversion.
- **Record** the sinus rhythm in the same leads.
- **Stabilize** the patient and obtain a history.
- **Diagnose** by close examination of the tracings with and without the tachycardia.
- **Refer** for radiofrequency ablation if CMT or refractory AVNRT is diagnosed.

IMPORTANCE OF RECORDING MULTIPLE LEADS DURING TACHYCARDIA

1. A delta wave is not always present in the electrocardiogram (ECG) of patients with Wolff-Parkinson-White (WPW) syndrome. However, the diagnosis can often be made from the ECG during the tachycardia.
2. P waves are small and not always seen in all leads; therefore in the absence of a 12-lead ECG at least five leads (I, II, III, V_1, V_6) are needed. Lead I is an excellent diagnostic lead in cases of left- and right-sided accessory pathways. In such cases the P′ wave is either negative (left-sided) or positive (right-sided). The partially hidden P′ waves of AVNRT are best seen in leads II, III, and V_1.
3. It is helpful to know what the clinical arrhythmia is before performing electrophysiologic studies, because rhythms that are not clinically relevant can be elicited during the studies.

4. The axis of the P′ wave during the tachycardia indicates the location of the accessory pathway and provides a guide to the electrophysiologist (Table 12-2).
5. An identification of the tachycardia mechanism in the emergency setting guarantees proper referral.

METHODS OF VAGAL STIMULATION

Stimulation of the vagus nerve causes a release of acetylcholine, which in turn lengthens the refractory period of the AV node and thus terminates PSVT. Carotid sinus massage (see the following section) and the gag reflex are strong vagal maneuvers in the hospital setting. Immersion of the face in cold water is particularly useful in infants. Patients can be instructed in several other vagal maneuvers such as coughing, assuming a recumbent position with legs elevated against the wall, and the Valsalva maneuver, in which in addition to gagging there is blowing against a closed glottis or squatting.

CAROTID SINUS MASSAGE

The carotid sinus is located at the bifurcation of the carotid artery at the angle of the jaw (not in the neck). Carotid sinus stimulation is an excellent diagnostic or therapeutic vagotonic maneuver. Massaging this area elevates pressure in the carotid sinus so that there is reflex slowing of AV conduction. This maneuver is diagnostic only when the tachycardia is confined to the atria (e.g., atrial flutter) and the AV block created by stimulation of the carotid sinus allows the examiner to see the flutter waves.

Carotid sinus massage may have no effect on the tachycardia because of the dominance of the sympathetic nervous system. It may temporarily slow the ventricular rate, or it may terminate the tachycardia. The effects on the different mechanisms of supraventricular tachycardia are as follows[4]:

- **Sinus tachycardia.** Gradual and temporary slowing of the heart rate
- **Paroxysmal atrial tachycardia.** No effect, or the tachycardia may cease
- **"Incessant" atrial tachycardia.** Temporary slowing of the ventricular rate or no effect
- **Atrial fibrillation.** Temporary slowing of the ventricular rate or no effect
- **PSVT (CMT or ANVRT).** Termination of the tachycardia or no effect

TABLE 12-2   LOCATING THE ACCESSORY PATHWAY USING P′ WAVE AXIS

LOCATION	LEAD	POLARITY
Left ventricle	I	Negative
Septal	II and III	Negative
Lateral	II and III	Equiphasic or positive
Right ventricle	I	Positive or biphasic
	II	Positive or equiphasic
	III	Positive
	V_1	Negative or biphasic
Posteroseptal	aV_R and aV_L	P′ in aV_R > P′ in aV_L

Caution

- Do not use carotid sinus massage if there is a history of transient ischemic attacks, if carotid artery stenosis is found on palpation, or if carotid bruits are present.
- Do not apply pressure for longer than 5 seconds.
- Do not use carotid sinus massage on patients over 65 years of age; sinus pauses of 3 to 7 seconds have been reported under such circumstances. With aging there is a normal development of the parasympathetic nervous system, which is exacerbated by carotid sinus massage.

Procedure for Carotid Sinus Massage

1. Place the patient in a supine position with the neck extended (small pillow or your arm under the patient's shoulders).
2. Turn the patient's head away from the side to be massaged.
3. Locate the bifurcation of the carotid artery just below the angle of the jaw.
4. If the patient is not hypersensitive (begin with slight pressure), press the carotid sinus against the lateral processes of the cervical vertebra with a massaging action for no more than 5 seconds.
5. Monitor the effect on the ECG; if an ECG monitor is not available, listen to the heart with the stethoscope while massaging the carotid sinus.

BEDSIDE DIAGNOSIS

- Regular pulse
- Blood pressure constant
- Constant intensity of S_1
- The "frog sign"[3] (rapid, regular expansion of the neck veins [the *a* wave] as the atria contract against closed AV valves)

Other symptoms of PSVT depend on the duration and rate of the tachycardia and the presence or absence of structural heart disease. Symptoms include feelings of palpitations, nervousness, polyuria (typically with rates >120 beats/min for 10 to 30 minutes in 20% to 50% of patients), anxiety, angina, heart failure, syncope, and shock.

AV NODAL REENTRANT TACHYCARDIA

Definition

In its common form, AVNRT is a narrow QRS PSVT that is usually initiated by an atrial premature beat (APB) and supported by a reentry circuit that uses a slowly conducting inferior atrionodal pathway in the anterograde direction and a more rapidly conducting superior atrionodal pathway in the retrograde direction. This mechanism has been identified as the most common in symptomatic PSVT.[1]

Anatomy

A circuit that repeatedly reenters the AV node is based on a model of dual AV nodal pathways that are functionally and anatomically distinct.[5] A so-called "fast" pathway flows from the atrial septum near the tendon of Todaro to the superior approaches to the compact AV node. A slow pathway flows from the os of the coronary sinus to the inferior approaches to the compact node in the posteroseptal right atrium (Figure 12-1; see p. 158).

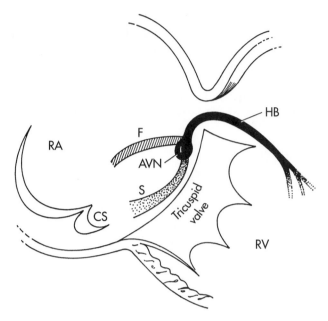

FIGURE 12-1 A so-called "fast" *(F)* anterior pathway and "slow" *(S)* inferior pathway that approach the AV node *(AVN)*. The fast pathway has a longer refractory period than the slow pathway. *CS*, Coronary sinus; *HB*, His bundle; *RA*, right atrium; *RV*, right ventricle. (Modified from Keim S, Werner P, Jazayeri M et al: Localization of the fast and slow pathways in atrioventricular nodal reentrant tachycardia by intraoperative ice mapping, *Circulation* 86:919, 1992.)

Mechanism

The onset of a sustained reentry circuit using the slow and fast atrionodal pathways illustrated in Figure 12-1 is possible because the refractory periods in the two pathways differ. Because the fast pathway has the longer refractory period, a very early APB is likely to be blocked in that pathway, while gaining entrance to the ventricles through the slow pathway. In Figure 12-2, *A*, note that once the impulse reaches the compact AV node it can now proceed in both directions—up to the atria and down to the ventricles. Initial retrograde atrial activation has been recorded by a His bundle catheter; it occurs at the *low septal right atrium* (the location of the fast pathway).[6] As shown in Figure 12-2, *B*, the repetition of this reentry circuit results in PSVT. Note that the P′ wave is buried within the QRS complex because atrial and ventricular activation are simultaneous. The P′ wave often distorts the terminal part of the QRS complex, especially in leads II, III, and aV$_F$, where the end of the negative P′ wave peeks out of the QRS complex like an S wave and in fact is called a "pseudo S wave." The retrograde P′ is positive in lead V$_1$ and often looks like an r′ wave distorting the end of the QRS complex. The pattern in lead V$_1$ is called a "pseudo right bundle branch block" (RBBB) pattern.

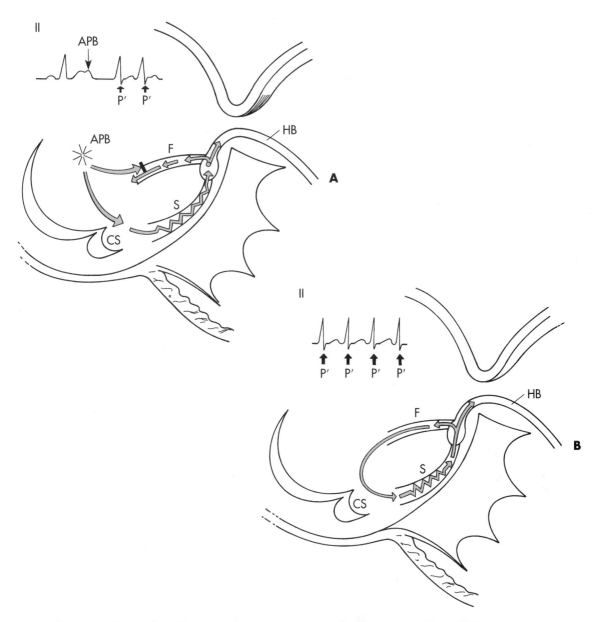

FIGURE 12-2 A, The onset of AV nodal reentrant tachycardia. An early atrial premature beat *(APB),* in the T wave of the first beat, finds the fast pathway *(F)* refractory and the slow pathway *(S)* nonrefractory. Thus ventricular activation is through the slow pathway, which results in a long P′R interval. Within the compact AV node, the impulse moves back to the atria and down to the ventricles simultaneously, causing the P′ wave to be located within the QRS complex. The P′ wave distorts the end of the QRS complex, which causes a pseudo S wave in the inferior leads. **B,** The reentry circuit described in **A** is sustained. *CS,* Coronary sinus; *HB,* His bundle.

ECG Recognition

- **Heart rate.** 170 to 250 beats/min
- **Rhythm.** Regular or slightly irregular in cases of changing conduction velocities through the AV node
- **Initiating P'R interval.** Approximately 0.38 seconds (slow pathway conduction time)
- **Location of the P' waves.** Buried within the QRS complex; either distorts the end of the QRS complex or is not seen at all
- **Polarity of the P' waves.** Negative in leads II, III, and aV_F; positive in lead V_1
- **QRS complex.** Narrow but often distorted by the P' wave, causing a pseudo S wave in the inferior leads and/or a pseudo r' wave in lead V_1
- **Conduction ratio.** 1:1
- **Aberrant ventricular conduction.** Uncommon
- **Distinguishing features.**
  Paroxysmal, narrow QRS tachycardia
  Often with pseudo S waves in inferior leads and/or pseudo r' waves in V_1
  Usually initiated by an APB
  Figure 12-3 is an example of AVNRT as seen in five leads. The P' waves are clearly evident in these tracings if the mechanism is understood. The P' waves are the pseudo S waves in leads II, III, and V_6 and the r' waves (pseudo RBBB pattern) in lead V_1.

Clinical Implications

- Usually benign and self-limiting
- Easily terminated by a vagal maneuver (patient should be taught several vagal maneuvers)
- Occasionally refractory to vagal maneuvers and referred for radiofrequency ablation

Treatment

The emergency response to PSVT has been discussed earlier in this chapter (see p. 155). For the long term, when AVNRT cannot be controlled by the patient (vagal maneuvers), radiofrequency ablation of the slow atrionodal pathway is considered and in experienced hands is very successful.[7] The risk of complete heart block exists because of the danger of damage to the AV node or damage to an atypically located fast atrionodal pathway.[5] Because of the delicacy of the procedure for ablating a slow atrionodal pathway, the patient is advised that a repeat procedure may be necessary before block of the slow pathway is complete.

ORTHODROMIC CIRCUS MOVEMENT TACHYCARDIA
Definition

In its common form, CMT is a paroxysmal supraventricular narrow QRS tachycardia. It is usually initiated by an APB and supported by an atrioventricular reentry circuit that uses the AV node anterogradely and a rapidly conducting accessory pathway retrogradely. CMT is the second most common mechanism of PSVT.[1]

Anatomy

The presence of an extra muscle fiber (accessory pathway) that connects the atrium and ventricle is a congenital anomaly. Such a connection is constructed of myocardial

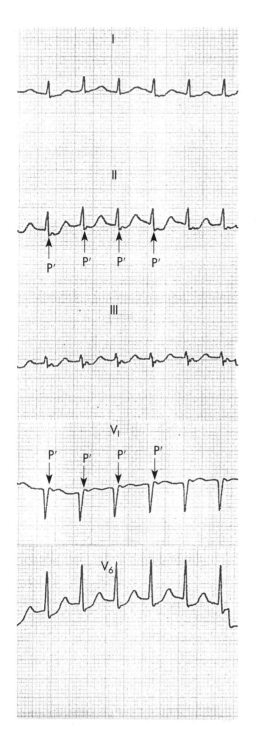

FIGURE 12-3 AV nodal reentrant tachycardia seen in five leads. With simultaneous activation of the atria and ventricles the P′ waves are buried in the QRS complexes and in this case distort the end of the QRS complexes *(arrows).* In the inferior leads this distortion is called a pseudo S wave; in V₁ it is called a pseudo R′ wave. (From Zimmerman FH: *Clinical electrocardiography,* New York, 1994, McGraw-Hill.)

tissue and is not protected by an AV node. Accessory pathways may conduct rapidly like normal myocardial fibers (most common) or slowly like the AV node (rare). Each type of accessory pathway has its own unique ECG presentation.

Mechanism
Wolff-Parkinson-White syndrome

During sinus rhythm in most individuals with accessory pathways, the normal sinus impulse gains entry to the ventricles prematurely (preexcitation) via the accessory pathway, which results in a short PR interval. Furthermore, the early activation of the ventricles in a location outside of the His-Purkinje system causes a depolarization wave that does not move as rapidly as it would had it entered the ventricles by the usual pathway of AV node–His-Purkinje axis. This phenomenon is reflected on the ECG by a slur at the beginning of the QRS complex *(delta wave)*.

Figure 12-4 illustrates the production of a delta wave. In this case, the QRS complex is actually a fusion beat as the sinus impulse enters the ventricles via the AV node in time to activate part of the ventricles. The ECG signs of short PR interval, broad QRS complex (because of the delta wave), and a tendency for PSVT comprise Wolff-

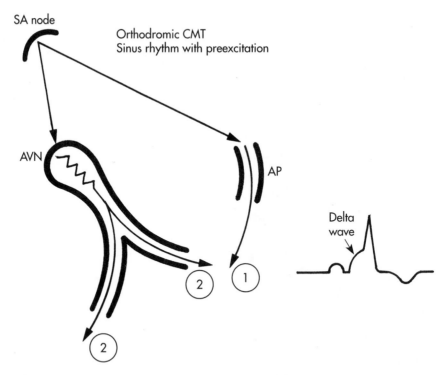

FIGURE 12-4 The production of a delta wave, a sign of preexcitation. The sinus impulse enters the accessory pathway *(AP)* first and activates the ventricles before the impulse can negotiate the slower-conducting AV node *(AVN)*. Such a sequence results in a fusion beat (the currents entering the ventricles by the AV node collide with those entering through the accessory pathway).

Parkinson-White syndrome. Not all individuals with accessory pathways have preexcitation (short PR), but they may present with symptomatic PSVT. Such individuals may have either a concealed or a latent accessory pathway. The *concealed accessory pathway* is capable of only retrograde conduction; the *latent accessory pathway* is capable of conduction in both directions.

Circus movement tachycardia (common form)

CMT differs from AVNRT in that in CMT each structure is activated in sequence (atria–AV node–ventricles–accessory pathway–atria), whereas in the common form of AVNRT the atria and ventricles are activated simultaneously.

Because of the two AV connections in individuals with accessory pathways, an AV reentry circuit is relatively easy to initiate. Figure 12-5, *A*, illustrates the initiation of CMT. An APB is blocked in the accessory pathway and travels down the AV node to produce a narrow QRS complex. (This direction of travel is called *orthodromic.*) It then returns to the atrium via the accessory pathway and continues the circuit repeatedly (Figure 12-5, *B*).

It is important to note that the P′ wave immediately *follows* the QRS complex. This is the common form of AV reentry using an accessory pathway. The P′ wave is in close proximity to the preceding QRS complex because of the fast conduction in the accessory pathway. Once the ventricles have been activated by the normal pathway, the impulse is quickly delivered back to the atrium at the location of the accessory pathway.

ECG Recognition

The ECG differential diagnosis between AVNRT and CMT is summarized in Table 12-3:

TABLE 12-3   ECG DIFFERENTIATION BETWEEN AV NODAL REENTRANT TACHYCARDIA AND CIRCUS MOVEMENT TACHYCARDIA

ECG SIGN	AVNRT	CMT
QRS alternans	Rare	Common
Initial P′R	Prolonged	Normal
P′ location	Within QRS complex; may look like terminal QRS (pseudo S wave in II, III, aV$_F$; pseudo r′ wave in V$_1$)	Separate from QRS complex (always)
P′ polarity	Negative in II, III, aV$_F$	Varies with AP location
		If negative in lead I, diagnostic of left-sided AP
Aberrancy	Rare	Common
HR during aberrancy compared with no aberrancy	Does not change	May slow with aberrancy (BBB same side as AP)
AV conduction	Usually 1:1	Always 1:1

AP, Accessory pathway; *AV,* atrioventricular; *BBB,* bundle branch block; *HR,* heart rate.

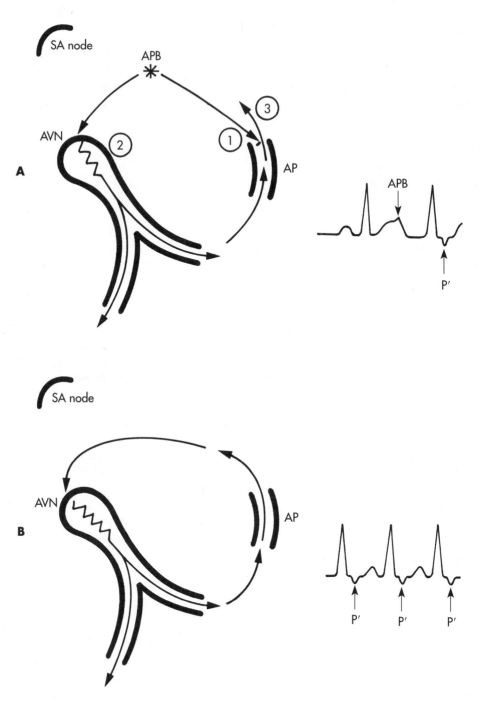

FIGURE 12-5 **A,** The initiation of a circus movement tachycardia using the AV node *(AVN)* in the anterograde (orthodromic) direction and an accessory pathway *(AP)* in the retrograde direction. An atrial premature beat *(APB)* finds the accessory pathway refractory and travels down only the AV node to the ventricles. Once the ventricles are activated the impulse can now return to the atrium, into which the accessory pathway is inserted. This location can be anywhere around the fibrous ring. Activation of the atria produces a separate P′ wave. **B,** The circus movement just described is maintained as the impulse repeatedly returns to the ventricles and the atrium in sequence, always producing a separate P′ wave.

- **Heart rate.** 170 to 250 beats/min
- **Rhythm.** Regular, but may be slightly irregular because of changing conduction through the AV node
- **Initiating P′R interval.** Not prolonged
- **Location of P′ waves.** Always separate from the QRS complex
- **Polarity of P′ waves.** Depends on the atrial insertion of the accessory pathway; left free wall location causes a negative P′ in lead I and is diagnostic of an accessory pathway
- **QRS complex.** Normal unless there is aberrant ventricular conduction; QRS alternans is present in approximately 30% of cases
- **Conduction ratio.** Always 1:1
- **Aberrant ventricular conduction.** Common
- **Heart rate during aberrancy.** Slower with aberrancy than without if the accessory pathway is on the same side as the BBB; this is a diagnostic sign (Figure 12-6); if accessory pathway is located on opposite ventricle from the BBB, rate is the same with and without aberrancy
- **QRS alternans.** Common
- **Distinguishing features.**
  Initial P′R not prolonged
  Narrow QRS complex
  Begins and ends abruptly
  P′ waves closely *follow* QRS complex
  Negative P′ in lead I if left-sided accessory pathway (diagnostic)
  QRS alternans common
  Aberrant ventricular conduction common

Figure 12-7 is an example of CMT using a left-sided accessory pathway. The heart rate is only 150 beats/min, but the position of the P′ waves relative to the QRS complex and their negativity in lead I leave little doubt as to the mechanism. The P′ waves immediately follow the QRS complex in leads I, aV_L, II, III, aV_F, and V_1. Note that the P′ waves are also negative in the inferior leads and in aV_L.

Figure 12-8 shows CMT with QRS alternans, a common finding and a helpful clue in the differential diagnosis of PSVT. The P′ wave is separate from and immediately follows the QRS complex.

Figure 12-9 illustrates the ECG and mechanism of a ventricular premature beat that initiates PSVT. When this happens, the mechanism is usually CMT because the ventricular impulse easily enters the atria via the rapidly conducting accessory pathway. After activating the atria, the impulse passes down the AV node to the ventricles, and a reentry circuit is established.

Figure 12-10 shows CMT being initiated by sinus tachycardia. When the sinus rhythm reaches a critical rate, anterograde conduction in the accessory pathway is blocked. Conduction proceeds down the AV node and is able to return to the atria via the accessory pathway to establish a reentry circuit.

Clinical Implications

- May lead to life-threatening atrial fibrillation, with heart rates >200 beats/min and sometimes 300 beats/min
- Repeated bouts of PSVT may result in cardiomyopathy
- A cure is available at centers skilled in the use of radiofrequency ablation

Text continued on p. 171

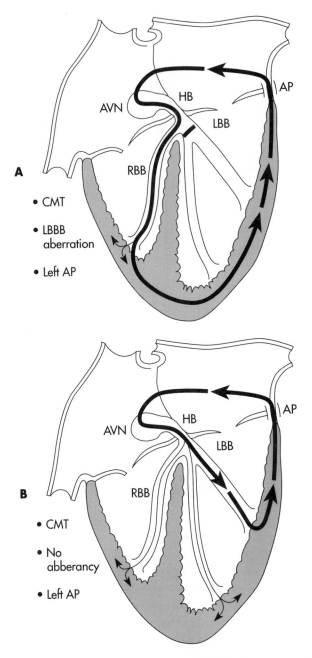

FIGURE 12-6 Circus movement tachycardia using a left-sided accessory pathway *(AP)* with **(A)** and without **(B)** left bundle branch block aberration. When the bundle branch block is on the same side of the heart as the accessory pathway, the journey through the ventricles to activate the accessory pathway retrogradely is longer than if the impulse were able to travel through the left bundle branch *(LBB)*. *AVN,* Atrioventricular node; *HB,* His bundle; *RBB,* right bundle branch.

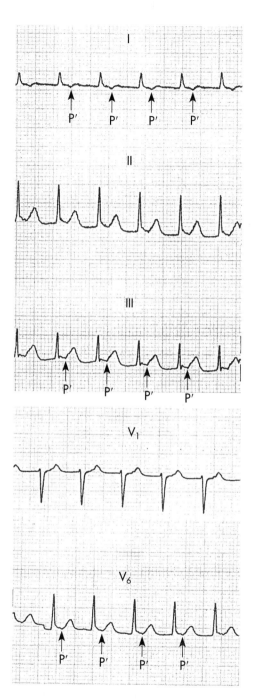

FIGURE 12-7 Circus movement tachycardia using a left-sided accessory pathway. Note the negative P′ wave immediately following the QRS complex in lead I. Negative P′ waves can also be seen in leads II, III, aV$_L$, aV$_F$, V$_5$, and V$_6$. (Leads aV$_L$, aV$_F$, V$_5$, and V$_6$ are not illustrated here.) (From Zimmerman FH: *Clinical electrocardiography,* New York, 1994, McGraw-Hill.)

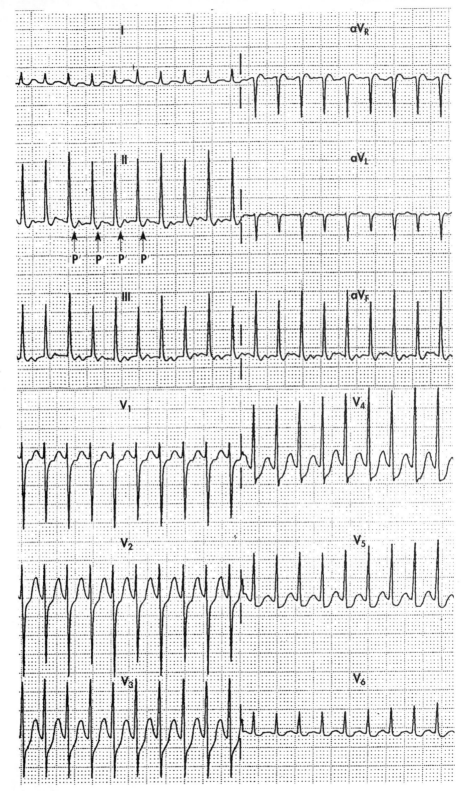

FIGURE 12-8 An example of QRS alternans in a 12-year-old girl complaining of light-headedness when presenting in the emergency department. In this case, QRS alternans, a common and very useful sign of circus movement tachycardia, is present in seven leads (II, III, aV$_R$, aV$_L$, aV$_F$, V$_1$, and V$_2$).

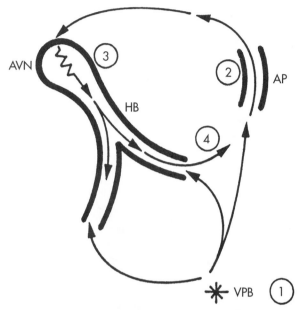

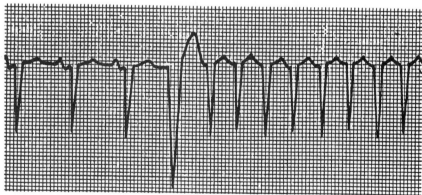

FIGURE 12-9 The ECG and mechanism of a ventricular premature beat that initiates PSVT. *1,* The ventricular premature beat *(VPB)* gains easy access to an atrium *(2)* through the accessory pathway *(AP).* The ventricles are reactivated when the current returns down the AV node *(AVN) (3, 4).* *HB,* His bundle. (Courtesy Hein JJ Wellens, MD, The Netherlands.)

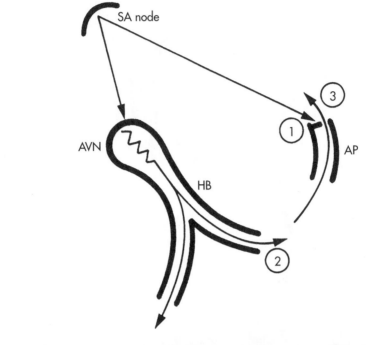

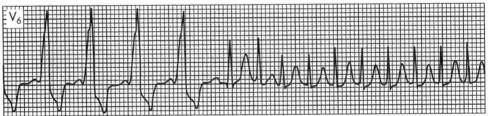

FIGURE 12-10 Sinus tachycardia in a patient with Wolff-Parkinson-White syndrome initiates circus movement tachycardia. Note the signs of WPW syndrome at the beginning of the tracing (short PR and wide QRS complex during sinus rhythm). At a sinus rate of approximately 150 beats/min, the refractory period of the accessory pathway *(AP)* is exceeded, and anterograde conduction is blocked *(1)*. However, the AV node *(AVN)* continues to conduct the sinus impulse. Once in the ventricles *(2)*, the depolarization wave can now return to the atrium where the AP is located *(3)* and establish a sustained rapid circus movement. *HB,* His bundle. (Courtesy Hein JJ Wellens, MD, The Netherlands.)

Treatment

The emergency response to PSVT has been discussed earlier in this chapter (see p. 155) and is the same for the two common forms of this condition. Long-term treatment of CMT is curative (i.e., radiofrequency ablation of the accessory pathway).

ATYPICAL AV NODAL REENTRANT TACHYCARDIA
Definition

In its uncommon form, AVNRT is a narrow QRS PSVT that is supported by a reentry circuit that travels in a direction opposite to the common form of AVNRT. In the more common form, which has already been discussed, anterograde conduction travels down the slow atrionodal pathway and retrograde conduction uses the fast atrionodal pathway. This conduction causes the P′ waves to be hidden within or to peek out just beyond the QRS complex. In the uncommon form of AVNRT, anterograde conduction occurs through the fast atrionodal pathway and retrograde conduction through the slow pathway. This type of conduction not only separates the P′ wave from the QRS complex but also distances it (RP′ > P′R). This type of PSVT resembles the so-called "incessant" junctional tachycardia (a CMT using a slowly conducting accessory pathway).

Mechanism

The atypical form of AVNRT is usually initiated by an APB and uses the rapidly conducting inferior atrionodal pathway in the anterograde direction and the slowly conducting superior atrionodal pathway in the retrograde direction. Intraatrial recordings have localized the earliest retrograde atrial activation to the slow atrionodal pathway near the coronary sinus ostium.[8]

ECG Recognition
- **Heart rate.** 170 to 250 beats/min
- **Rhythm.** Regular or slightly irregular in cases of changing conduction velocities through the AV node
- **Location of P′ waves.** RP′ interval longer than the P′R interval
- **Polarity of P′ waves.** Negative in leads II, III, and aV_F; positive or isoelectric in lead I; negative in leads V_5 and V_6[8]
- **QRS complex.** Narrow
- **Distinguishing features.**
  Paroxysmal, narrow QRS tachycardia
  RP′ interval longer than P′R interval
  Positive P′ wave in lead I (differentiates atypical AVNRT from incessant junctional tachycardia)[8]
  Does not dominate the patient's life as does incessant junctional tachycardia

Figure 12-11 is an example of atypical AVNRT. Note the long RP′ interval and the positive P′ wave in lead I. Figure 12-12 shows the onset of long RP′ tachycardia. Lead I is not available, but the mechanism is probably atypical AVNRT because the tachycardia occurs infrequently. This patient could terminate the PSVT by lying on the floor with his or her feet on the wall; a cough or a Valsalva maneuver does not work. Note that the tachycardia is initiated by APBs and that the P′ waves are negative in the modified V_1 and V_5 leads.

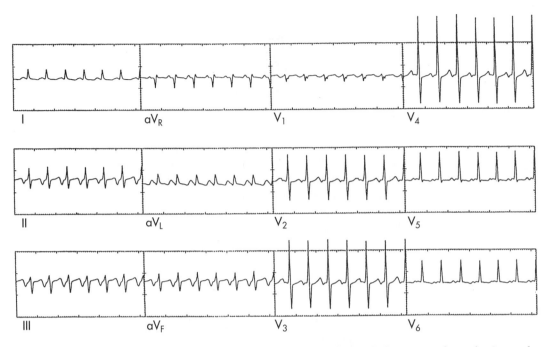

FIGURE 12-11 Atypical AV nodal reentrant tachycardia in which anterograde conduction to the ventricles occurs through the fast atrionodal pathway and retrograde conduction occurs via the slow atrionodal pathway. This conduction causes the P′ wave to be separated further from the QRS complex than with the typical AV nodal reentrant tachycardia, in which atrial and ventricular activation are simultaneous. (From Ng KS, Lauer MR, Young C et al: Correlation of P-wave polarity with underlying electrophysiologic mechanisms of long RP′ tachycardia, *Am J Cardiol* 77:1129, 1996.)

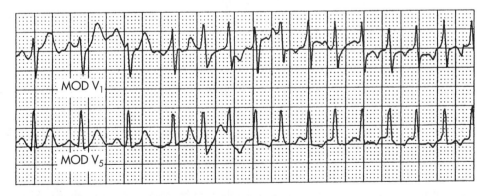

FIGURE 12-12 Holter monitoring leads show the onset of atypical AV nodal reentrant tachycardia in a symptomatic 30-year-old woman. The tachycardia is initiated with sinus tachycardia followed by atrial premature beats. In the last four beats, negative P′ waves with RP′ intervals that are longer than the P′R intervals are seen in the modified V_1 and V_5 leads. (Courtesy Julie Boudreau, BS.)

Clinical Implications
- Usually benign and self-limiting
- Usually terminated by a vagal maneuver; patient should be taught several vagal maneuvers

Treatment

The emergency response to PSVT has been discussed earlier in this chapter. If the tachycardia cannot be controlled by the patient with vagal maneuvers, radiofrequency ablation of the slow atrionodal pathway is considered.

INCESSANT JUNCTIONAL TACHYCARDIA (ATYPICAL ORTHODROMIC CIRCUS MOVEMENT TACHYCARDIA)
Definition and Mechanism

Unfortunately, the term *incessant junctional tachycardia* is misleading and inaccurate and requires a lengthy parenthetical qualification. The tachycardia is present more than 12 hours a day and alternates with brief periods of sinus rhythm; therefore the condition is not truly incessant. Neither is the term *permanent* acceptable because it is not clear if the term refers to the tachycardia per se (never abates) or to the permanent condition of *frequently recurring episodes* (what it actually is). Furthermore, because there is not a focus in the AV junction, this condition is not junctional in the usual sense. One source has simply grouped this tachycardia with others under the title "long RP′ tachycardia," which accurately describes the ECG picture.[8]

The misnomers aside, it is important to know that this debilitating condition is *easily curable* with radiofrequency ablation, a fact that places a grave responsibility on those who interpret ECG tracings. The mechanism is an orthodromic CMT (down the AV node) that uses a slowly conducting accessory pathway for return to the atrium and places the P′ wave at a distance from the QRS complex. The tachycardia itself commonly recurs, is refractory to treatment, and results in tachycardia-related cardiomyopathy. The accessory pathway is usually located in the posterior septal region near the coronary sinus os. Left-sided, slowly conducting accessory pathways have also been described.[8,9]

ECG Recognition
- **Heart rate.** 130 to 200 beats/min
- **Rhythm.** Regular
- **Location of P′ waves.** RP′ interval is longer than the P′R interval
- **Polarity of P′ waves.** Negative in leads II, III, aV$_F$, and V$_4$ to V$_6$; negative or biphasic in lead I[8,9]
- **QRS complex.** Narrow
- **Distinguishing features.**
  Paroxysmal narrow QRS tachycardia
  RP′ interval longer than P′R interval
  Negative P′ waves present in leads II, III, aV$_F$, and V$_4$ to V$_6$
  Negative or biphasic P′ wave in lead I (differentiates it from atypical AVNRT, which has a positive P′ wave in lead I)[8]

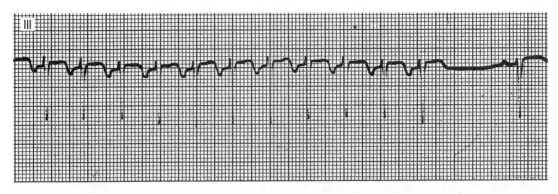

FIGURE 12-13 Atypical circus movement tachycardia using a slowly conducting accessory pathway. Note the long RP′ interval and the negative P′ wave in lead III.

Present more than 12 hours a day

Narrow QRS tachycardia alternating with brief periods of sinus rhythm

Result of tachycardia-related cardiomyopathy

Figure 12-13 is an example of atypical CMT using a slowly conducting accessory pathway. Note the long RP′ interval and the negative P′ wave in lead III.

Clinical Implications

- Usually benign and self-limiting
- Usually terminated by a vagal maneuver; patient should be taught several vagal maneuvers

Treatment

Because atypical orthodromic CMT is usually refractory to antiarrhythmic drugs, radiofrequency ablation is considered early in the management of these patients. Improvement of the tachycardia-related left ventricular dysfunction usually occurs after the arrhythmia has been cured.[9]

DIFFERENTIATING THE RECIPROCATING SUPRAVENTRICULAR TACHYCARDIAS

Electrophysiologists have adduced the following clues to help differentiate the various types of supraventricular tachycardia:

1. The more common type of AVNRT, which uses the slow pathway anterogradely and the fast pathway retrogradely, results in a P′ wave that usually coincides with the QRS complex and is therefore not seen at all or distorts the terminal QRS complex (Figure 12-14, *A*).
2. An uncommon form of AVNRT uses the fast pathway anterogradely and the slow pathway retrogradely, which results in a P′ wave that is closer to the following QRS complex than it is to the preceding QRS complex (RP′ > P′R) (see Figure 12-14, *A*).

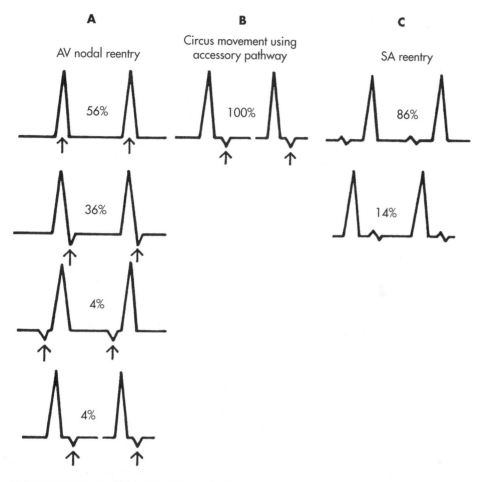

FIGURE 12-14 Location of the P′ wave in the common mechanisms of PSVT. (Courtesy Hein JJ Wellens MD, The Netherlands.)

3. In CMT using an accessory pathway, the atria and ventricles are activated in sequence because of the relatively wide physical separation of the anterograde and retrograde pathways. Anterograde conduction usually occurs through the AV node and His bundle, which takes longer than retrograde conduction through the rapidly conducting accessory pathway and results in P waves that immediately follow the QRS complex (RP′ < P′R) (Figure 12-14, *B*).

4. In SA nodal reentry tachycardia P waves precede rather than follow QRS complexes (Figure 12-14, *C*). Conduction to the ventricles is not a necessary link in the maintenance of this reentry circuit as it is with the tachycardia using an accessory pathway.

5. In the atypical orthodromic CMT using a slowly conducting accessory pathway (the so-called incessant or permanent junctional tachycardia) there is slow retrograde conduction over an accessory pathway, which causes the RP′ to be greater than the P′R.

PEDIATRICS
Neonate and Infant

CMT using an accessory pathway is the most common arrhythmia in the neonate and accounts for most of the PSVTs that occur in infants. Of 112 infants studied at Children's Hospital, Harvard Medical School, 86 had an an accessory pathway, 10 had AVNRT, 11 had intraatrial reentry, and 5 had an ectopic focus in the atria.[10] WPW syndrome is overt in 50% of cases and concealed in the others.[11] Although 30% of children with overt WPW syndrome lose their delta wave in the first year of life and 50% of them no longer have PSVT after that time, the SVT returns by age 20.[12] Until then, no treatment is required.[11]

Treatment depends on the clinical setting. Of the 112 infants in the Harvard study, 106 were treated pharmacologically, 9 of whom failed medical management and required radio frequency ablation. The study reported that antiarrhythmic drug therapy appears to be effective and safe in infants with SVT. Radiofrequency ablation should be reserved for those rare infants who fail aggressive medical regimens or for situations that are complicated by ventricular dysfunction, severe symptoms, or complex congenital heart disease.[11]

Fetus

Mechanisms in the fetus include intraatrial reentry and CMT. The diagnosis is usually made during random fetal heart rate monitoring, when a heart rate of 300 beats/min is noted. Rarely, the mother reports a decrease in fetal movements. The diagnosis may also be made during fetal sonograms by visualizing the atrial and ventricular contractions and/or the movement of the AV valves. In the fetus, a rate of 300 beats/min results in hydrops fetalis in just a few hours. A rate of 300 beats/min is well tolerated in infants up to 1 year of age.

SUMMARY

The two most common forms of paroxysmal supraventricular tachycardia are AV nodal reentrant tachycardia (50%) and orthodromic circus movement tachycardia (40%).[1] The ECGs of these two conditions differ mainly because of the position of the P′ wave relative to the QRS complex. The emergency treatment is the same.

All uncommon forms of narrow QRS PSVT (SA nodal reentrant tachycardia, intraatrial reentrant tachycardia, atypical AVNRT, and atypical CMT using a slow accessory pathway) have a long RP′ interval for different reasons. All of these conditions can be cured by radiofrequency ablation.

REFERENCES

1. Josephson ME, Wellens HJJ: Differential diagnosis of supraventricular tachycardia, *Cardiol Clin* 8:411, 1990.

2. Mayer AG: Rhythmical pulsation in scyphomedusae. II. *In Papers from the Tortugas Laboratory of the Carnegie Institution of Washington,* Pub no 102, Part 7, 1908.

3. Wellens HJJ, Conover M: *The ECG in emergency decision making,* Philadelphia, 1992, WB Saunders.

4. Wellens HJJ, Brugada P, Büar F: Diagnosis and treatment of the regular tachycardia with a narrow QRS complex. In Kulbertus HE, editor: *Medical management of cardiac arrhythmias,* Edinburgh, 1986, Churchill Livingstone.

5. Engelstein ED, Stein KM, Markowitz SM, Lerman BB: Posterior fast atrioventricular node pathways: implications for radiofrequency catheter ablation of atrioventricular node reentrant tachycardia, *J Am Coll Cardiol* 27:1098, 1996.

6. Wu D: Dual atrioventricular nodal pathways: a reappraisal, *PACE* 5:72, 1982.

7. Morady F, Strickberger SA, Man KC et al: Reasons for prolonged or failed attempts at radiofrequency catheter ablation of accessory pathways, *J Am Coll Cardiol* 27:683, 1996.

8. Ng KS, Lauer MR, Young C et al: Correlation of P-wave polarity with underlying electrophysiologic mechanisms of long RP' tachycardia, *Am J Cardiol* 77:1129, 1996.

9. Gaita F, Haissaguerre M, Giustetto C et al: Catheter ablation of permanent junctional reciprocating tachycardia with radiofrequency current, *J Am Coll Cardiol* 25:648, 1995.

10. Weindling SN, Saul JP, Walsh EP: Efficacy and risks of medical therapy for supraventricular tachycardia in neonates and infants, *Am Heart J* 131:66, 1996.

11. Gillette PC, Zeigler VL, Case CL: Pediatric arrhythmias: are they different? In Zipes DP, Jalife J, editors: *Cardiac electrophysiology from cell to bedside,* ed 2, Philadelphia, 1995, WB Saunders.

12. Gillette PC, Blair HL, Crawford FA: Preexcitation syndromes. In Gillette PC, Garson A Jr, editors: *Pediatric arrhythmias: electrophysiology and pacing,* Philadelphia, 1990, WB Saunders.

CHAPTER 13

Digitalis Dysrhythmias

Digitalis glycosides 179
Mortality in undiagnosed digitalis toxicity 179
Cellular basis for digitalis dysrhythmias 179
Triggered activity 180
Digitalis and K+ derangements 180
Factors that interact with digoxin 182
Serum digoxin concentration 182
ECG effects of therapeutic digoxin 183
Systematic approach to the ECG 183
Clinical alert to digitalis toxicity 184
ECG recognition of digitalis dysrhythmias 185
Treatment 198

DIGITALIS GLYCOSIDES

Digitalis is derived from the dried leaf of the foxglove plant, *Digitalis purpurea.* Digoxin, the digitalis compound most widely used clinically, is derived from the *Digitalis lanata* plant. Digitoxin, which is metabolized by an enterohepatic route and has a serum half-life of 5 to 6 days, is derived from both of these plants.

Digitalis glycosides are the only group of positive inotropic drugs that persistently increase the ejection fraction during long-term administration in patients with heart failure, thus decreasing their symptoms and increasing their exercise capacity. Although the clinical efficacy of these drugs in the different stages of heart failure remains undefined, recent evidence indicates that their therapeutic benefit is comparable to diuretics and angiotensin converting enzyme (ACE) inhibitors in symptomatic heart failure.[1] Digoxin also increases vagal activity, slowing conduction through the AV node, and is therefore useful in controlling the ventricular response to atrial tachyarrhythmias.

MORTALITY IN UNDIAGNOSED DIGITALIS TOXICITY

In the patients studied by Dreifus and colleagues,[2] 100% (7:7) died when atrial tachycardia with block went unrecognized and digitalis was continued; when digitalis was discontinued, there was a 6% mortality rate (1:16). When junctional tachycardia was not recognized as a digitalis dysrhythmia, 81% died (25:31). When the diagnosis was made and digitalis discontinued, the mortality rate was 16% (7:43).

CELLULAR BASIS FOR DIGITALIS DYSRHYTHMIAS

Digitalis intoxication should be ruled out in any patient with arrhythmias who is taking this drug, especially in patients with a diseased heart. Digitalis concentrations that have no effect on normal Purkinje fibers can enhance arrhythmias in ischemic Purkinje fibers. Digitalis also suppresses phase 4 depolarization in normal pacemaker cells.[3] The time required for the development of toxic changes in the action potential depends on the drug concentration and the heart rate.[4] Studies show that although low levels of digitalis may have little or no effect on the action potential, higher levels can cause the appearance of delayed afterdepolarizations and bursts of triggered activity.[4]

The only known receptor of cardiac glycosides is Na$^+$-K$^+$–ATPase (adenosinetriphosphatase), which is present in the membranes of most cells of higher organisms and directly or indirectly controls many essential cellular functions. Regulation of this enzyme and ion transporter is believed to play a key role in the etiology of some pathologic processes.[5] The following steps lead to the inotropic, vagal, and toxic effects of digitalis on the human heart:

1. Digitalis competes with K^+ for a binding site on the cell membrane, interfering with the sodium pump (Na^+-K^+–ATPase).[3,6]
2. This competition impairs Na^+ efflux and results in an accumulation of intracellular Na^+, which in turn stimulates the Na^+-Ca^{2+} exchanger to work in reverse, bringing Ca^{2+} into the cell.[6]
3. The increase in the Ca^{2+} pool of the sarcoplasmic reticulum causes a net gain in intracellular Ca^{2+} and a positive inotropic effect. After intravenous bolus administration of digoxin, the peak vagal effects on atrioventricular (AV) conduction occur early, and the positive inotropic effects increase progressively for at least 27 minutes with little or no effect on the electrical activity of the heart or its cells.[4,7]
4. Higher dosages (toxic levels) of digoxin lead to spontaneous calcium release from the sarcoplasmic reticulum and high concentrations of free intracellular calcium.[8]
5. The resultant high concentration of intracellular Ca^{2+} stimulates a transient inward Na^+ current—the cause of the tachycardias of digitalis toxicity.

As illustrated by the solid line in Figure 13-1, this transient inward Na^+ current occurs during electrical diastole (after full repolarization), causing a *delayed afterdepolarization.*[3] If the delayed afterdepolarization does not reach threshold potential, it cannot cause ectopic beats or rhythms on the surface electrocardiogram (ECG). Important factors that cause the delayed afterdepolarization to reach threshold potential are K^+ derangements, shortening of the cycle length, and/or increased catecholamines.

TRIGGERED ACTIVITY

The cellular electrical activity that results from afterdepolarizations (early or delayed) is called *triggered activity* or a *triggered rhythm* because it is not automatic. It does not result from normal enhanced automaticity or abnormal automaticity but is dependent on the preceding beat. A triggered beat is illustrated by the dashed line in Figure 13-1.

The triggered rhythm caused by delayed afterdepolarizations is self-perpetuating in that each triggered beat is followed by its own afterdepolarization. This afterdepolarization is guaranteed to reach threshold potential because of the short cycle preceding it and because of the catecholamine production a tachycardia will generally be elicited in the body. The rhythm finally terminates itself when the rapid rate causes an increase of intracellular Na^+. This increase stimulates the Na^+ pump to work faster, which in turn causes the cell to become more negative (hyperpolarization), thus terminating the tachycardia.

DIGITALIS AND K^+ DERANGEMENTS
Hypokalemia

Hypokalemia is an arrhythmogenic mechanism on its own and sets the stage for abnormal automaticity and slow conduction. When digitalis is administered to a patient with hypokalemia, arrhythmogenesis is compounded. This compounding occurs because the binding of digitalis to its K^+ receptor site on the membrane is facilitated by the lack of K^+, which promotes the development of delayed afterdepolarizations and triggered activity.

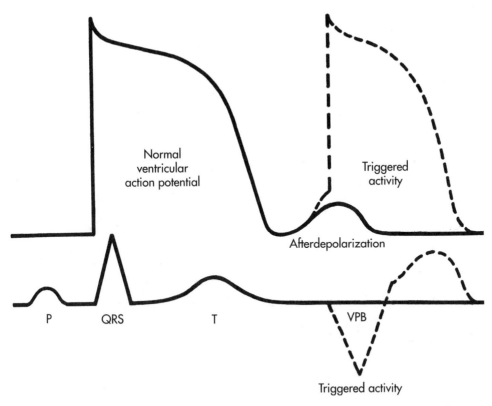

FIGURE 13-1 Myocardial action potential and delayed afterdepolarization as they relate to the surface ECG. Dashed lines represent the sequence of events that result when an afterdepolarization reaches threshold potential. (From Conover M: *Understanding electrocardiography,* ed 7, St Louis, 1996, Mosby.)

Hypokalemia can potentially influence cardiac glycoside sensitivity at multiple levels:
1. It directly increases the affinity of cardiac glycosides for Na^+ pumps by decreasing competition with K^+.
2. It decreases the efficiency of the cardiac Na^+ pump, which may already be compromised secondary to heart failure itself and cardiac glycoside inhibition.
3. It decreases the efficiency of skeletal muscle Na^+ pumps, which influences the relative tissue and plasma distributions of cardiac glycosides.[9]

Hyperkalemia

Because of the competitive relationship between digitalis and K^+ for binding sites on the membrane, the inhibitory effects of digitalis on the Na^+ pump are partially reversed when extracellular K^+ concentration is elevated.[3] However, an elevation in extracellular K^+ to more than approximately 5 mM has the same end result as hypokalemia of less than 3 to 4 mM. Although the extra K^+ in the extracellular compartment reduces the binding of digitalis to the cellular membrane, it also accelerates repolarization and lowers the resting membrane potential, which slows or blocks conduction.[3] Because both hypokalemia and hyperkalemia exacerbate digitalis dysrhythmias, the goal during digitalis therapy is to maintain serum K^+ levels within the physiologic range.[3]

In conditions of extreme digitalis toxicity, digitalis can cause a loss of K^+ from skeletal muscle as it replaces K^+ on the cell. This loss may be sufficient to produce significant hyperkalemia.[4]

FACTORS THAT INTERACT WITH DIGOXIN
Factors That May Require a Decrease in Digoxin Dosage

Factors that require a decrease in dosage of digoxin are renal disease, old age, hypothyroidism, small stature, chronic pulmonary disease, hypokalemia, hypomagnesemia, congestive heart failure, myocardial ischemia, and hypercalcemia.

Quinidine, amiodarone, verapamil, and diltiazem interact with digoxin to cause an increase in serum digoxin.[10,11] Procainamide, disopyramide, mexiletine, flecainide, ethmozine, and nifedipine do not appear to affect digoxin concentration.[12]

Quinidine and verapamil

Digoxin is secreted by P-glycoprotein located on the luminal membrane of renal tubular epithelial cells. Clinically important interactions with quinidine and verapamil are caused by the inhibition of P-glycoprotein.[13] The digoxin-quinidine interaction significantly increases digitalis toxicity, even in the therapeutic range of serum digoxin levels.[14] Therefore if quinidine is added to digoxin therapy, the dose of digoxin should be decreased by approximately 50%.[15]

Amiodarone

In one study there was a mean increase in plasma digoxin concentration of 70% when amiodarone (600 mg/day) was administered along with the digoxin. This result is caused by a decrease in renal and nonrenal clearance of digoxin and by an increase in half-life.[10,15]

Diltiazem

A 22% increase in steady-state plasma digoxin concentration occurs when diltiazem (180 mg/day) is added to digoxin. In two patients, the use of high-dose calcium channel blocker therapy (diltiazem) with digoxin was reported to have potentially serious drug interactions in the treatment of pulmonary hypertension. Even in the approved normal dosages for the treatment of angina and hypertension, calcium channel blockers are known to cause significant changes in the metabolism of other drugs.[16]

Factors That May Require an Increase in Digoxin Dosage

Factors that require an increase in digoxin dosage are malabsorption, antacids, neomycin, cholestyramine, cholestipol, hyperthyroidism, hyperkalemia, reserpine, youth, and hypocalcemia.[17]

SERUM DIGOXIN CONCENTRATION

Although the monitoring of serum levels of digoxin has reduced the incidence of digitalis toxicity, there is considerable overlap of levels between the groups of patients with and without toxicity, and digitalis intoxication remains a significant problem.[18] It is therefore important that serum digoxin levels be used in combination with an ECG evaluation and an informed assessment of the patient's symptoms.

During digitalization, approximately 13% of the skeletal muscle digitalis glycoside receptors are occupied with digoxin. In light of the large skeletal muscle contribution to body mass, the skeletal muscle Na^+-K^+–ATPase pool constitutes a major volume of distribution for digoxin during digitalization.[19] Because it takes many hours for the body stores of digitalis to reach a steady state, the physician should specify that blood be obtained at least 6 hours after the previous dose of digoxin (intravenous or oral). Serum digoxin concentration obtained earlier than this is usually 2 to 4 ng/ml and does not reflect steady-state serum concentration.[20]

After the drug has been distributed to the tissues, a serum level of 2.5 to 3 ng/ml confirms digitalis toxicity; a serum level of 1.5 to 2.5 ng/ml suggests the possibility of digitalis toxicity. Although levels below 1.5 ng/ml suggest that digitalis toxicity is unlikely, the possibility should not be excluded.[21] The positive inotropic effect of digitalis is maximal at concentrations of 1.5 to 2.0 ng/ml.[20] The measurement of serum digoxin levels is indicated particularly when digoxin is being given in combination with drugs that can raise serum digoxin levels (quinidine, verapamil, diltiazem, propafenone, amiodarone), when there is moderate or marked renal insufficiency, and when a rapid ventricular response to atrial fibrillation is not responding to the usual doses of digoxin. Serum digoxin levels may also be useful in the elderly, who have variable dosage requirements and are especially vulnerable to toxicity.[21]

ECG EFFECTS OF THERAPEUTIC DIGOXIN

Scooping of the ST segment and flattening of the T wave are the characteristic therapeutic effects of digoxin on the ECG in leads in which the QRS complex is predominately positive; scooping when the QRS complex is negative indicates toxicity. Prolongation of the PR interval during normal sinus rhythm is not significant unless there is AV nodal disease; neither is the QRS complex changed by digoxin. A slowing of the sinus rate during digoxin administration is usually observed only in patients who have a reduction in sympathetic tone secondary to sinus (sinoatrial [SA]) node dysfunction or congestive heart failure.[20]

SYSTEMATIC APPROACH TO THE ECG

At first glance, the arrhythmias of digitalis toxicity look either extremely basic or very complicated. However, digitalis toxicity arrhythmias are seldom "basic." If a systematic approach is not adhered to, the diagnosis can be missed and lead to catastrophic consequences. Although digitalis toxicity arrhythmias are usually complicated, they are not as complex as they may first seem if a systematic approach is used.

Evaluating the Events in the Atria First

Look for P waves in lead II, determine the rate, and commit to a diagnosis of the atrial condition. If no P waves are seen (atrial fibrillation), evaluate for AV dissociation (regular or group beating) and switch to V_1 to evaluate the shape of the QRS complex.

Monitoring

Informed ECG monitoring is important. Lead II should be used if the patient is in sinus rhythm. It is in this lead that typical atrial tachycardia is first seen. The P′ waves look very similar to sinus P waves and are easily differentiated from P waves from a low atrial origin.

In cases of atrial fibrillation, monitor the patient in V_1 because the shape of the QRS complex is important. In this lead it is easy to distinguish between a junctional rhythm (rS) and a fascicular rhythm (rSR′). Observe also for additional signs of digitalis toxicity such as regularization or group beating.

Evaluating for AV Conduction

If atrial tachycardia is present, assess AV conduction. If there is AV conduction, the diagnosis is determined and that is the end of the ECG assessment. If there is AV dissociation, switch to lead V_1 to determine the origin of the subsidiary pacemaker. It will usually be either junctional escape, accelerated junctional rhythm, junctional tachycardia, or fascicular tachycardia, all of which are determined by the rate and shape of the ventricular complex.

It is important to resist the temptation to evaluate AV conduction first. Once Wenckebach conduction, 2:1 conduction, or AV dissociation is noticed, the events in the atria often go without comment, and a diagnosis of digitalis toxicity is not made. If a diagnosis of atrial tachycardia is made, the patient will probably not receive the incorrect treatment, even if the AV dissociation and accelerated junctional rhythm that are also present are missed. However, there is a widespread tendency to stop the cognitive process and do nothing after diagnosing AV dissociation.

CLINICAL ALERT TO DIGITALIS TOXICITY

Watch for the following signs of digitalis toxicity:
- Neurologic symptoms (headache; malaise; neuralgic pain; pseudodementia such as disorientation, memory lapses, hallucinations, nightmares, restlessness, insomnia, and listlessness).
- Changes in the quality of color vision, especially red and green
- Gastrointestinal symptoms such as anorexia, nausea, and vomiting that are mediated by chemoreceptors in the medulla
  Bradycardia
  Sinus
  SA block
  AV block
- Tachycardia
  Atrial tachycardia with block
  Junctional tachycardia
  Fascicular ventricular tachycardia
- Regularity in atrial fibrillation
  Junctional tachycardia
  AV block with junctional escape
- Group beating in atrial fibrillation
  Junctional tachycardia with Wenckebach exit block

- Group beating in sinus rhythm
  Ventricular bigeminy
  SA Wenckebach
  AV Wenckebach
- Atrial flutter with AV dissociation or high-degree AV block (bradycardia)

ECG RECOGNITION OF DIGITALIS DYSRHYTHMIAS
Sinus Bradycardia and Junctional Tachycardia

Digitalis intoxication causes bradycardia, pacemaker shifts, and conduction disturbances in the SA node. When SA nodes isolated from guinea pig atrial tissue were perfused in vitro with ouabain and digoxin, the SA node was quickly intoxicated by calcium overload. This intoxication caused marked conduction disturbances and fractionation of SA node activity.[22] Figure 13-2 illustrates a threefold effect of digitalis toxicity: sinus bradycardia, junctional tachycardia, and a minor degree of AV block.

SA Block

Digitalis can impair the conduction of the sinus impulse to the atrial tissue, even in therapeutic doses.[23] Such a block can be of the Wenckebach type. SA Wenckebach is recognized by the following:
- Sinus rhythm
- Group beating
- Shortened PP intervals
- Pauses less than twice the shortest PP cycle

The bigeminal rhythm in Figure 13-3 represents 3:2 SA Wenckebach. The possibility of this being atrial bigeminy is excluded because the P waves have identical shapes.

AV Block

Digitalis prolongs the refractory period of AV nodal cells by vagal stimulation and by its direct effect on AV nodal cells. Often it is this precise effect that the clinician is seeking when attempting to slow the ventricular response to a rapid atrial rhythm (paroxysmal supraventricular tachycardia, atrial fibrillation, or atrial flutter). However, the AV node is influenced not only by vagal tone but also by sympathetic tone, which enhances AV conduction. Often the emergency setting of supraventricular tachycardia is associ-

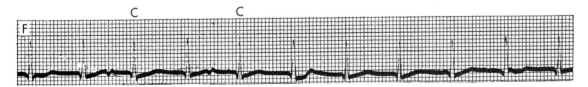

FIGURE 13-2 Sinus bradycardia (rate = 55 beats/min) with some degree of AV block and junctional tachycardia, all a result of digitalis. The third and fifth beats end slightly shorter cycles and are presumably conducted (capture; *C*) with prolonged PR intervals; otherwise the two rhythms are dissociated.

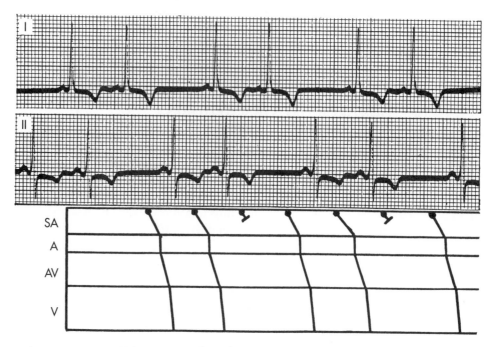

FIGURE 13-3 Sinus rhythm with 3:2 SA Wenckebach.

ated with increased sympathetic tone; digoxin alone is ineffective in slowing the ventricular response.[24] This is also true for the chronic administration of digitalis. In some patients the sympathetic nervous system may override the vagal effect of digitalis during exercise. To achieve control of the ventricular rate during daily activity, it is necessary for these patients to combine digitalis with another drug.

In toxic doses, AV conduction can be compromised enough to cause symptomatic bradycardia, or it may fail completely (third-degree AV block). Figure 13-4 illustrates a profound life-threatening bradycardia caused by high-grade AV block in an acute digitalis overdose (suicide attempt). The top tracing was recorded at admission. The bottom tracing shows conduction improvement with treatment.

Atrial Tachycardia

Atrial tachycardia caused by digitalis toxicity is often associated with AV block, secondary not only to the rapid atrial rate but also to the lengthening of the AV nodal refractory period. The ECG is typical.[12,17,25]

ECG recognition

- **Atrial rate.** Dose-related in the range of 130 to 250 beats/min.
- **AV conduction.** Usually 2:1 but sometimes manifests Wenckebach periods. When digitalis is discontinued, conduction improves before the tachycardia converts to sinus rhythm. Thus there is usually a transient period of 1:1 conduction.

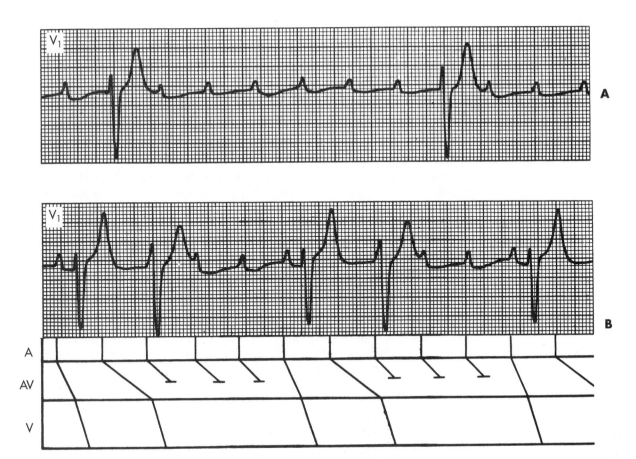

FIGURE 13-4   Profound AV block in a patient with acute digitalis toxicity (attempted suicide). **A,** Conduction ratio is 7:1. **B,** Situation has improved with a conduction ratio of 5:2. (From Conover M: *Cardiac arrhythmias,* St Louis, 1974, Mosby.)

- **Rhythm.** At times (60%) there is ventriculophasic behavior of P′P′ intervals (i.e., the P′P′ interval containing the R wave is shorter than the P′P′ interval without an R wave).[25] In some cases this behavior is so marked that it may resemble bigeminal non-conducted atrial premature beats. The mechanism of ventriculophasic changes in P′P′intervals is the same as that seen in complete heart block. Peak sympathetic activity occurs just before the upstroke of the aortic pressure (shortly after the onset of the QRS complex), which causes the atrial cycle to shorten. Sympathetic activity decreases sharply; vagal tone increases, which causes the next atrial cycle to lengthen.[17]
- **P′ wave shape.** The shape of the P′ waves is identical or almost identical to the sinus P waves.
- **Best lead.** Lead II; in this lead the typical atrial focus of digitalis toxicity produces a positive P′ wave, which can easily be differentiated from low atrial foci.
- **Mortality.** 100%.

Figure 13-5 is a remarkable example of the development, recognition, and treatment of digitalis toxicity more than 40 years ago, published by Mervin J. Goldman, MD, a man ahead of his time.[26]

In Figure 13-5, *C*, the reason for the increase in the atrial rate after the original manifestation of toxicity is that the atrial rate increases in a dose-related fashion. The upright P′ waves in lead aV$_F$ do indeed indicate a high right atrial focus (the usual location for the atrial tachycardia of digitalis toxicity), which produces the positive P′ wave in lead II. *Ventriculophasic P′P′ intervals* are also seen in this lead and are typical of atrial tachycardia with 2:1 conduction.

In Figure 13-5, *D*, a typical scenario develops when the digitalis is discontinued. Conduction improves, which causes the heart rate to increase. At this point there is sometimes confusion and the mistaken belief that digitalis should be started again. However, it is usually only necessary to prescribe bed rest and closely monitor the patient. As long as there is hemodynamic stability and no renal problems, the digitalis is excreted in a timely fashion. The patient finally returns to sinus rhythm 3 days after discontinuing the digitalis.

Figure 13-6 is an example of atrial tachycardia with varying AV block produced by digitalis. Note the upright P′ waves in lead II. The sagging ST segments are characteristic of the digitalis effect.

Figure 13-7 illustrates a case of an accidental overdose of digoxin. The tracing is taken from a 30-year-old woman with postpartum cardiomyopathy who was mistakenly given 2 mg digoxin intravenously with disturbing results: atrial tachycardia with varying block interspersed with ventricular extrasystoles.

Junctional Tachycardia

In the strict sense of the word *tachycardia*, the junctional rhythms resulting from digitalis toxicity must be divided under two groups: (1) accelerated junctional or idiojunctional rhythm when the rate is 60 to 99 beats/min, and (2) junctional tachycardia when the rate is at least 100 beats/min. One is simply a worsening of the other, and both are caused by the same mechanism, with rates that are faster than junctional pacemakers are supposed to beat. Clinically, digitalis overdose has long been considered the most common cause of junctional tachycardia. Other causes are acute myocardial infarction, cardiac surgery, rheumatic fever, chronic obstructive pulmonary disease, and hypokalemia.

During junctional tachycardia, Wenckebach conduction from the junctional pacemaker can occur. The result on the ECG is group beating, an event that may be missed if there is also atrial fibrillation. It is important to recognize the first signs of digitalis toxicity in atrial fibrillation (i.e., regularization of the rhythm or group beating, both of which are junctional rhythms, one with and one without exit block).[27]

ECG recognition

- **Junctional rate.** 70 to 140 beats/min; increases with exercise but rarely exceeds 140 beats/min. Carotid sinus massage has no effect, or there may be nodoventricular block.
- **Retrograde conduction.** Conduction from the junctional focus to the atria is usually absent because of the AV block created by the digitalis; therefore AV dissociation is usually present.

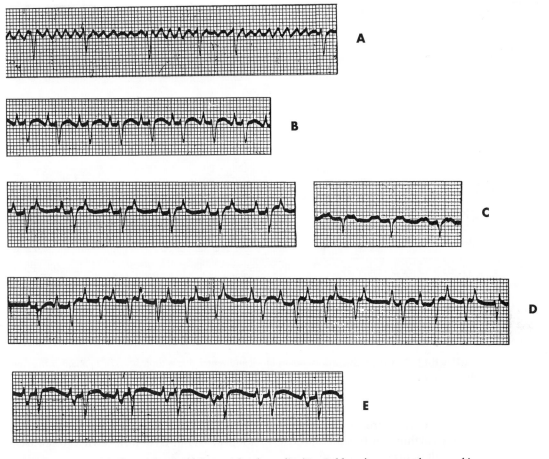

FIGURE 13-5 Digitalis toxicity producing atrial tachycardia. (Dr. Goldman's exact words are used in the legend. Concepts that either are more known about or have changed since 1964 are italicized and discussed in the text.) **A,** 2/6/53: Atrial fibrillation. The patient is receiving digitalis. **B,** 2/12/53 AM: An atrial tachycardia with 1:1 conduction has appeared; the rate is 160. This sudden appearance of an atrial tachycardia during digitalis therapy for atrial fibrillation should always make one suspicious of digitalis intoxication. *This was not appreciated, and more digitalis was given.* **C,** 2/12/53 PM: Four hours after the last dose of digitalis. The extra digitalis has increased the AV block, producing atrial tachycardia with 2:1 block. *The direct effect of digitalis on atrial conduction has increased the atrial rate to 200 beats/min.* The P′ waves are upright in aV$_F$, *indicating a high atrial ectopic focus.* **D,** 2/13/53: Digitalis has been discontinued and potassium and quinidine therapy begun. The atrial rhythm remains regular at a rate of 177 beats/min, but the ventricular response is irregular. One notices a progressive increase in the PR interval and finally a failure of ventricular response. Thus this is an atrial tachycardia with a Wenckebach type of AV block. **E,** 2/16/53: Further quinidine therapy. The rhythm has been reverted to regular sinus. The sinus P waves are diphasic in contrast to the tall, upright P′ waves of the tachycardia. (From Goldman MJ: *Principles of clinical electrocardiography,* Los Altos, Calif, 1964, Lange Medical Books.)

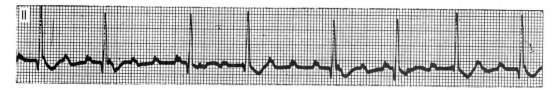

FIGURE 13-6 Atrial tachycardia with variable conduction. Note the upright P′ waves in lead II.

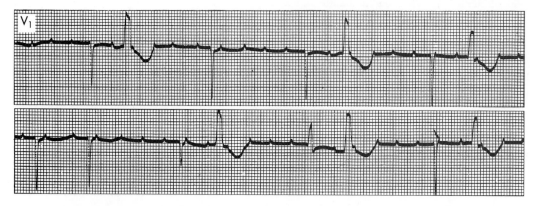

FIGURE 13-7 Atrial tachycardia with 4:1 block and ventricular ectopic beats in a patient with acute digitalis toxicity.

- **Rhythm.** Nonparoxysmal accelerated junctional rhythm (gradual onset); the underlying rhythm may be sinus, atrial fibrillation, atrial flutter, or atrial tachycardia (itself a result of digitalis toxicity).
- **Best lead.** V_1; in this lead junctional tachycardia (rS pattern) can be differentiated from fascicular ventricular tachycardia (VT) (rSR′ pattern).
- **Mortality.** 80%.

Figure 13-8 illustrates a slightly irregular accelerated idiojunctional rhythm with a rate of 88 beats/min. There is isorhythmic AV dissociation (i.e., the sinus rate is approximately the same as the junctional rate). In the bottom strip the sinus rhythm accelerates and conducts to the ventricles. During atrial fibrillation in patients who are taking digitalis, it is important to look for the two ECG signs of digitalis toxicity: regularization of the ventricular rhythm and group beating.

Figure 13-9 illustrates atrial fibrillation with regularization of the ventricular rhythm caused by junctional tachycardia. A regular ventricular rhythm in the presence of atrial fibrillation is a sign of AV dissociation.

Figure 13-10 illustrates a tracing from a 12-year-old girl who required a mitral commissurotomy. After successful surgery her digitalis dosage was not reduced, and signs of intoxication soon developed in the form of the accelerated idiojunctional rhythm seen in this tracing. Note the AV dissociation in the same tracing.

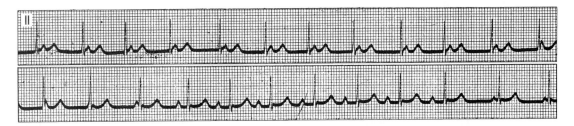

FIGURE 13-8 A slightly irregular accelerated idiojunctional rhythm (88 beats/min) is beating at approximately the same rate as the SA node, resulting in isorhythmic AV dissociation.

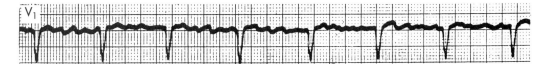

FIGURE 13-9 Atrial fibrillation with a regular ventricular rhythm caused by an accelerated junctional rhythm and digitalis toxicity.

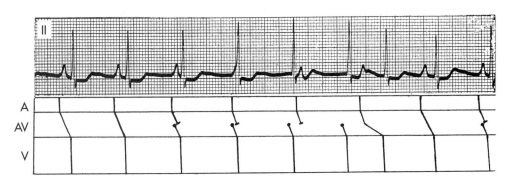

FIGURE 13-10 Accelerated idiojunctional rhythm (rate = 78 beats/min) in digitalis toxicity usurps control from a sinus rhythm (rate = 70 to 75 beats/min). The seventh beat is a ventricular capture conducted with a prolonged PR interval.

Fascicular Ventricular Tachycardia

With digitalis toxicity, ventricular arrhythmias are thought to originate in one of the fascicles of the left bundle branch, producing a pattern that resembles incomplete right bundle branch block (RBBB) with axis deviation.

ECG recognition

- **QRS width.** Narrower than usual (usually approximately 0.12 seconds).
- **QRS pattern.** Right bundle branch block pattern (rSR' in V$_1$), but not the pathologic condition. Competition for the pacing role may exist among the Purkinje fibers, which causes the QRS configuration during the tachycardia to be inconsistent.[17,25,28]
- **QRS axis.** Left or right; a focus in the anterosuperior fascicle produces right axis deviation; a focus in the posteroinferior fascicle produces left axis deviation.
- **Rate.** Usually 90 to 160 beats/min.
- **Mortality.** 100%.

Figure 13-11 illustrates fascicular VT in a patient with atrial fibrillation. Because of the location of the focus in the His-Purkinje system, this VT mimics a supraventricular tachycardia with aberrant ventricular conduction. It has a typically narrow QRS complex of less than 0.14 second, a RBBB pattern, and right axis deviation, indicating an origin in the anterior fascicle of the left bundle branch. Patients with this degree of digitalis intoxication are usually symptomatic and require digitalis-specific Fab fragments (Digibind). Note the digitalis effect of a scooped down ST segment.

Figure 13-12, *A*, illustrates atrial fibrillation and fascicular VT. The fibrillatory line is evident, and the regular rhythm with the RBBB pattern leads to the diagnosis. Figure 13-12, *B*, is taken from a patient who was being relentlessly nudged toward his death by repeated intravenous doses of digoxin. Hypokalemia and/or hypomagnesemia may also have been factors. Fascicular VT is present (note the RBBB pattern). When the cycle lengthens in the bottom strip, VT resembling torsades de pointes follows. Torsades de pointes is associated with a long QT interval and is precipitated by a lengthening of the cycle (short-long-short), which exacerbates the already long QT interval.

The profound and progressive effects of acute digitalis intoxication can be seen in Figure 13-13, which was taken from a 50-year-old woman with acute inferior infarction and in whom sinus tachycardia developed at a rate of 130 beats/min. She was given 0.75 mg of digoxin intravenously, and the dose was repeated 1 hour later. During the subsequent several hours many manifestations of digitalis intoxication appeared, including severe vomiting and the cardiotoxic effects shown.

Bifascicular Ventricular Tachycardia

Bifascicular VT is a life-threatening form of ventricular tachycardia and is a manifestation of severe digitalis intoxication. The two fascicles of the left bundle branch alternate pacing the ventricles, resulting in a unique ECG pattern.

FIGURE 13-11 Fascicular ventricular tachycardia resulting from digitalis toxicity. Note the relatively narrow QRS complex of 0.12 second, the right bundle branch block pattern, and the axis deviation. (Courtesy Hein JJ Wellens, MD, The Netherlands).

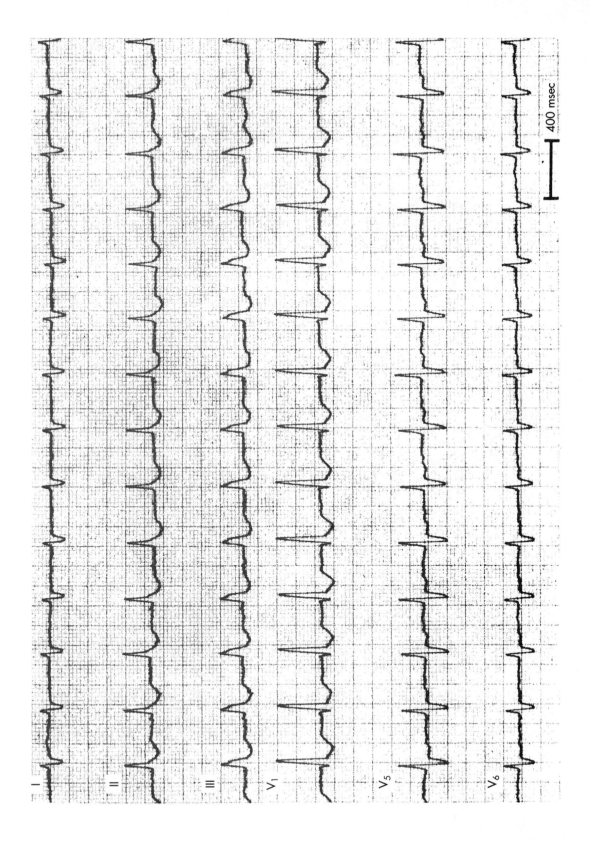

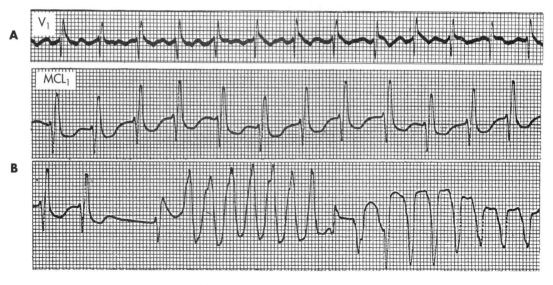

FIGURE 13-12 A, Atrial fibrillation with fascicular ventricular tachycardia (140 beats/min). Note the QRS complex of 0.10 second and the right bundle branch pattern. **B,** The strips are continuous. Atrial fibrillation with fascicular ventricular tachycardia (125 beats/min) suddenly terminates and gives way to a polymorphous ventricular tachycardia.

ECG recognition

- **QRS width.** Narrower than usual (usually about 0.12 second).
- **QRS pattern.** RBBB pattern, but not the pathologic condition (rSR′ in V_1). There is QRS alternans in V_1 caused by the alternating axes (right and left).
- **QRS axis.** Alternating right and left.
- **Rate.** Usually 90 to 160 beats/min.
- **Mortality.** 100%.

Figure 13-14 illustrates the characteristic digitalis-induced bidirectional VT with a relatively narrow QRS complex with RBBB configuration and alternating right and left axis deviation. The QRS alternans is the result of the axis swings.

Double Tachycardia

Digitalis toxicity is the most common cause of "double tachycardia," or the simultaneous existence of two rapidly firing but independent foci. Figure 13-15 illustrates simultaneous atrial and junctional tachycardia. The slight irregularity of the ventricular rhythm is the result of occasional ventricular capture, which in this figure occurs in pairs. The captured beats are identified because of the slightly shorter cycle length. However, capture is not the only explanation for slight irregularities in digitalis toxicity tachycardias. It is not uncommon to find a slight irregularity as neighboring His-Purkinje fibers compete for dominance. The pattern of the shortened cycles is so consistent in this tracing that there is little doubt that AV conduction has occurred.

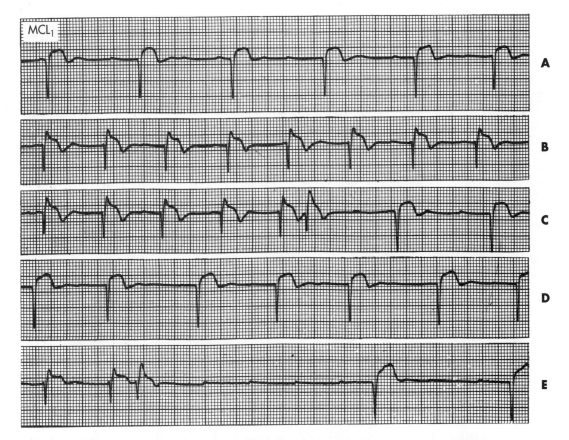

FIGURE 13-13 Strips are not continuous but were selected during several hours of severe digitalis intoxication in a patient with acute inferior infarction who received 1.5 mg of digoxin intravenously in 1 hour. **A,** Sinus tachycardia (rate = 135 beats/min) with significant AV block and junctional escape rhythm (rate = 50 beats/min). **B,** The incomplete right bundle branch block pattern is rate dependent. **C,** Cessation of fascicular rhythm after two closely linked beats; junctional escape rhythm follows. **D,** AV Wenckebach period with junctional escape rhythm. **E,** When the fascicular rhythm fails again, so does the junctional escape rhythm. There is now complete heart block.

Ventricular Bigeminy

Ventricular extrasystoles are the most common cardiac manifestation of digitalis overdosage in adults. Supraventricular ectopics are more common in children. However, ventricular arrhythmias are in no sense diagnostic of digitalis intoxication. They are common in both health and disease of any type, with ventricular bigeminy most commonly seen in patients with coronary artery disease.[17] Furthermore, digitalis is often effective in reducing or eliminating ventricular extrasystoles not caused by the drug. Ventricular bigeminy has long been regarded as a common manifestation of digitalis toxicity. Because Purkinje fibers compete for the pacing role, the ventricular ectopic beats often have different configurations, even though the coupling interval is fixed.

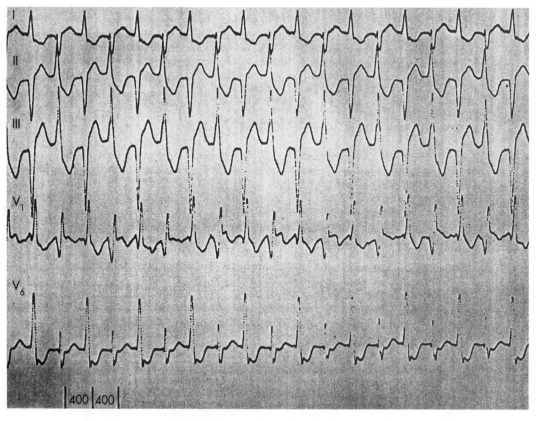

FIGURE 13-14 Bifascicular ventricular tachycardia typically caused by digitalis toxicity. Note its characteristic features. Leads I and II: alternating left and right axis. Lead V_1: RBBB pattern with a QRS duration of approximately 0.12 second. The QRS alternans is the result of the alternating axis. (Courtesy Hein JJ Wellens, MD, The Netherlands.)

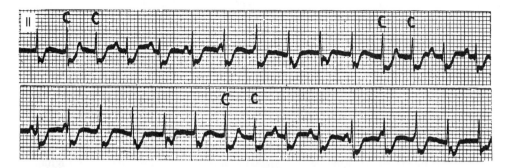

FIGURE 13-15 A double tachycardia seen in a continuous tracing. There is simultaneous but independent atrial tachycardia (172 beats/min) and junctional tachycardia (154 beats/min) in a patient taking digitalis.

Figure 13-16 is an example of a bigeminal rhythm in a case of accidental digitalis overdose. Following mitral valve surgery, a 10-year-old boy was mistakenly maintained on a double dose of digitalis. He developed an accelerated idioventricular rhythm that was dissociated from his sinus rhythm; ventricular bigeminy was also present. Four days later, after discontinuing the digitalis, he reverted to sinus rhythm. As in most cases of advanced digitalis toxicity, the rhythm is complicated. Apart from the obvious ventricular bigeminy, note that the PR intervals become progressively shorter as an accelerated idioventricular rhythm with its bigeminal partner takes over.

Concealed Ventricular Bigeminy

Sometimes the bigeminy caused by digitalis is intermittently concealed; bigeminal runs may be seen, and all interectopic intervals contain only odd numbers of sinus beats.[29] Figure 13-17 is an example of concealed ventricular bigeminy in which two runs of bigeminy are seen and the number of sinus beats intervening between consecutive ectopic beats is always an odd number.

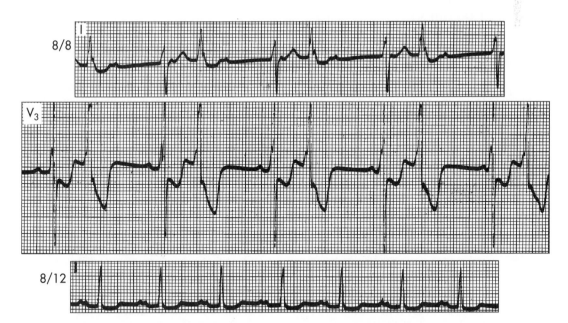

FIGURE 13-16 AV block, accelerated idioventricular rhythm, ventricular bigeminy. ECG is taken from a 10-year-old boy who was mistakenly maintained on a double dose of digitalis after mitral valve surgery. On 8/8 he developed an accelerated idioventricular rhythm (rate = 64 beats/min) with ventricular bigeminy dissociated from his sinus rhythm (rate = 90 beats/min). There is also some degree of AV block; the P waves in the T waves in lead I should be conducted but are not. Digitalis was discontinued, and 4 days later he reverted to sinus rhythm (rate = 80 beats/min) with residual first-degree AV block. Note the P-mitrale in lead I.

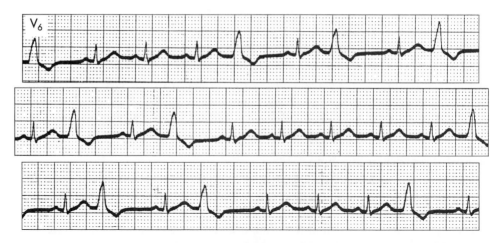

FIGURE 13-17 Concealed ventricular bigeminy. A short sample of a much longer strip in which the number of sinus beats intervening between consecutive ectopics is always an odd number. The tendency for bigeminy is apparent in this sample, in which the intervening sinus beats consecutively number 3,1,1,1,1,5,1,1,3.

TREATMENT
Early Stages

When early signs of digitalis excess are noted it may be sufficient to temporarily withdraw the drug until the patient is stabilized.[23] A more aggressive management is needed when the arrhythmias become more obtrusive and/or the patient manifests symptoms. In addition to discontinuing the drug, bed rest is important because sympathetic stimulation aggravates the condition. Electrolyte abnormalities are corrected. Ventricular pacing is indicated in cases of symptomatic bradycardia. The condition becomes life-threatening if hemodynamic instability develops. If phenytoin is used, a pacing wire is in place.

Life-Threatening Digitalis Toxicity

The clinical findings that indicate the necessity for digoxin-specific antibody Fab fragments (Digibind) after massive digitalis ingestion include hemodynamic instability, hyperkalemia, AV block, and malignant ventricular tachyarrhythmias. Reasons for partial responses and nonresponses have been identified as a misdiagnosis of digitalis toxicity, a dose of Fab fragments that is too low, and treatment of moribund patients.[30]

Digibind is a highly purified antidigoxin Fab fragment that is purified from the immunoglobulin G produced in sheep; it has become standard therapy for life-threatening digitalis toxicity.[18] Fragmentation of the antibody reduces immunogenicity and nonspecific effects of the antibody and enhances distribution and elimination.[18] The first clinical report of treatment of advanced digoxin toxicity with Fab fragments was published in 1976.[31]

Fab fragments have a stronger digoxin-binding affinity than do biologic membranes and can sequester tissue-bound and intracellular digoxin in the extracellular spaces, resulting in a rapid increase in digoxin serum concentrations in the central compartment. Because the majority of digoxin is bound by Fab, it cannot interact with its biologic receptor, and digoxin toxicity is reversed.

After the administration of digoxin-specific Fab, free digoxin concentrations fall rapidly, rebound upward within 12 to 24 hours, and decline again depending on the renal and nonrenal routes of elimination. During this time period, Fab retains its capability of binding digoxin while residing in plasma. There is no evidence to support a dissociation of the Fab-digoxin complex over extended periods of time as a cause of the rebound; it has been suggested that distribution from the vascular spaces is the likely cause.[32]

Fab fragments in renal failure

In patients with renal impairment and end-stage renal disease, the elimination half-life for the digoxin-Fab complex is prolonged up to tenfold, and the rebound of free digoxin is delayed by 12 to 130 hours, increasing the risk of recurrence of toxicity and necessitating prolonged clinical monitoring.[33] The high molecular weight of digoxin and digoxin-Fab complex prevents its elimination by hemodialysis or continuous arteriovenous hemofiltration.[34] Monitoring free digoxin following the administration of Fab fragments may be of value in selected patients to guide additional Fab fragment dosing, confirm possible rebound toxicity, or guide the reinitiation of digoxin therapy.[35]

Fab fragments in oleander poisoning

Digoxin-specific FAB antibody fragments are also successful in reversing life-threatening oleander poisoning.[36] Oleander *(Nerium oleander)* is an ornamental plant whose toxicity to humans results from a mixture of nondigitalis cardiac glycosides. The clinical manifestations of oleander poisoning combine cardiac and gastrointestinal symptoms and are similar to those of a digitalis overdose. Clinicians must include oleander poisoning in the differential diagnosis of bradyarrhythmias, particularly in children and young people without known cardiovascular disease and in areas in which this plant is either used as a herbal medicine or known as poisonous.[37] Curiously enough, in a case of intentional overdose with homemade foxglove extract, Fab therapy resulted in a temporary improvement but not a shortened clinical course as would be expected in the setting of commercial glycoside product poisoning.[38]

SUMMARY

In the SA node, digitalis intoxication causes marked conduction disturbances because of calcium overload and leads to the fractionation of SA node activity. Digitalis also causes AV block because of its vagomimetic effect and abnormal impulse formation, particularly in the high right atrium, AV node–His bundle region, and fascicles of the left bundle. The tachycardias are often typical and are caused by delayed afterdepolarizations that precipitate triggered activity. The clinician can usually make a correct diagnosis using a combination of knowledge about the patient's symptoms and digoxin levels and an informed evaluation of the ECG. Any new arrhythmia or any change from one type of arrhythmia to another in patients who are taking digitalis should be suspected of being digitalis-induced. The challenge lies in a systematic approach to the ECG and an informed response when toxicity is discovered.

REFERENCES

1. Erdmann E: Digitalis—friend or foe? *Eur Heart J Suppl* F:16, 1995.
2. Dreifus LS et al: Digitalis intolerance, *Geriatrics* 18:494, 1963.
3. Rosen MR: Cellular electrophysiology of digitalis toxicity, *J Am Coll Cardiol* 5:22A, 1985.
4. Cranefield PF, Aronson RS: *Cardiac arrhythmias: the role of triggered activity and other mechanisms,* Mount Kisco, NY, 1988, Futura.
5. Rose AM, Valdes R Jr: Understanding the sodium pump and its relevance to disease, *Clin Chem* 40:1674, 1994.
6. Katz AM: Effects of digitalis on cell biochemistry: sodium pump inhibition, *J Am Coll Cardiol* 5:16A, 1985.
7. Powell AC, Horowitz JD, Hasin Y et al: Acute myocardial uptake of digoxin in humans: correlation with hemodynamic and electrocardiographic effects, *J Am Coll Cardiol* 15:1238, 1990.
8. Charlemagne D: Molecular and cellular level of action of digitalis, *Herz* 18:79, 1993.
9. McDonough AA, Wang J, Farley RA: Significance of sodium pump isoforms in digitalis therapy, *J Mol Cell Cardiol* 27:1001, 1995.
10. Marcus FI: Pharmacokinetic interactions between digoxin and other drugs, *J Am Coll Cardiol* 5:82A, 1985.
11. Eisenman DP, McKegney FP: Delirium at therapeutic serum concentrations of digoxin and quinidine, *Psychosomatics* 35:91, 1994.
12. Wellens HJJ, Conover M: *The ECG in emergency decision making,* Philadelphia, 1991, WB Saunders.
13. Hori R, Okamura N, Aiba T, Tanigawara Y: Role of P-glycoprotein in renal tubular secretion of digoxin in the isolated perfused rat kidney, *J Pharmacol Exp Ther* 266:1620, 1993.
14. Mordel A, Halkin H, Zulty L et al: Quinidine enhances digitalis toxicity at therapeutic serum digoxin levels, *Clin Pharmacol Ther* 53:457. 1993.
15. Freitag D, Bebee R, Sunderland B: Digoxin-quinidine and digoxin-amiodarone interactions: frequency of occurrence and monitoring in Australian repatriation hospitals, *Clin Pharm Ther* 20:179, 1995.
16. Clarke WR, Horn JR, Kawabori I, Gurtel S: Potentially serious drug interactions secondary to high-dose diltiazem used in the treatment of pulmonary hypertension, *Pharmacotherapy* 13:402, 1993.
17. Vanagt EJ, Wellens HJJ: The electrocardiogram in digitalis intoxication. In Wellens HJJ, Kulbertus HE, editors: *What's new in electrocardiography,* The Hague, 1981, Martinus Nijhoff.
18. Azrin MA: The use of antibodies in clinical cardiology, *Am Heart J* 124:753, 1992.
19. Schmidt TA, Holm-Nielsen P, Kjeldsen K: Human skeletal muscle digitalis glycoside receptors (Na, K-ATPase): importance during digitalization, *Cardiovasc Drugs Ther* 7:175, 1973.
20. Johnson JH, Jadonath RL, Marchlinski FE: Digoxin. In Podrid PJ, Kowey PR, editors: *Cardiac arrhythmia mechanisms, diagnosis, and management,* Baltimore, 1995, Williams & Wilkins.
21. Marcus FI: Use and toxicity of digitalis, *Heart Dis Stroke* Jan/Feb:27, 1992.
22. Gonzalez MD, Vassalle M: Role of oscillatory potential and pacemaker shifts in digitalis intoxication of the sinoatrial node, *Circulation* 87:1705, 1993.
23. Smith TW, Braunwald E, Kelly RA: The management of heart failure. In Braunwald E, editor: *Heart disease,* ed 4, Philadelphia, 1995, WB Saunders.
24. Ewy GA: Urgent parenteral digoxin therapy: a requiem, *J Am Coll Cardiol* 15:1248, 1990.
25. Wellens HJJ: The electrocardiogram in digitalis intoxication. In Yu PN, Goodwin JF, editors: *Progress in cardiology,* Philadelphia, 1976, Lea & Febiger.
26. Goldman MJ: *Principles of clinical electrocardiography,* Los Altos, Calif, 1964, Lange Medical Books.

27. Zipes DP: Specific arrhythmias: diagnosis and treatment. In Braunwald E, editor: *Heart disease,* ed 4, Philadelphia, 1992.

28. Wellens HJJ: The electrocardiogram 80 years after Einthoven, *J Am Coll Cardiol* 7:484, 1986.

29. Schamroth L, Marriott HJL: Concealed ventricular extrasystoles, *Circulation* 27:1043, 1963.

30. Antman EM, Wenger TL, Butler VP et al: Treatment of 150 cases of life-threatening digitalis intoxication with digoxin-specific Fab antibody fragments: final report of a multicenter study, *Circulation* 81:1744, 1990.

31. Smith TW, Haber E, Yeatman L, Butler VP Jr: Reversal of advanced digoxin intoxication with Fab fragments of digoxin-specific antibodies, *N Engl J Med* 294:797, 1976.

32. Ujhelyi MR, Robert S: Pharmacokinetic aspects of digoxin-specific Fab therapy in the management of digitalis toxicity, *Clin Pharmacokinet* 28:483, 1995.

33. Ujhelyi MR, Robert S, Cummings DM et al: Disposition of digoxin immune Fab in patients with kidney failure, *Clin Pharmacol Ther* 54:388, 1993.

34. Berkovitch M, Akilesh MR, Gerace R et al: Acute digoxin overdose in a newborn with renal failure: use of digoxin immune Fab and peritoneal dialysis, *Ther Drug Monit* 16:531, 1994.

35. Ujhelyi MR, Robert S, Cummings DM et al: Influence of digoxin immune Fab therapy and renal dysfunction on the disposition of total and free digoxin, *Ann Intern Med* 119:273, 1993.

36. Safadi R, Levy I, Amitai Y, Caraco Y: Beneficial effect of digoxin-specific Fab antibody fragments in oleander intoxication, *Arch Intern Med* 155:2121, 1995.

37. Nishioka S de A, Resende ES: Transitory complete atrioventricular block associated with ingestion of Nerium oleander, *Rev Assoc Med Bras* 41:60, 1995.

38. Rich SA, Libera JM, Locke RJ: Treatment of foxglove extract poisoning with digoxin-specific Fab fragments, *Ann Emerg Med* 22:1904, 1993.

CHAPTER 14

Exacerbation of Arrhythmias by Antiarrhythmic Drugs

History of awareness of
proarrhythmia in the
postinfarction period 204
Clinical manifestations 205
Predictors of arrhythmia
aggravation 205
Drugs that are
proarrhythmic 206
Mechanisms 206
The membrane chan-
nel 207
Fast sodium channel
blockade by local
anesthetic antiarrhyth-
mics 208
Abnormal conduction 210

V ENTRICULAR ARRHYTHMIA IS OBSERVED IN 5% TO 10% OF ALL PATIENTS RECEIVING quinidine and other class Ia antiarrhythmic agents for the treatment of cardiac arrhythmias. Approximately half of the patients who develop torsades de pointes while taking quinidine have quinidine plasma concentrations less than 1 μg/ml, and most of them have serum potassium concentrations below 4 mEq/L.[1]

The induction of unexpected and sometimes fatal reactions to cardiac or noncardiac drugs at therapeutic or subtherapeutic levels has been a cause for great concern ever since Selzer and Wray published the first description of "quinidine syncope" occurring concomitantly with low blood levels of this drug.[2] It is now known that the paroxysmal ventricular fibrillation described by these authors was in fact torsades de pointes (i.e., the polymorphous ventricular tachycardia [VT] associated with a long QT interval) (see Chapter 18). Arrhythmogenesis can be an unwanted side effect of any antiarrhythmic drug and is commonly referred to as *proarrhythmia*, the dichotomy that exists between arrhythmia suppression and patient mortality.[3]

Not included under the classification of proarrhythmic drugs are those that are given inappropriately or in excess (overdosage). For example, when verapamil is given for atrial fibrillation with conduction down an accessory pathway or for VT in a diseased heart, the resultant ventricular fibrillation would not be unexpected.[4] The ventricular fibrillation would not be a proarrhythmic response but rather mismanagement and culpable practice. Such a case is illustrated in Figure 14-1, a tracing that was originally published under the title "Proarrhythmic Responses."

Antiarrhythmic drugs act by binding to specific sites on the cell membrane. For example, fast sodium channels are blocked by class I drugs, slow calcium channels are blocked by verapamil, and potassium channels are blocked by class Ia and class III drugs. Potassium channels are modified by drugs such as quinidine; the electrophysiologic function of the heart is changed by β-adrenergic blockers; digitalis binds to the membrane in place of the potassium in the enzyme Na$^+$-K$^+$–ATPase (adenosinetriphosphatase); and vagal input to the heart is enhanced either directly by digitalis, which increases acetylcholine release, or indirectly by edrophonium, which inhibits acetylcholinesterase and thus reduces the breakdown of acetylcholine. These actions may be both antiarrhythmic and proarrhythmic. The risk of aggravating arrhythmias is lowest for amiodarone and is probably related to the complex electrophysiologic profile of this drug. The incidence of

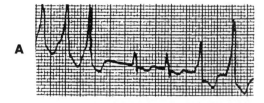
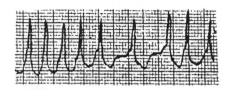

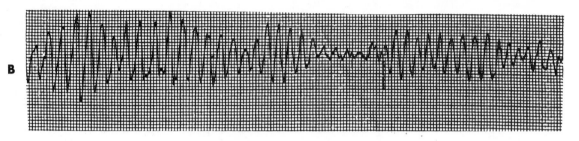

FIGURE 14-1 A, Atrial fibrillation with conduction over an accessory pathway. **B,** Ventricular fibrillation 5 minutes after the administration of verapamil. This result cannot be classified as proarrhythmic because the verapamil should not have been given in the first place; the acceleration of the rate and development of ventricular fibrillation is not unexpected. (From Falk RH: Atrial fibrillation. In Podrid PJ, Kowey PR, editors: *Cardiac arrhythmia mechanisms, diagnosis, and management,* Baltimore, 1995, Williams & Wilkins.)

torsades de pointes with sotalol increases with dose and the baseline values of the QT interval. The fact that D-sotalol increases mortality in postinfarction patients suggests that it may possibly be a common property of most, if not all, pure class III compounds.[5] Indeed, it seems that the patients at greatest risk for developing life-threatening arrhythmias are those most at risk for the proarrhythmic effects of antiarrhythmics.

There is a high incidence of ventricular arrhythmia and sudden death in patients with heart failure. Unfortunately, currently available antiarrhythmic agents have only limited efficacy and may result in proarrhythmia and hemodynamic deterioration in these patients. However, it has been demonstrated that intravenous magnesium chloride reduces the frequency of ventricular arrhythmias in patients with symptomatic heart failure.[6]

HISTORY OF AWARENESS OF PROARRHYTHMIA IN THE POSTINFARCTION PERIOD

More than 30 years ago class I antiarrhythmic drugs were first used in an attempt to reduce mortality rates in survivors of myocardial infarction. It was not until 1988 that this concept was tested in the Cardiac Arrhythmia Suppression Trial (CAST), with stunning results.[7,8] After a 10-month average follow-up, the study was prematurely terminated by the safety committee because in the encainide and flecainide treatment groups there was a significant increase in the incidence of lethal arrhythmias and nonfatal cardiac arrests. The study was continued with the moricizine-placebo component (CAST-

II) and was also discontinued because of an increased incidence of cardiac arrests during the first 2 weeks of moricizine therapy.[9]

CLINICAL MANIFESTATIONS

- Lightheadedness
- Syncopal episodes
- Hemodynamic deterioration
- Cardiac arrest or death

PREDICTORS OF ARRHYTHMIA AGGRAVATION

Although drug toxicity is the cause of many arrhythmias (e.g., digitalis dysrhythmias and torsades de pointes), proarrhythmia does not necessarily occur because of toxicity or because blood levels of the drug are too high; it may simply be a result of the known therapeutic action of the drug on borderline arrhythmogenic foci. Arrhythmias caused by digitalis and by drugs that lengthen the QT interval can be anticipated because of their obvious effects on the surface ECG and, in the case of digitalis, typical physical symptoms. The arrhythmias that are difficult to identify as drug-related are those that result from a change in vulnerable period and conduction velocity.

Patients with a history of a sustained ventricular arrhythmia, especially when left ventricular dysfunction is present, are at high risk for the development or aggravation of arrhythmia. In one retrospective case-controlled study, patients who presented with either sustained ventricular tachycardia or ventricular fibrillation were 3.4 times more likely to have arrhythmia aggravation as compared with patients presenting with nonsustained ventricular tachycardia or ventricular premature beats.[10] Patients with a left ventricular ejection fraction less than 35% were 2.2 times more likely to develop this drug complication as compared with patients with an ejection fraction greater than 35%. There was no association between other clinical parameters and the aggravation of arrhythmias. That is, in this study electrocardiographic intervals, ventricular arrhythmia density, drug dose, and drug levels did not aggravate arrhythmias. In addition, an aggravated response to one drug did not predict its occurrence with another drug of the same class.

Other predictors of proarrhythmia include the following:

- Organic heart disease (class Ic drugs, encainide or flecainide)
- The combination of atrial fibrillation, organic heart disease, and a decreased left ventricular ejection fraction
- VT vs benign premature ventricular contractions (PVCs) (incidence 11% vs 2%)
- Supraventricular tachycardia (SVT) or ventricular fibrillation treated with encainide or flecainide
- Prolonged QT interval before treatment
- Prolonged QT interval during treatment associated with hypokalemia, hypomagnesemia, postectopic pauses, or bradycardia
- Increased amplitude or altered polarity of U waves
- Prolonged QT interval in patients with prior myocardial infarction (risk of sudden death increases 2.16 times); appears to be multifactorial (autonomic nervous system, abnormal electrophysiology, mechanical changes)[3]
- Atrial arrhythmia

DRUGS THAT ARE PROARRHYTHMIC

Most of the drugs that have been reported to cause arrhythmias produce either QT prolongation or an increase in adrenergic tone. These cardiac drugs include the following antiarrhythmics:

- **Class Ia agents.** Quinidine, procainamide, disopyramide; primarily block sodium channels
- **Class Ib agents.** Mexiletine, tocainide, aprindine; moderately proarrhythmic when used to treat benign or potentially lethal ventricular arrhythmias
- **Class Ic agents.** Flecainide, encainide, propafenone, moricizine; very effective antiarrhythmic agents with high proarrhythmic effects, especially when there is decreased left ventricular function or lethal ventricular arrhythmias
- **Class III agents.** Amiodarone, sotalol; primarily block potassium channels
- **Coronary vasodilators.** Prenylamine, lidoflazine, bepridil
- **Inotropics.** Amrinone, milrinone, dobutamine, digitalis

The list of noncardiac drugs that cause arrhythmias is not well defined; reports are based on single cases. These drugs include some antimicrobial, psychotropic, peripheral vasodilator, and antihistamine medications.[3]

MECHANISMS

The proarrhythmic action of class I antiarrhythmic drugs results from the combination of drug-induced and ischemia-induced slow conduction and from a prolonged refractory period.

Slow Conduction

Antiarrhythmic drugs may further depress conduction and disarm troublesome tissue. By the same mechanism they may also change slightly depressed cells into active foci for abnormal automaticity or reentry circuits and thus be proarrhythmic.

Class I drugs increase the incidence of VT and ventricular fibrillation because they slow conduction through injured myocardium but do not produce overt conduction block or inexcitability. Figure 14-2 provides an example of the exacerbation of nonsustained VT. When procainamide was taken orally the VT was sustained for a longer period.

One of the mechanisms that classifies class I drugs as antiarrhythmic is their ability to slow conduction, which causes two-way block in depressed fibers and eliminates the possibility of reentry. However, by the same mechanism these drugs, especially class Ic drugs with their lack of selectivity for ischemic tissue, can change a minimally depressed fiber that is adjacent to the myocardial injury and causing no trouble into a markedly depressed fiber that is capable of supporting a reentry circuit and facilitating lethal arrhythmias.[11]

Prolonged Refractory Period

Class Ia agents, quinidine being the prototype, are also antiarrhythmic because they lengthen the refractory period either by blocking I_K currents that mediate repolarization or by producing postrepolarization refractoriness.[12,13] This action may elicit tachycardia by afterdepolarizations or by reentry. When the relative refractory period is prolonged, conduction can be slowed at shorter cycle lengths, facilitating the induction and perpetuation of reentry (the "leading circle" and reflection; see Chapter 5).[1]

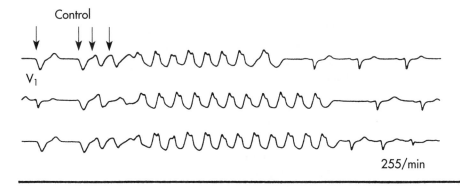

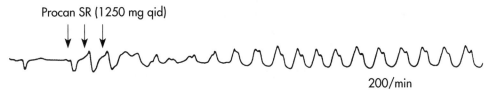

FIGURE 14-2 Conversion of inducible nonsustained ventricular tachycardia to inducible ventricular tachycardia sustained at a slower rate by procainamide. Before administration of procainamide, repeated attempts to induce tachycardia with ventricular pacing and two extrasystoles *(arrows)* resulted in nonsustained ventricular tachycardia at a slower rate (200 beats/min). (From Patterson E, Szabo B, Scherlag BJ, Lazzara R: Arrhythmogenic effects of antiarrhythmic drugs. In Zipes DP, Jalife J, editors: *Cardiac electrophysiology from cell to bedside,* ed 2, Philadelphia, 1995, WB Saunders.)

Starmer, Romashko, and Reddy et al[14] have suggested that reduction of the I_K repolarizing currents is directly coupled with a proarrhythmic property: destabilizing the spiral core of a stationary reentrant wave front, causing it to become unstable and to drift and resulting in a polymorphic process (torsades de pointes). The wave front fragments may annihilate one another, producing a nonsustained tachycardia, or multiple wavelets may arise (spirals), causing fibrillation and sudden cardiac death.

Roden and Hoffman[15] have demonstrated that relatively low concentrations of quinidine elicit early afterdepolarizations when associated with a low extracellular potassium concentration and long cycle lengths. Others have shown that when potassium ion channels are blocked by cesium, prolonged repolarization is associated with early afterdepolarizations of Purkinje fibers during phase 2 and phase 3, tachycardia-dependent delayed afterdepolarizations, and oscillations of 5 to 10 mV during phase 4.[1]

THE MEMBRANE CHANNEL

Membrane channels can be thought of as specialized protein pores that provide a transmural pathway through the lipid bilayer of the cell membrane.[16] Water-soluble ions cannot easily pass through the bilayer without these special aqueous pathways.

A *selectivity filter* lies near the outside of the pore, and gates lie toward the inside; the binding site for local anesthetic drugs is found between these two structures. A diagrammatic representation of the membrane channel and its structures is illustrated in Figure 14-3. The selectivity filter permits ions to pass according to their size, shape, and charge; the fast sodium channel admits mainly Na$^+$ and some H$^+$.

As discussed in Chapter 2, the gates guarding the membrane channels are designated *m* and *h,* which open and close in response to voltage and time, admitting or blocking the entrance of Na$^+$:

- **Closed state.** The excitable (resting) phase of the cell is electrical diastole, during which time the m gate is closed and the h gate is open; the channel is closed.
- **Open state.** The m gate is the activation gate; the channel is in the open state when the m gate opens, which occurs when the membrane voltage reaches threshold potential. At this time there are strong Na$^+$ concentration gradients and electrical gradients that rapidly draw Na$^+$ into the cell (phase 0 of the action potential).
- **Inactivated state.** The voltage-dependent h gate closes when the cell becomes positive on the inside. The channel is inactivated and cannot respond to a stimulus until negative voltage is restored.

FAST SODIUM CHANNEL BLOCKADE BY LOCAL ANESTHETIC ANTIARRHYTHMICS

Local anesthetic drugs block the fast sodium channels; their antiarrhythmic effect is attributed to this action. Clinically useful agents do not usually block resting channels but have a preference for the activated and/or inactivated state. If this were not the case, the drug would be arrhythmogenic because it would cause conduction block in nor-

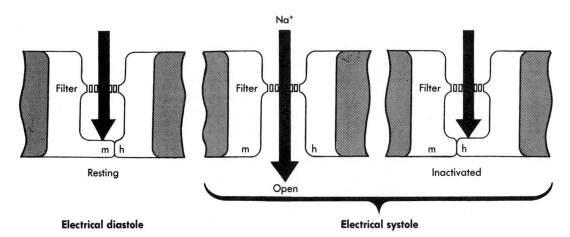

FIGURE 14-3 States of the fast sodium channel during different phases of the action potential. The resting state is seen during phase 4 of the action potential and constitutes electrical diastole. Both the open state and the inactivated state occur during electrical systole; the open state occurs during phase 0, and the inactivated state occurs during phase 2 and part of phase 3. The selectivity filter determines the size and shape of molecule that will be admitted; the m and h gates open and close in response to voltage and time. (Modified from Rosen MR, Wit AL: Arrhythmogenic actions of antiarrhythmic drugs, *Am J Cardiol* 59[11]:10E, 1987.)

mal tissue. For example, quinidine blocks activated (open) channels, amiodarone blocks inactivated channels, and lidocaine blocks both.[17] This function in turn determines which tissue will be affected relative to action potential duration. A drug that mostly blocks open channels, although strongly voltage dependent, is not affected by action potential duration because its only entry into the channel occurs during phase 0. On the other hand, a drug that blocks inactivated channels exerts its effect for a longer time (during the plateau of the action potential). Therefore this drug would have more effect on Purkinje fibers, in which the action potential duration is longest, than on atrial tissue, in which the action potential duration is shortest.

In addition to these considerations, the effectiveness of channel blockade depends on (1) whether the plasma molecule of the drug is uncharged or ionized, (2) the membrane potential, (3) whether there is acidosis, and (4) the molecular weight and shape of the drug.

Given a physiologic pH, drugs exist in the extracellular space in both the nonionized and ionized forms. Within the membrane sodium channel between the selectivity filter and the gates is a "locus" where local anesthetic agents bind. However, an anesthetic agent is too big to be admitted through the selectivity filter that guards the membrane sodium channel. Instead it gains access to binding sites in the channel directly through the lipid bilayer of the membrane. The ease with which it does this depends on the lipid solubility of the drug and whether or not it is ionized.

Figure 14-5 illustrates how the local anesthetic drugs gain access to the locus within the channel. In the nonionized form these drugs have high lipid solubility and can traverse the lipid bilayer of the cell membrane and reach binding sites between the selectivity filter and the channel gates from both directions—straight through the lipid bilayer and channel protein and also through the lipid bilayer into the cytosol and through the gates when they are briefly open during phase 0 of the action potential (Figure 14-4, *B*).

On the other hand, an ionized local anesthetic drug does not have the high lipid solubility of the nonionized molecule and must move slowly through the lipid bilayer toward the cytosol, in which it can move freely. Thus the ionized form of the drug reaches its binding site from an intracellular position during electrical systole, when the gates are briefly open (Figure 14-4, *B*); access is closed to the ionized molecule at all other times in the cardiac cycle (Figure 14-4, *A* and *C*). Such a drug would be more effective during tachycardia than during bradycardia because during tachycardia there are more electrical systoles per minute and more opportunities for the drug to "use" the channel and bind at its locus. The terms *frequency-dependent* or *use-dependent* express this fact. That is, drug-induced reduction of channel availability is caused by use of the channels by the ionized molecules. The term *tonic-blocking actions* applies to the uncharged molecules that gain access to their channel-binding sites directly through the lipid bilayer and channel protein, regardless of the position of the gates. Tonic block can occur in both open and inactivated channels.

Some of the variables that influence channel blockade are (1) membrane potential, (2) pH, and (3) molecular weight and structure[16]:

1. Blockage of transmembrane ionic channels is both time- and voltage-dependent. Lidocaine, for example, binds more readily to the channel when the membrane is depressed, which explains its greater effectiveness in depressing conduction in in-

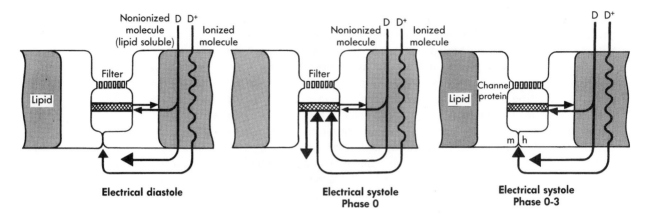

FIGURE 14-4 Access of local anesthetics to their binding site *(cross-hatched area)*. *D* represents nonionized molecules, which easily gain access to the channel binding site from both directions and during all channel states (resting, open, and inactivated). *D⁺* represents ionized molecules, which traverse the lipid bilayer poorly. After gaining access to the aqueous cytosol, these ionized molecules can readily enter the channel when it is open but not when it is closed. (Modified from Rosen MR, Wit AL: Arrhythmogenic actions of antiarrhythmic drugs, *Am J Cardiol* 59[11]:10E, 1987.)

farcted tissue and suppressing arrhythmias in diseased (depolarized) tissue while having only minimal effects on conduction in normal cardiac tissue.[16]

2. Most local anesthetic antiarrhythmics are weak bases that exist in both cationic and neutral forms at physiologic pH. However, acidosis as it occurs in ischemic tissue increases the proportion of the ionized form of the drug molecule and causes it to dissociate more slowly from the channel receptor site. Thus the drug selectively depresses conduction in acidotic tissue at any given heart rate. If the pH changes, so do the actions of the drug. For example, if the plasma becomes alkaline, the neutral form of the drug dominates, and sodium channel blockade is reduced.[17]

3. Drugs with higher molecular weight bind to the channel more persistently than do those with lower molecular weight.[18]

ABNORMAL CONDUCTION

Class I drugs induce arrhythmias by blocking fast sodium channels (unlike ischemia) and by prolonging the vulnerable period (like ischemia). Stimulation during the cardiac vulnerable period results in unidirectional block. Thus class I agents inherently amplify the probability of initiating reentry when prematurely stimulated.[19-21]

Sodium Channel Blockade

Blocking the fast sodium channels causes slow conduction and one-way conduction, rendering a fiber capable of supporting a reentry mechanism. Whereas cardiac ischemia may cause failure of the Na^+-K^+–ATPase pump and K^+ loss because of the effects of lactate and phosphate generated by the ischemic cell, antiarrhythmic drugs depolarize the fiber by blocking the fast sodium channels. Conduction velocity slows in both cases.[22]

Therapeutically, an antiarrhythmic drug causes a two-way block in an area of one-way conduction and thus obliterates the reentry circuit. Figure 14-5, *A,* illustrates the modification of conduction by lidocaine and lidocaine-like drugs. In the arrhythmogenic state there is a depressed fast-response action potential in an area of ischemia, which results in anterograde block through the area, slow one-way conduction in the retrograde direction, and a reentry circuit, resulting in tachycardia. The lidocaine further depresses the area and terminates the tachycardia. Lidocaine-like drugs can also further slow conduction without blocking it, producing new arrhythmias. In Figure 14-5, *B*, there is another area of ischemia that is not as depressed as that in Figure 14-5, *A*. Conduction has been slowed but anterograde conduction persists; no arrhythmia results. The administration of the antiarrhythmic drug further blocks the fast sodium channels in the borderline tissue and depresses the fiber, modifying conduction so that reentry results and a new arrhythmia appears.

Prolonging the Refractory Period

Besides the effect on borderline arrhythmogenic foci, there is another way by which drugs can alter conduction velocity: as a secondary effect of prolongation of the vulnerable period. The antiarrhythmic property of sodium channel blockade is the prolongation of the recovery of excitability. However, as in ischemia this action leads to a prolongation of the vulnerable period. Thus class I antiarrhythmic agents inherently amplify the probability of initiating reentry following a premature beat. Sodium channel blockade, like ischemia, causes slow conduction and one-way conduction following a premature beat by prolonging the cardiac vulnerable period.[14,19-21,23,24]

Figure 14-6 illustrates two possible effects of lengthening the vulnerable period, as would occur with the use of quinidine and quinidine-like drugs. In Figure 14-6, *A*, an ectopic beat occurs during phase 3 repolarization, causing conduction velocity to be slow through that area of the heart; reentry circuits may result. When the refractory period is lengthened, the ectopic focus is suppressed. In Figure 14-6, *B*, the ectopic beat occurs during diastole. Although it is premature, it propagates normally. When the refractory period is lengthened by the antiarrhythmic drug, the ectopic firing occurs during phase 3 repolarization, creating the same arrhythmogenic situation that existed in Figure 14-6, *A*.

Drugs that lengthen the vulnerable period are capable of not only modifying conduction velocity but also causing early afterdepolarizations that can initiate triggered activity. Even quinidine concentrations within the therapeutic range are capable of this effect.[15,22] Early afterdepolarizations and triggered activity are discussed in Chapter 5.

SUMMARY

Local anesthetic antiarrhythmic drugs act by blocking membrane channels; other antiarrhythmics prolong refractory periods or cause triggered activity. Many factors such as myocardial state and preexisting arrhythmias work together to contribute to the proarrhythmic actions or toxicity of antiarrhythmic drugs. Other factors such as pH, heart rate, and the molecular size and shape of the drug influence the binding and release of the local anesthetic antiarrhythmic drugs at their receptor sites. The arrhythmias promoted by antiarrhythmic drugs are not unlike those induced by myocardial disease and ischemia, but the mechanisms differ. Through the very mechanism that causes an antiarrhythmic drug to suppress an arrhythmogenic focus, it is possible for such a drug to cause arrhythmias by converting adequately propagating ectopic foci

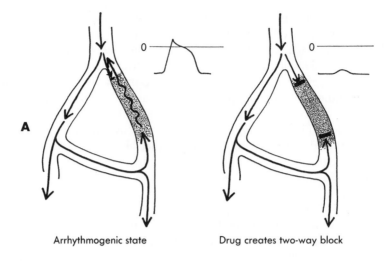

A

Arrhythmogenic state   Drug creates two-way block

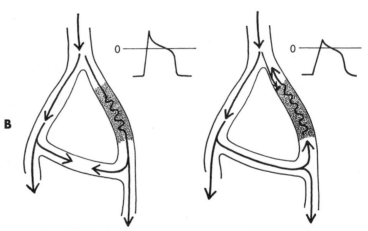

B

Borderline arrhythmogenic state   Drug creates arrhythmogenic state

FIGURE 14-5 Modification of conduction by an antiarrhythmic drug. **A,** In the arrhythmogenic state a reentry circuit and tachyarrhythmia are established through depressed fibers because of an area of slow, one-way conduction. The drug further depresses the fibers, producing two-way block and interrupting the reentry circuit. **B,** The fiber on the left is only slightly depressed; conduction is slow but adequate. The antiarrhythmic drug further depresses the fiber, creating the arrhythmogenic state seen in **A.** (Modified from Rosen MR, Wit AL: Arrhythmogenic actions of antiarrhythmic drugs, *Am J Cardiol* 59[11]:10E, 1987.)

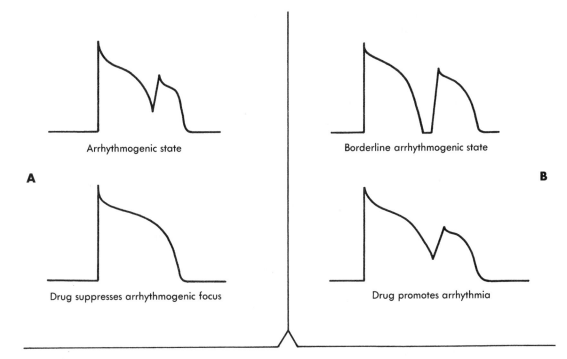

A

B

FIGURE 14-6 Modification of transmembrane potential characteristics by prolonging repolarization. **A,** An arrhythmogenic state exists because an ectopic focus discharges during phase 3 when the membrane potential is depressed, which contributes to slow conduction. When the refractory period is lengthened by an antiarrhythmic drug, the premature action potential is obliterated. **B,** A premature beat propagates normally. When an antiarrhythmic drug is given to lengthen the refractory period, the premature beat arrives during phase 3 and propagates abnormally. (Modified from Rosen MR, Wit AL: Arrhythmogenic actions of antiarrhythmic drugs, *Am J Cardiol* 59[11]:10E, 1987.)

into more depressed, slowly propagating tissue. Information about the proarrhythmic mechanisms presented in this chapter has been derived from the latest in cellular electrophysiology and clinical evidence. Much work is still needed to prove the relationship between drug toxicity, long QT intervals, and triggered activity. Unfortunately, arrhythmias are aggravated by the very factors that require antiarrhythmic intervention (i.e., acute ischemia, existing arrhythmia, and poor ventricular function).

REFERENCES

1. Patterson E, Szabo B, Scherlag BJ, Lazzara R: Arrhythmogenic effects of antiarrhythmic drugs. In Zipes DP, Jalife J: *Cardiac electrophysiology from cell to bedside,* ed 2, Philadelphia, 1995, WB Saunders.
2. Selzer A, Wray HW: Quinidine syncope: paroxysmal ventricular fibrillation occurring during treatment of chronic atrial fibrillation, *Circulation* 30:17, 1964.
3. Kerin NZ, Somberg J: Proarrhythmia: definition, risk factors, causes, treatment, and controversies, *Am Heart J* 128:575, 1994.

4. Falk RH: Proarrhythmic responses to atrial antiarrhythmic therapy. In Falk RH, Podrid PJ, editors: *Atrial fibrillation: mechanisms and management,* New York, 1992, Raven Press.

5. Hohnloser SH, Singh BN: Proarrhythmia with class III antiarrhythmic drugs: definition, electrophysiologic mechanisms, incidence, predisposing factors, and clinical implications, *J Cardiovasc Electrophysiol* 6(10;pt 2):920, 1995.

6. Sueta CA, Clarke SW, Dunlap SH et al: Effect of acute magnesium administration on the frequency of ventricular arrhythmia in patients with heart failure, *Circulation* 89:660, 1994.

7. The Cardiac Arrhythmia Suppression Trial (CAST) Investigators: Preliminary report: effect of encainide and flecainide on mortality in a randomized trial of arrhythmia suppression after myocardial infarction, *N Engl J Med* 321:406, 1989.

8. Echt DS, Liebson PR, Mitchell LB et al: Mortality and morbidity in patients receiving encainide, flecainide, or placebo: the cardiac arrhythmia suppression trial, *N Engl J Med* 324:781, 1991.

9. Greene HL, Roden DM, Katz RJ et al: The cardiac arrhythmia suppression trial: first CAST . . . then CAST-II, *J Am Coll Cardiol* 19:894, 1992.

10. Slater W, Lampert S, Podrid PJ, Lown B: Clinical predictors of arrhythmia worsening by antiarrhythmic drugs, *Am J Cardiol* 61:349, 1988.

11. Carson DL, Cardinal R, Savard P et al: Relationship between an arrhythmogenic action of lidocaine and its effects on excitation patterns in acutely ischemic porcine myocardium, *J Cardiovasc Pharmacol* 8:126, 1986.

12. Roden DM, Bennett PB, Snyders DJ et al: Quinidine delays I_K activation in guinea pig ventricular myocytes, *Circ Res* 62:1055, 1988.

13. Lazzara R, Hope RR, El-Sherif N et al: Effects of lidocaine on hypoxic and ischemic cardiac cells, *Am J Cardiol* 41:872, 1978.

14. Starmer CF, Romashko DN, Reddy RS et al: Proarrhythmic response to potassium channel blockade: numerical studies of polymorphic tachyarrhythmias, *Circulation* 92:595, 1996.

15. Roden DM, Hoffman BF: Action potential prolongation and induction of abnormal automaticity by low quinidine concentrations in canine Purkinje fibers: relationship to potassium and cycle length, *Circ Res* 56:857, 1985.

16. Rosen MR: Fast response action potential. In Podrid PJ, Kowey PR, editors: *Cardiac arrhythmia mechanisms, diagnosis, and management,* Baltimore, 1995, Williams & Wilkins.

17. Hondeghem LM: Antiarrhythmic agents: modulated reception applications, *Circulation* 75:514, 1987.

18. Courtney KR: Review: quantitative structure/activity relations based on use-dependent block and repriming kinetics in myocardium, *J Mol Cell Cardiol* 19:319, 1987.

19. Starmer CF, Lastra AA, Nesterenko VV, Grant AO: Proarrhythmic response to sodium channel blockade: theoretical model and numerical experiments, *Circulation* 84:1364, 1991.

20. Starmer CF, Lancaster AR, Lastra AA, Grant AO: Cardiac instability amplified by use-dependent Na channel blockade, *Am J Physiol* 262:H1305, 1992.

21. Starobin J, Zilberter YI, Starmer CF: Vulnerability in one-dimensional excitable media, *Physica D* 70:321, 1994.

22. Rosen MR, Wit AL: Arrhythmogenic actions of antiarrhythmic drugs, *Am J Cardiol* 59:10E, 1987.

23. Nesterenko VV, Lastra AA, Rosenshtraukh LV, Starmer CF: A proarrhythmic response to sodium channel blockade: modulation of the vulnerable period in guinea pig ventricular myocardium, *J Cardiovasc Pharmacol* 19:810, 1992.

24. Starmer CF, Biktashev VN, Romashko DN et al: Vulnerability in an excitable medium: analytical and numerical studies of initiating unidirectional propagation, *Biophys J* 65:1775, 1993.

CHAPTER 15

Aberrant Ventricular Conduction

Mechanisms 215
Rate-dependent and
  critical rate bundle
  branch block 220
Patterns of aberration 223
Additional helpful
  clues 226
Aberrancy in atrial
  fibrillation 230
Ashman's phenomenon
  230
Aberrancy in atrial
  tachycardia 231
Alternating aberrancy 233
Clinical implications 233

A S EARLY AS 1910, SIR THOMAS LEWIS[1] DESCRIBED ABERRANT VENTRICULAR CON-
duction of atrial premature beats (APBs) and during atrial fibrillation and flutter. He stated, "I term the . . . beats aberrant because they are caused by impulses
which have gone astray." Since that time *aberrancy, aberrant ventricular conduction,* and
ventricular aberration have become interchangeable terms.

Lewis also illustrated bundle branch block (BBB) as a form of permanent ventricular aberration. Although the term *aberration* is now usually reserved for transient BBB,
these early studies correctly identified the mechanism.

Further delineating the type of BBB involved in ventricular aberration, Wellens,
Bär, and Lie[2] found that out of 70 episodes of aberration, 69% were right bundle
branch block (RBBB). Sandler and Marriott[3] have reported that the incidence of
RBBB aberration is as high as 80% to 85%. In a relatively sick population (e.g., in a
coronary care facility) left bundle branch block (LBBB) aberration assumes greater
prominence and accounts for perhaps one third of the aberrant conduction encountered; Wellens, Bär, and Lie[2] found that 31% were LBBB aberration. In the study
by Kulbertus, de Laval-Rutten, and Casters et al[4] RBBB accounted for a smaller-than-
expected proportion of the aberration produced experimentally, whereas left posterior hemiblock occurred with surprising frequency. By inducing APBs in 44 patients,
116 aberrant configurations were produced. The results of this study are presented in
Table 15-1.

MECHANISMS

The following three mechanisms are responsible for aberrant ventricular conduction:
1. Stimulation during phase 3 of the action potential (phase 3 aberration)
2. Retrograde concealed conduction, a common mechanism (see Chapter 6)
3. Stimulation during phase 4 of Purkinje fiber action potentials (phase 4 aberration)

Phase 3 Aberration

Among other things, conduction velocity depends on the rate of rise of phase 0 of the
action potential (dV/dt) and the height to which it rises (V_{max}). These factors in turn depend on the membrane potential at the time of stimulation. The more negative the
membrane potential, the more fast sodium channels available, and the greater the influx
of Na^+ into the cell during phase 0.

215

TABLE 15-1   RELATIVE FREQUENCY OF EXPERIMENTAL ABERRATION

ABERRATION	PERCENTAGE
RBBB	24
RBBB + LAHB	18
LAHB	15
RBBB + LPHB	10
LPHB	9
LBBB	9
ILBBB	5
Trivial changes	6
Marked anterior displacement	4
Totals	
RBBB	52
LAHB	33
LPHB	19
LBBB	14

Modified from Kulbertus HE, de Laval-Rutten F, Casters P et al: Vectorcardiographic study of aberrant conduction, *Br Heart J* 38:549, 1976.
ILBBB, Incomplete left bundle branch block; *LAHB,* left anterior hemiblock; *LPHB,* left posterior hemiblock.

Figure 15-1 illustrates that if a stimulus occurs during phase 3 of the action potential, the membrane potential at the time of stimulation is reduced and conduction is compromised—hence the term *phase 3 aberration.* In Figure 15-1, the ECG shows an APB conducted with aberration. The action potential of the right bundle branch (RBB) is shown above the electrocardiogram (ECG) and indicates that aberration occurs because the stimulus reaches the RBB during phase 3—when the membrane potential is −65 mV. At this time only approximately half of the fast sodium channels are available for activation. The resulting action potential is a slow channel response, and conduction fails.

Functional or physiologic phase 3 aberration (BBB) can occur in normal fibers if the impulse is premature enough to reach the fiber during electrical systole of the preceding beat—when the membrane potential is still reduced. This is the common form of aberration that often accompanies very early APBs.

Phase 3 aberration may also occur pathologically if electrical systole and/or the refractory period are abnormally prolonged and the involved fascicle is stimulated at a relatively rapid rate. Thus the terms *systolic block* or *tachycardia-dependent BBB* are sometimes used. In the case of abnormal prolongation of the refractory period, refractoriness extends beyond the action potential duration or the QT interval.

Although the supernormal period is a part of phase 3, very early premature beats can occur before the period of supernormal excitability. This property is not exhibited by all fibers (see Chapter 21). Figure 15-2 illustrates the abrupt onset of supernormal excitability and the small portion of the action potential actually involved. Spear and

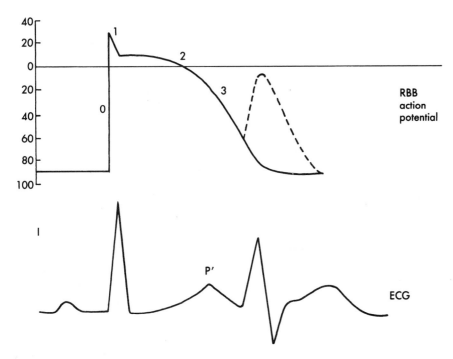

FIGURE 15-1 Action potentials and corresponding ECG representation of phase 3 aberration. An early atrial premature beat arrives during the relative refractory period of the right bundle branch *(RBB)* and produces an action potential that does not propagate. The impulse is successfully conducted down the left bundle branch to produce an RBBB pattern.

Moore[5] found that intraventricular conduction times of very early premature beats could be both decreased and increased.

Figure 15-3 illustrates examples of phase 3 RBBB aberration after an APB. In these cases it is often difficult or impossible to distinguish between physiologic phase 3 BBB and a pathologic one involving lengthening of the refractory period.

Phase 4 Aberration

The principles governing phase 4 aberration are the same as those for phase 3 aberration (i.e., conduction velocity depends on the steepness and height of phase 0 of the action potential [dV/dt; V_{max}]), which are in turn dependent on the negativity of the membrane potential at the time of stimulation. Figure 15-4 illustrates that if a stimulus occurs late during phase 4 of a pacemaker cell action potential, the membrane potential at the time of stimulation is reduced and conduction is compromised—hence the term *phase 4 aberration*. Aberration occurs for the same reason as during phase 3 (activation at a reduced membrane potential) but in a different setting. Instead of incomplete repolarization being the cause of aberration as it is in the phase 3 type, the reduction of the membrane potential by the pacemaker current is responsible for phase 4 aberration. In Figure 15-4, the ECG shows a long cycle ending with RBBB. The action poten-

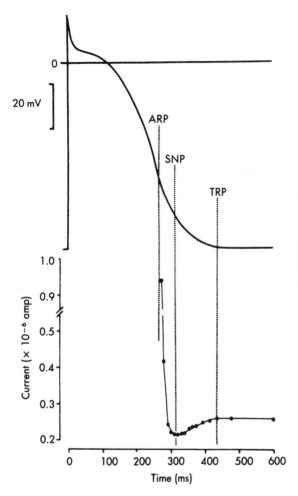

FIGURE 15-2 Excitability determination in a canine Purkinje fiber. The excitability curve is displayed beneath the action potential and represents the minimum depolarizing current necessary to evoke a response at the time indicated. *ARP,* Absolute refractory period; *SNP,* minimal current requirements to excite the fiber during the supernormal period; *TRP,* total refractory period. (From Spear JF, Moore N: In Wellens HJJ, Lie KI, Janse MJ, editors: *The conduction system of the heart,* Philadelphia, 1976, Lea & Febiger.)

tial of the RBB indicates enhanced automaticity; by the time the impulse arrives in the RBB, the membrane potential has been reduced. The resulting action potential is a slow channel response, and conduction fails.

Phase 4 aberration is one of the theories offered to explain the development of abnormal intraventricular conduction at the end of a lengthened cycle. Because better conduction is expected at the end of a longer diastole, this form of aberration is known as the *paradoxical critical rate.* It is also sometimes referred to as *bradycardia-dependent BBB,* but this term is unsatisfactory as an inclusive term because it is not always necessary to achieve a rate that merits the designation *bradycardia.*

Phase 4 block occurs late in diastole and is associated with the cyclical reduction in resting membrane potential that is typical of latent pacemaker cells. If these cells are activated when their membrane potential is reduced, conduction disturbances can result like those that develop when activation occurs during phase 3.[6-8]

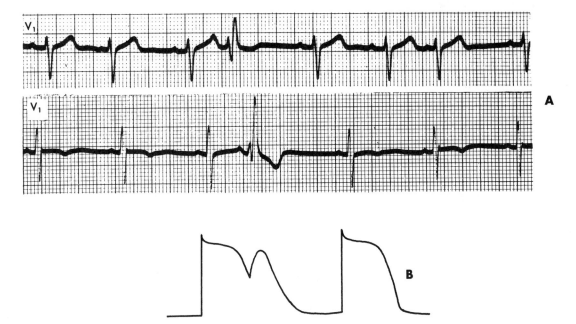

FIGURE 15-3 Phase 3 bundle branch block. **A,** After three normally conducted beats, an atrial extrasystole arises, and its impulse arrives at the right bundle branch, when it is still refractory. It is therefore conducted with RBBB aberration. The second and seventh beats are also extrasystoles, but they are less premature and are therefore conducted normally. **B,** The action potentials illustrate the mechanism.

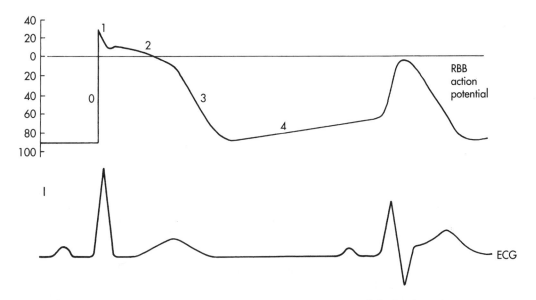

FIGURE 15-4 Action potentials and corresponding ECG representation of phase 4 aberration. During a long pause the fibers of the His-Purkinje system begin to depolarize in an effort to reach threshold potential. By the time the late sinus beat reaches the ventricles, not all His-Purkinje fibers are negative enough to propagate. In this representation, the fibers of the right bundle branch *(RBB)* are activated by the supraventricular impulse but do not propagate, which leaves the task of activating the ventricles to the left bundle branch. As a result, an RBBB pattern is produced on the ECG.

Phase 4 aberration would be expected in the setting of bradycardia or enhanced normal automaticity (enhanced automaticity of pacemaker cells). However, in spite of the fact that bradycardia is common and cells with phase 4 depolarization are abundant, phase 4 block is not commonly seen; most reported cases are associated with organic heart disease. Singer and Cohen[8] offer the following explanation: In normal fibers conduction is well maintained at membrane potentials greater than −70 to −75 mV. Significant conduction disturbances are first manifested when the membrane potential is below −70 mV at the time of stimulation; local block appears at −65 to −60 mV. Because the threshold potential for normal His-Purkinje fibers is −70 mV, spontaneous firing occurs before the membrane can actually be reduced to the potential necessary for conduction impairment or block. Phase 4 block is therefore always pathologic when it does occur, and it requires one or more of the following situations:

1. The presence of slow diastolic depolarization, which need not be enhanced
2. A decrease in excitability (a shift in threshold potential toward zero) so that, in the presence of significant bradycardia, enough time elapses before the impulse arrives for the bundle branch fibers to reach a potential at which conduction is impaired
3. A deterioration in membrane responsiveness so that significant conduction impairment develops at −75 mV instead of −65 mV; this occurrence would also negate the necessity for such a long cycle before conduction falters

Membrane responsiveness is determined by the relationship of the membrane potential at excitation to the maximum height of phase 0. Hypopolarization (the loss of maximum diastolic potential) is an important factor in phase 4 block because it itself causes both a decrease in excitability and enhanced automaticity.[9]

Two examples of phase 4 BBB are illustrated in Figure 15-5. In Figure 15-5, *A*, the longer sinus cycles end with LBBB; in Figure 15-5, *B*, the lengthened postextrasystolic cycles end with RBBB conduction.

RATE-DEPENDENT AND CRITICAL RATE BUNDLE BRANCH BLOCK

Rate-dependent bundle branch block is the term used when the block comes and goes with changes in heart rate. *Critical rate* is the term given to the rate at which BBB develops during acceleration or disappears during slowing. It is of interest that rate-dependent BBB develops at a critical rate faster than the rate at which it disappears. Note in Figure 15-6 that although rate-dependent BBB develops when the rate reaches 66 beats/min (cycle length = 91), normal conduction is not restored until the rate falls to 56 beats/min (cycle length = 108).

There are two reasons for this phenomenon. As the heart rate accelerates, the refractory period shortens; normal conduction tends to be preserved because of this response. Conversely, the refractory period lengthens as the heart rate slows. It is thus necessary for the heart rate to slow down more than would be expected to reestablish normal intraventricular conduction.

Second and more important is the fact that once BBB is established, the actual cycle for the blocked bundle does not begin until approximately halfway through the QRS complex. For example, in the case of rate-dependent LBBB it takes approximately 0.06 second for the impulse to negotiate the unaffected right bundle and septum and to reach the depressed left bundle (Figure 15-7). Therefore the left bundle actually

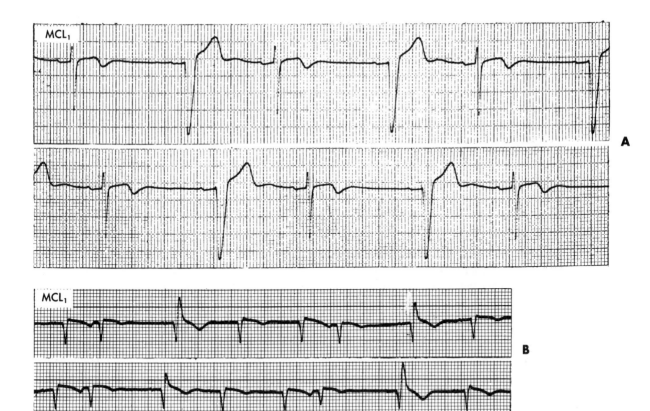

FIGURE 15-5 Paradoxical critical rate. **A,** All of the longer cycles (range = 138 to 142 ms) end with LBBB, whereas the shorter cycles (range = 107 to 110 ms) end with improved, virtually normal, intraventricular conduction. The alternate longer and shorter sinus cycles are presumably caused by a 3:2 sinus Wenckebach period. **B,** Sinus rhythm is repeatedly interrupted by atrial extrasystoles. All conducted beats that end the lengthened postextrasystolic cycles show RBBB, whereas the shorter sinus cycles and the even shorter extrasystolic cycles show more normal intraventricular conduction.

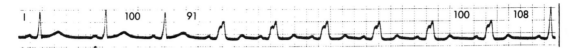

FIGURE 15-6 Rate-dependent left bundle branch block. As the sinus rhythm accelerates, LBBB develops when the rate exceeds 60 beats/min (cycle length <100 ms). For normal conduction to resume, the rate must fall below 60 beats/min (cycle length >100 ms).

begins its cycle 0.06 second after the right bundle. For normal conduction to resume, the cycle during deceleration (as measured from the beginning of one QRS complex to the beginning of the next) must be longer than the "critical" cycle during acceleration by at least 0.06 second.

Figure 15-8 illustrates two more examples of phase 3 BBB. This time the fact that the BBB is rate-dependent is revealed only because of the pause following ventricular premature beats (VPBs) in Figure 15-8, *A*, and a nonconducted APB in Figure 15-8, *B*. In each case the complex that ends the pause achieves better intraventricular conduction.

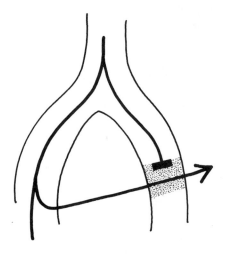

FIGURE 15-7 One of the two mechanisms responsible for the fact that the "critical rate" is different (faster) during acceleration than it is during deceleration (see text).

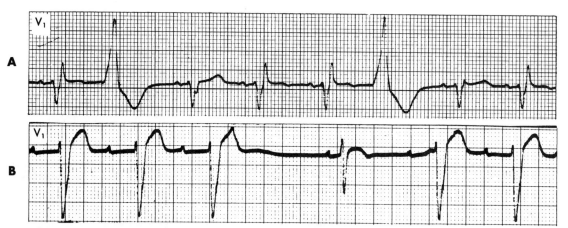

FIGURE 15-8 Examples of postextrasystolic revelation of rate-dependent bundle branch block. **A,** After each of the ventricular extrasystoles, the returning sinus beat manifests a lesser degree of RBBB than do the sinus beats ending the normal (shorter) sinus cycles. **B,** After three sinus beats conducted with first-degree AV block and LBBB, a nonconducted atrial extrasystole results in a prolonged ventricular cycle. At the end of this cycle the returning sinus beat is conducted with normal PR and normal intraventricular conduction, which demonstrates that both the AV delay and the LBBB are rate-dependent.

PATTERNS OF ABERRATION

Because aberrant ventricular conduction is either RBBB and/or hemiblock or LBBB, recognizing it depends on the ability to recognize the typical ECG patterns in these conditions. The patterns of RBBB and LBBB aberration are discussed in the following sections. The differential diagnosis of broad QRS tachycardia with application of all of the current and past rules is discussed in Chapter 16.

RBBB Aberration

In 1965 and 1970 the RBBB pattern in V_1 (rSR′) was described as 10:1 in favor of aberration.[3,10] RBBB aberration is recognized because of the classical triphasic rSR′ pattern in V_1 and qRS pattern in V_6 (Figure 15-9). Note the narrow little q wave in V_6, which reflects normal septal activation. This q wave is a strong indicator of RBBB aberration if the pattern in V_1 is positive. It is important not to apply this rule to V_6 when the complex in V_1 is negative.

The studies by Wellens and associates[2,11] show the third and fourth complexes to be strongly in favor of aberration (Table 15-2). This phenomenon was also demonstrated by Gulamhusein, Yee, Ko, and Klein,[12] who studied patients with atrial fibrillation.

Note the first complex in Table 15-3. This classical triphasic RBBB pattern in V_6 (qRs) is strong evidence of aberration when the complex is upright in V_1.

LBBB Aberration

The classical pattern of LBBB in V_1 and V_2 is a good clue to the presence of LBBB aberration.[13] The typical pattern of LBBB is also seen in lead V_6 (no Q and no S). If an r wave is present in either V_1 or V_2, it is narrow in LBBB aberration (<0.03 second), and the downstroke of the S wave is clean and swift (no slurs or notches). Because of the narrow r and/or the clean downstroke, the distance from the beginning of the QRS complex to the nadir of the S wave is 0.06 second or less. Figure 15-10 illustrates the typical LBBB patterns that can be used to diagnose aberrant ventricular conduction. Hemiblock aberration is diagnosed by axis deviation with or without RBBB aberration.

The shapes of right and left bundle branch aberration in lead V_1 and V_2 are nicely compared in Figure 15-11. In Figure 15-11, *A,* note the rSR′ pattern typical of RBBB, and in Figure 15-11, *B,* note the narrow little r wave and the swift, clean downstroke of the S wave typical of LBBB. These are examples of critical-rate BBB secondary to a pathologic prolongation of the action potential and/or refractory period in the respective bundle branches.

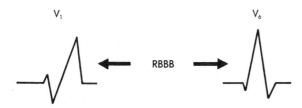

FIGURE 15-9   Classic right bundle branch block pattern in V_1 and V_6.

TABLE 15-2   THE DIFFERENTIAL DIAGNOSIS IN WIDE QRS TACHYCARDIA USING
QRS PATTERNS IN LEAD V_1

COMPLEX	V_1	ABERRANT	VENTRICULAR TACHYCARDIA
1		—	15
2		11	17
3		19	3
4		38	3
5		—	7
6		1	16
7		—	4
Total		69	65

From Wellens HJJ, Bär FWHM, Lie KI: The value of the electrocardiogram in the differential diagnosis of a tachycardia with a widened QRS complex, *Am J Med* 64:27, 1978; and Wellens HJJ, Bär
FWHM, Vanagt EJDM, Brugada P: Medical treatment of ventricular tachycardia: considerations in
the selection of patients for surgical treatment, *Am J Cardiol* 49:187, 1982.

TABLE 15-3   THE DIFFERENTIAL DIAGNOSIS IN WIDE QRS TACHYCARDIA USING QRS PATTERNS IN LEAD V_6

COMPLEX	V_6	ABERRANT	VENTRICULAR TACHYCARDIA
1		44	3
2		21	15
3		4	27
4		—	16
5		—	3
6		—	1
Total		69	65

From Wellens HJJ, Bär FWHM, Lie KI: The value of the electrocardiogram in the differential diagnosis of a tachycardia with a widened QRS complex, *Am J Med* 64:27, 1978; and Wellens HJJ, Bär FWHM, Vanagt EJDM, Brugada P: Medical treatment of ventricular tachycardia: considerations in the selection of patients for surgical treatment, *Am J Cardiol* 49:187, 1982.

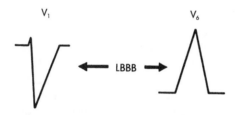

FIGURE 15-10   Classic left bundle branch pattern in V_1 and V_6.

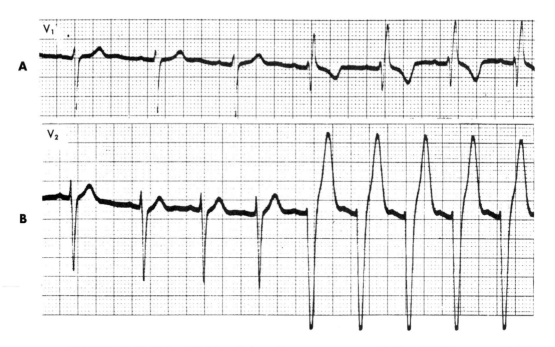

FIGURE 15-11 Right and left bundle branch patterns are compared. Note the rSR′ pattern of RBBB in lead V_1 compared with the rS pattern of LBBB seen here in lead V_2. An r wave that is present in lead V_1 or V_2 in uncomplicated LBBB will be narrow and small as illustrated here. The S downstroke is swift and clean (no slurs or notches). **A,** From a 19-year-old student nurse. As the sinus rate accelerates and the cycle shortens in response to gentle exercise, progressively increasing degrees of RBBB develop ("critical-rate" or "rate-dependent" RBBB). **B,** From a 64-year-old man with severe coronary disease. As the sinus rate accelerates, the cycles shorten. LBBB develops at a critical rate of slightly more than 100 beats/min.

ADDITIONAL HELPFUL CLUES

In addition to the classical RBBB and LBBB patterns in V_1, V_2, and V_6, other signs that support aberration are a QRS complex of less than 0.14 second, preceding atrial activity, an anomalous second-in-the-row beat and, in the RBBB pattern, an initial deflection in V_1 identical to that of conducted beats. Atrioventricular (AV) dissociation, the shape of ectopic beats, the patient history and physical examination, and other clues useful in the differential diagnosis of broad QRS tachycardia are discussed in Chapter 16.

QRS Duration

A QRS complex of 0.14 second or less supports but is not diagnostic of aberration.[2,11] As discussed in Chapter 19, exceptions to this rule are the ventricular tachycardias (VTs) that look like supraventricular tachycardia (SVT):
- Fascicular VT (RBBB pattern; QRS complex <0.14 second)
- Idiopathic VT (RBBB or LBBB pattern; relatively narrow QRS complex)
- Bundle branch reentry VT (usually LBBB pattern; relatively narrow QRS complex)

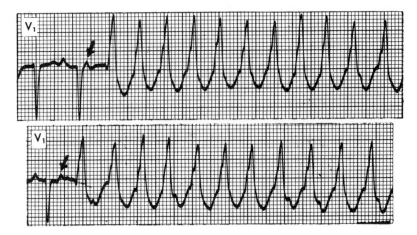

FIGURE 15-12 This broad QRS tachycardia begins with an atrial premature beat *(arrows)*. However, the QRS pattern is that of ventricular tachycardia, which indicates one of two possibilities: ventricular tachycardia or antidromic circus movement tachycardia.

Preceding Atrial Activity

Ectopic P waves before the broad complex in question may be helpful in differentiating aberration from ectopy as long as this clue is used in combination with QRS morphology. However, because atrial ectopic beats can initiate VT, SVT with aberration, and antidromic circus movement tachycardia (using an accessory pathway in the anterograde direction), the value of this clue is somewhat limited.[14-21] Figure 15-12 is a case in point. Although APBs *(arrows)* can clearly be seen initiating this broad QRS tachycardia, the QRS pattern is that of VT (R wave in V_1), which raises the possibility that it is truly VT or an SVT that looks like VT. When a supraventricular impulse gains entrance to the ventricles solely through an accessory pathway, the QRS pattern is that of VT.

Figure 15-13 provides another example of APBs initiating a broad QRS tachycardia. In this case the QRS pattern is that of LBBB aberration—a narrow r wave (first complex of the broad QRS series), a swift clean downstroke, and a relatively narrow QRS complex (0.12 second). Therefore it is clear that all possible clues must be used, because an initiating APB alone is not diagnostic of SVT.

Initial Deflection Identical with That of Conducted Beats

The initial deflection in the ECG is identical to that of conducted beats only with RBBB aberration because the initial forces in uncomplicated RBBB are normal (septal) and are best seen in V_1 and in the lateral leads I, aV_L, and V_6. Figure 15-14 contains both RBBB and LBBB aberrations. Note that the initial deflections of the RBBB aberration are almost the same as the sinus-conducted beats. The QRS patterns, their relatively narrow width, and the presence of P′ waves in front of the anomalous complexes secure the diagnosis of aberration.

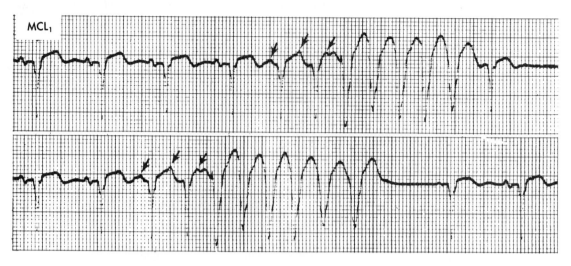

FIGURE 15-13 Each strip contains a brief run of supraventricular tachycardia with LBBB aberration. The diagnosis can be made because of antecedent P′ waves *(arrows)*, the width of the QRS (0.12 second), and the QRS pattern.

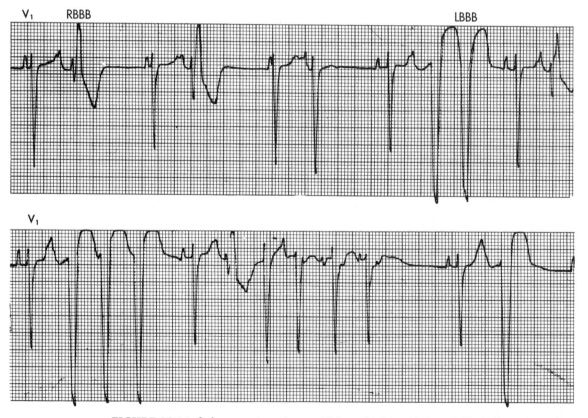

FIGURE 15-14 Strips are not continuous. Right and left bundle branch block aberration. When the aberration is RBBB, the initial deflection is often identical to that of the conducted sinus beats. Note the atrial premature beats in front of the aberrant beats.

Second-in-the-Row Anomaly

The second-in-the-row beat of rapid beats is most likely to be aberrant because it is the only one that ends a relatively short cycle preceded by a relatively long one. The duration of the action potential (and hence the refractory period) is directly related to the cardiac cycle. As the cycle lengthens or shortens, so does the refractory period (this is reflected in the QT interval, which shortens as the heart rate increases).

Figure 15-15 illustrates short, five-beat bursts of atrial tachycardia in which only the first beat of the tachycardia (second-in-the-row, counting the preceding sinus beat) is anomalous. The first premature beat shortens the cycle, causing itself to be conducted with RBBB aberration. The aberrant beat ends a relatively short cycle, which creates a short refractory period for itself and gives the next beat a better chance for normal conduction. Unfortunately, according to the rule of bigeminy,[22] a lengthened cycle tends to precipitate a VPB; therefore the longer-shorter cycle sequence is inconclusive. The QRS pattern and the presence of a P′ wave preceding the onset of tachycardia are clearly more helpful in making the diagnosis.

In Figure 15-16 the alternative mechanism is illustrated—a VPB initiates paroxysmal supraventricular tachycardia (PSVT). In this tracing the second-in-the-row beat is also

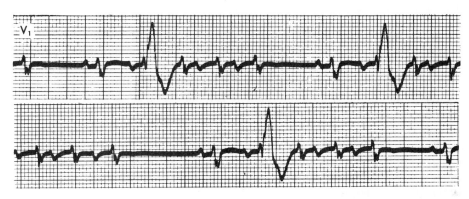

FIGURE 15-15 Strips are continuous. Three short bursts of supraventricular tachycardia in which only the first beat (second-in-the-row) develops ventricular aberration.

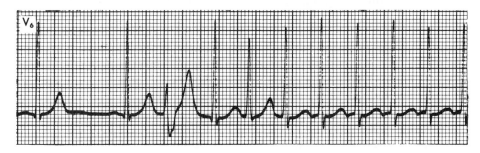

FIGURE 15-16 A ventricular premature beat initiates paroxysmal supraventricular tachycardia. This tracing illustrates another reason that the second-in-the-row beat is anomalous.

anomalous. However, the pattern of the anomalous beat in V_6 (RS) and the absence of visible ectopic atrial activity strongly support a diagnosis of a VPB that is initiating PSVT. Because the P′ wave is located before the QRS complex instead of immediately following or hidden within it, the mechanism of the SVT could be (1) the uncommon fast-slow form of AV nodal reentry (down the fast atrionodal pathway and up the slow pathway), or (2) the uncommon form of circus movement tachycardia using a slowly conducting accessory pathway for retrograde conduction to the atria. In the latter case the RP′ is greater than the P′R.

ABERRANCY IN ATRIAL FIBRILLATION

Because there is always preceding atrial activity in atrial fibrillation, ECG patterns are relied on heavily to distinguish between aberration and ectopy. This reliance is justified by the His bundle studies[23] examining 1100 abnormal QRS complexes (750 ectopic, 350 aberrant) in patients with chronic atrial fibrillation. V_1 was the most helpful lead in differentiating aberration from ectopy, with the rSR′ pattern affording 24:1 odds in favor of aberration. Gulamhusein, Yee, Ko, and Klein[12] arrived at the same conclusion in 1985.

ASHMAN'S PHENOMENON

In 1947 Gouaux and Ashman[24] defined the mechanism of ventricular aberration by relating it to the refractory period and cycle length in atrial fibrillation. Although the cycle length of the bundle branches during atrial fibrillation cannot be determined from the surface ECG because of the prevalence of concealed conduction into the bundle branches, the concept of the long-short phenomenon is still valid (less so when applied to atrial fibrillation). Thus their statement was correct: "Aberration occurs (may occur) when a short cycle follows a long one because the refractory period varies with cycle length."[24] Much to their credit, Gouaux and Ashman concluded through deductive reasoning that RBBB aberration is the more common form because the RBB has a longer refractory period than the LBB. This fact was later verified by the experimental studies of Moe, Mendez, and Han.[25]

Pauses do lengthen the refractory period of the terminating beat. This concept is well applied to rhythms with P waves, such as the onset of torsades de pointes. However, the application of Ashman's phenomenon in atrial fibrillation is precarious for two reasons. First, by the rule of bigeminy a lengthened cycle also tends to precipitate a ventricular extrasystole.[22] Second, because of concealed conduction, it is never known from the surface ECG exactly when a bundle branch is activated. It is known that the rampant electrical activity that occurs during atrial fibrillation incompletely penetrates the His bundle and bundle branches (concealed conduction); one result is the irregular ventricular rhythm during atrial fibrillation. Thus there are often pauses that are longer than the actual refractory period of the AV conduction system. If an aberrant beat does end a long-short cycle sequence during atrial fibrillation, it may be because of refractoriness of a bundle branch secondary to concealed conduction into it rather than because of changes in the length of the ventricular cycle.

In more than 400 cases of chronic atrial fibrillation and 1100 anomalous beats, Vera et al[23] did not find Ashman's phenomenon helpful in differentiating aberration from

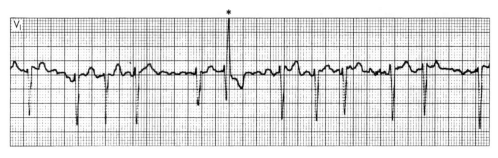

FIGURE 15-17 RBBB aberration *(asterisk)* following a long-short sequence during atrial fibrillation.

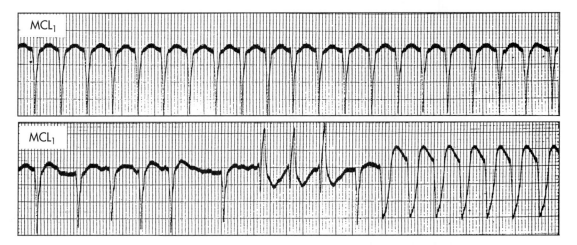

FIGURE 15-18 PSVT *(top)* precipitates atrial fibrillation in this patient. In the bottom tracing RBBB aberration follows a long-short sequence during atrial fibrillation. The three beats with RBBB are followed by one normally conducted beat and LBBB aberration.

ectopy. Gulamhusein, Yee, Ko, and Klein[12] examined 1068 wide QRS complexes in chronic atrial fibrillation and did not find Ashman's phenomenon specific for SVT. These studies and the examples in Figures 15-17 to 15-19 should put to rest the use of Ashman's phenomenon in the differential diagnosis between aberrancy and ectopy during atrial fibrillation. Figures 15-17 and 15-18 show atrial fibrillation in which aberrant beats end a long-short sequence; Figure 15-19 shows atrial fibrillation in which ventricular ectopic beats end a long-short sequence.

ABERRANCY IN ATRIAL TACHYCARDIA

Figure 15-20 illustrates aberration that was misdiagnosed and led to gross mismanagement. The top strip shows the patient's rhythm on admission: atrial tachycardia with 2:1 AV conduction (note the nonconducted P waves partially hidden in the ventricular

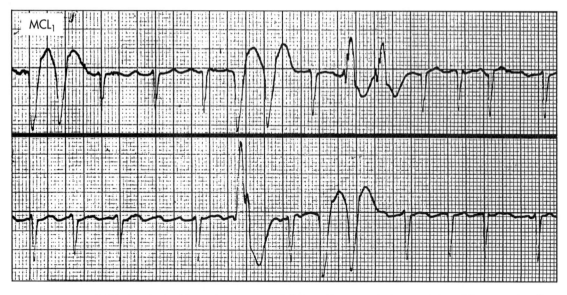

FIGURE 15-19 A long-short sequence is followed by a ventricular ectopic beat. The top tracing illustrates atrial fibrillation with LBBB and RBBB aberration. In the bottom tracing the one ventricular ectopic beat (fifth complex) is easily identified by its "rabbit ear" pattern in lead V_1, the left one being taller.

complexes). This patient was started on digitalis and by the next morning (second strip) frequently manifested 4:1 conduction ratios. Because of this satisfactory "impairment" of conduction, digitalis was discontinued and quinidine was started. The bottom strip was obtained from the following morning and shows the situation that developed at approximately midnight and led to erroneous therapy for VT throughout the night. The strip represents atrial tachycardia with 1:1 AV conduction and RBBB aberration. The quinidine—perhaps partly through its antivagal effect but certainly through its slowing effect on the atrial rate (from 210 to 192 beats/min)—enabled the AV junction to conduct all the ectopic atrial impulses. The resulting much-increased ventricular rate (from approximately 90 to 192 beats/min) produced a dangerous hypotension from which the patient was finally rescued by administering a combination of a pressor agent and countershock.

In 1958 Rosenblueth[26] documented the effect of atrial rate on normal AV conduction by pacing the atria of normal dogs. He found that at an average rate of 257 beats/min the animals developed Wenckebach periods and began to drop beats; at an average rate of 285 beats/min they developed constant 2:1 conduction. Consider what this means in terms of ventricular rate. At an atrial rate of 286 beats/min the ventricular rate is 143 beats/min. If the atrial rate slows by only 30 beats/min (to 256 beats/min), conduction is 1:1 with a ventricular rate of 256 beats/min. Thus with slowing of the atrial rate by only 30 beats/min, the ventricular rate increases by 113 beats/min. This phenomenon explains

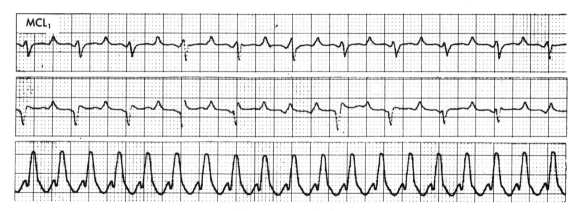

FIGURE 15-20 Strips are not continuous. Top strip (on admission) shows atrial tachycardia with 2:1 AV conduction. Middle strip (next day) shows 2:1 and 4:1 conduction. Bottom strip (24 hours later) shows a slower atrial rate with 1:1 conduction and RBBB aberration, which was mistaken for and treated for hours as ventricular tachycardia.

why it can be so dangerous to give atrial-slowing drugs such as lidocaine, quinidine, or even procainamide in the presence of atrial flutter or fibrillation when the ventricular response is already uncomfortably fast.[27] If atrial flutter at a rate of 300 beats/min is associated with a 2:1 response (which produces a ventricular rate of 150 beats/min) and a drug such as lidocaine is administered, the atrial rate may slow to 250 beats/min and AV conduction may increase to 1:1, producing a dangerous ventricular rate of 250 beats/min.

ALTERNATING ABERRANCY

It is not uncommon to see both RBBB and LBBB aberration in the same patient (Figure 15-21). An interesting feature of each of these tracings is the abrupt switch from one BBB form of aberration to the other after a single intervening, normally conducted beat. The mechanism of this phenomenon is unexplained but is sufficiently characteristic to assist in differentiating bilateral aberration from bifocal ectopy. It is of interest that the first published example of ventricular aberration (Lewis in 1910[1]) was alternating aberration complicating atrial bigeminy (Figure 15-22). Figure 15-23 illustrates a contemporary example of a similar alternating aberration.

CLINICAL IMPLICATIONS

RBB aberration is often considered physiologic (secondary to tachycardia or sudden shortening of the cycle). On the other hand, phase 4 and/or LBBB aberration are thought to indicate underlying cardiac disease. Whatever the cause, aberration is always secondary to another primary disturbance and never requires treatment.

It is important to recognize ventricular aberration because it may be mistaken for ventricular ectopy, which would lead to the administration of unnecessary drugs and a delay of the treatment and diagnosis of the mechanism of SVT.

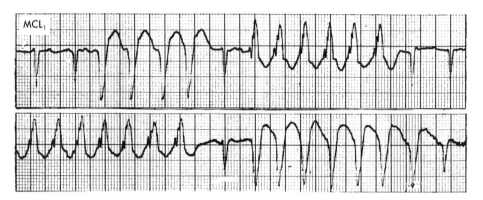

FIGURE 15-21 Both strips illustrate the abrupt change from one type of BBB aberration to the other, with a single intervening normally conducted beat.

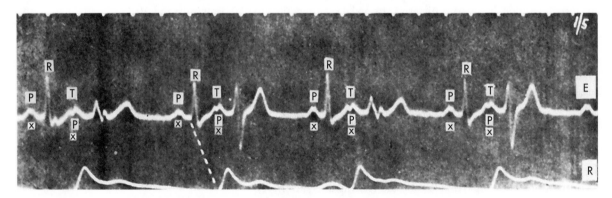

FIGURE 15-22 First published example of ventricular aberration (Lewis in 1910[1]). Sinus rhythm with atrial bigeminy; each extrasystole is conducted aberrantly, but the form of aberration alternates. E, Electrocardiogram; R, radial pulse.

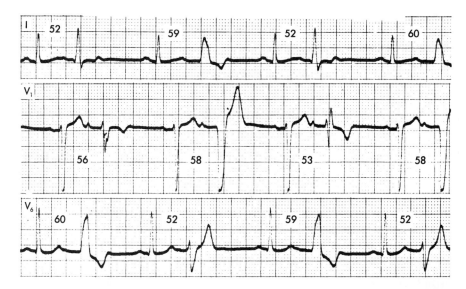

FIGURE 15-23 Sinus rhythm with atrial bigeminy. The shorter extrasystolic cycles end in some form of RBBB aberration, whereas the longer ones end with LBBB aberration. Beats with RBBB, as evidenced by the slightly increased height of the R waves in lead I and the rS pattern in V_6, presumably manifest bifascicular aberration (RBBB plus left anterior hemiblock). In V_1 the first atrial extrasystole shows only the earliest sign of RBBB, namely notching of the terminal upstroke.

SUMMARY

Aberrant ventricular conduction is a form of transient bundle branch block and/or hemiblock. It occurs most often as phase 3 aberration but also at times as phase 4 aberration. The morphologic clues that identify ventricular aberration are the classical forms of right and left bundle branch block as seen in leads V_1, V_2, and V_6. When the complex is mainly upright in V_1, an rSR′ or rR′ in that lead or a qRs complex in V_6 indicates RBBB aberration. When the complex is mainly negative in V_1, a sharp, narrow r (if one is present) and a smooth, quick downstroke to the S wave in leads V_1 and V_2 indicate LBBB aberration; in V_6 there is no Q wave of any size and no S wave. Other indicators of aberrant ventricular conduction are a QRS width of 0.14 second or less, preceding atrial activity, an initial deflection identical to that of conducted beats in the RBBB pattern, and second-in-the-row anomaly.

REFERENCES

1. Lewis T: Paroxysmal tachycardia, the result of ectopic impulse formation, *Heart* 1:262, 1910.
2. Wellens HJJ, Bär FWHM, Lie KI: The value of the electrocardiogram in the differential diagnosis of a tachycardia with a widened QRS complex, *Am J Med* 64:27, 1978.
3. Sandler IA, Marriott HJL: The differential morphology of anomalous ventricular complexes of RBBB type in lead V_1: ventricular ectopy versus aberration, *Circulation* 31:551, 1965.
4. Kulbertus HE, de Laval-Rutten F, Casters P et al: Vectorcardiographic study of aberrant conduction, *Br Heart J* 38:549, 1976.

5. Spear JF, Moore EN: Supernormal excitability and conduction. In Wellens HJJ, Lie KI, Janse MJ, editors: *The conduction system of the heart: structure, function, and clinical implications,* Philadelphia, 1976, Lea & Febiger.

6. Singer DH, Lazzara R, Hoffman BF: Interrelationships between automaticity and conduction in Purkinje fibers, *Circ Res* 21:537, 1967.

7. Singer KH, Yeh BK, Hoffman BF: Aberration of supraventricular escape beats, *Fed Proc* 23:158, 1967 (abstract).

8. Singer DH, Cohen HC: Aberrancy: electrophysiologic aspects and clinical correlations. In Mandel WJ, editor: *Cardiac arrhythmias,* Philadelphia, 1987, JB Lippincott.

9. Rosenbaum MB: Significance of phase 4 depolarization for clinical electrocardiography, *Eur J Cardiol* 3:253, 1975.

10. Marriott HJL: Differential diagnosis of supraventricular and ventricular tachycardia, *Geriatrics* 25:91, 1970.

11. Wellens HJJ, Bär FWHM, Vanagt EJDM, Brugada P: Medical treatment of ventricular tachycardia: considerations in the selection of patients for surgical treatment, *Am J Cardiol* 49:187, 1982.

12. Gulamhusein S, Yee R, Ko PT, Klein GJ: Electrocardiographic criteria for differentiating aberrancy and ventricular extrasystole in chronic atrial fibrillation: validation by intracardiac recordings, *J Electrocardiol* 18:41, 1985.

13. Kindwall E, Brown J, Josephson ME: Electrocardiographic criteria for ventricular tachycardia in wide complex left bundle branch block morphology tachycardia, *Am J Cardiol* 61:1279, 1988.

14. Wellens HJJ: Preexcitation. In Willerson JT, Cohn JN, editors: *Cardiovascular medicine,* New York, 1995, Churchill Livingstone.

15. Wellens HJJ, Schuilenberg RM, Durrer D: Electrical stimulation of the heart in patients with ventricular tachycardia, *Circulation* 46:216, 1972.

16. Guerot U et al: Tachycardie par re-entree de branch a branche, *Arch Mal Coeur* 67:1, 1974.

17. Wellens HJJ: Pathophysiology of ventricular tachycardia in man, *Arch Intern Med* 68:969, 1975.

18. Denes P, Wu D, Dhingra RC et al: Electrophysiological studies in patients with chronic recurrent ventricular tachycardia, *Circulation,* 54D:229, 1976.

19. Wellens HJJ, Duren DR, Lie KL: Observations on mechanisms of ventricular tachycardia in man, *Circulation* 54:237, 1976.

20. Myerburg RJ, Sung RJ, Gerstenblith G et al: Ventricular ectopic activity after premature atrial beats in acute myocardial infarction, *Br Heart J* 39:1033, 1977.

21. Zipes DP, Foster PR, Troup PJ, Pedersen DH: Atrial induction of ventricular tachycardia: reentry versus triggered automaticity, *Am J Cardiol* 44:1, 1979.

22. Langendorf LR, Pick A, Wintermitz M: Mechanisms of intermittent bigeminy. I. Appearance of ectopic beats dependent upon the length of the ventricular cycle, the "rule of bigeminy," *Circulation* 11:422, 1955.

23. Vera Z et al: His bundle electrography for evaluation of criteria in differentiating ventricular ectopy from aberrancy in atrial fibrillation, *Circulation* 46(suppl II):90, 1972.

24. Gouaux JL, Ashman R: Auricular fibrillation with aberration simulating ventricular paroxysmal tachycardia, *Am Heart J* 34:366, 1947.

25. Moe GK, Mendez C, Han J: Aberrant AV impulse propagation in the dog heart: a study of functional bundle branch block, *Circ Res* 16:261, 1965.

26. Rosenblueth A: Two processes for auriculoventricular and ventriculo-auricular propagation of impulses in the heart, *Am J Physiol* 194:495, 1958.

27. Marriott HJL, Bieza CF: Alarming ventricular acceleration after lidocaine administration, *Chest* 61:682, 1972.

CHAPTER 16

Aberrancy Versus Ectopy

Prevalence of misdiagnosis in broad QRS tachycardia 237
When in doubt use procainamide 237
What cannot be used in the differential diagnosis 238
Value of a baseline 12-lead ECG 238
Steps in the differential diagnosis 238
Importance of obtaining a history 238
Physical signs of AV dissociation 240
ECG signs of AV dissociation 240
ECG signs of VA conduction 241
QRS configuration 243
QRS width 253
Capture beats and fusion beats 253
Concordant pattern 253
Other findings 256

THE GREATEST NUMBER OF ERRORS IN THE DIAGNOSIS OF BROAD QRS TACHYCARdias are made because those responsible strive to prove aberration and are often unaware of the morphologic clues that identify ventricular tachycardia (VT). In addition, T waves are often mistaken for P waves, prompting the diagnosis of supraventricular tachycardia (SVT). A misdiagnosis of VT may result in immediate hemodynamic collapse in the acute stage of therapy; if the patient survives and continues to be misdiagnosed, subsequent mismanagement may result in death.

PREVALENCE OF MISDIAGNOSIS IN BROAD QRS TACHYCARDIA

Akhtar, Shenasa, and Jazayeri et al[1] analyzed the data from 150 consecutive patients with wide QRS tachycardia and found that 122 patients had VT, 21 had SVT with aberration, and 7 had accessory pathway conduction. One of the findings of this study was that only 39 of the 122 patients with VT were correctly diagnosed in the acute setting. The reasons for this shocking discovery were unclear, but several were suggested:

1. There is an erroneous perception that SVT with aberrancy is as common as VT.
2. In most patients presenting with wide complex tachycardia and hemodynamic stability, the clinician wrongly assumes that VT is unlikely.
3. The emergency nature of the clinical setting motivates the clinician to judge quickly rather than to analyze thoroughly the 12-lead electrocardiogram (ECG), obtain a history, and perform a physical examination. Certain findings on physical examination and on the ECG often swiftly provide a correct diagnosis.

WHEN IN DOUBT USE PROCAINAMIDE

When a patient presents with a broad QRS tachycardia, diagnostic errors can be avoided by remaining calm and systematically evaluating the patient. If the patient is in poor hemodynamic condition, cardiovert; otherwise, systematically evaluate the patient's history, the physical signs of AV dissociation, and the ECG signs outlined in this chapter.

Above all, when in doubt about the origin of the tachycardia, do not use verapamil; use intravenous procainamide unless torsades de pointes is suspected.[2] One study observed a 44% incidence (11 out of 25 patients) of severe hemodynamic deterioration after 5 to 10 mg intravenous verapamil was administered for sustained VT; immediate cardioversion was necessary.[3] Under less controlled conditions it is possible that hypotension precipitated by verapamil or other calcium channel blockers may render the arrhythmia impossible to cardiovert.

Do not administer digitalis or verapamil when confronted with a wide QRS tachycardia that is more than 200 beats/min and irregular; administer procainamide.[4] What is probably present is atrial fibrillation with conduction over an accessory pathway. If procainamide does not slow the rate and convert the rhythm, cardiovert and refer for evaluation for radiofrequency ablation.

Although both verapamil and procainamide have negative inotropic effects, procainamide slows the rate of the VT, partially compensating for the fall in blood pressure.[5,6] Procainamide also has advantages for both VT and SVT. In addition to being antifibrillatory and the drug of choice for nonischemic VT,[7] it also slows conduction in accessory pathways and in the retrograde fast AV nodal pathway and thus can terminate both circus movement tachycardia (which uses an accessory pathway) and the common form of AV nodal reentry (which uses a retrograde atrionodal fast pathway and an anterograde slow pathway).

WHAT CANNOT BE USED IN THE DIFFERENTIAL DIAGNOSIS

In the differential diagnosis of broad QRS tachycardia, hemodynamic status, age, and heart rate *should not be used*. VT can occur at all ages and at very rapid rates. Some patients are hemodynamically stable in spite of VT and are hemodynamically compromised during SVT. More emphasis should be placed on the patient's history, physical and ECG findings of AV dissociation, and ECG findings in broad QRS tachycardia than on the patient's age or hemodynamic status.

VALUE OF A BASELINE 12-LEAD ECG

To make a diagnosis on the basis of wave patterns, it is first necessary to record the tachycardia in as many of the 12 leads as possible; all 12 leads are ideal. If the system being used does not have the capability for recording multiple leads, begin sequentially to record leads V_1, V_2, and V_6 for morphologic clues and leads I and II or aV_F for axis clues.

A baseline 12-lead ECG is always advantageous, especially when there is preexisting bundle branch block (BBB) or ECG evidence of previous myocardial infarction. In patients with VT and preexisting BBB (right or left) the QRS pattern during the tachycardia is clearly different from that recorded during sinus rhythm.[1,8] In SVT the pattern is usually identical to that of the sinus rhythm (Figure 16-1).

STEPS IN THE DIFFERENTIAL DIAGNOSIS

- Obtain a history
- Look for the physical and ECG signs of AV dissociation
- Look for the ECG signs of VA conduction
- Evaluate the QRS configuration, width, and axis
- Look for precordial concordance, capture beats, and fusion beats

IMPORTANCE OF OBTAINING A HISTORY

The patient history is helpful in making a correct diagnosis and is essential in the prognosis and in making therapeutic decisions in the patient with VT. Tchou, Young, and Mahmud et al[9] found that the patient's history can be helpful in improving the clinical diagnosis of VT. Their study involved 31 consecutive patients referred for ECG documentation of sustained broad QRS tachycardia. Patients were asked if they have had a prior myocardial infarction and if the symptoms of tachycardia started only after the infarction. A "yes" answer to both questions prompted a diagnosis of VT. Of the 29 patients with VT, 28 were correctly diagnosed through the history alone.

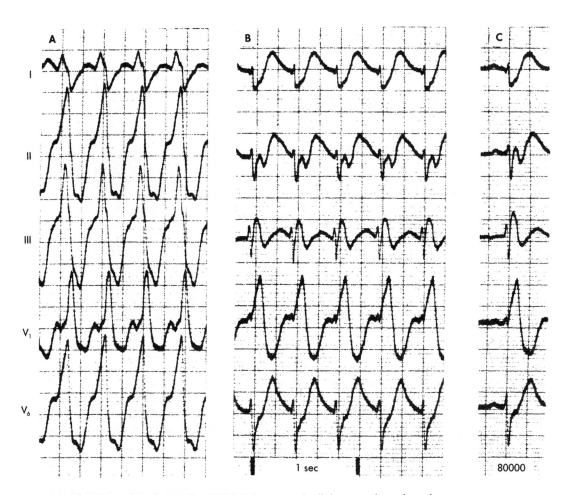

FIGURE 16-1 The value of a baseline ECG is demonstrated. All three panels are from the same patient. **A,** Ventricular tachycardia. **B,** Supraventricular tachycardia. **C,** Sinus rhythm with RBBB in the same patient. Note that the pattern in supraventricular tachycardia is identical to that in sinus rhythm, whereas the pattern in ventricular tachycardia differs from that of sinus rhythm. (From Wellens HJJ, Bär FWHM, Brugada P: Ventricular tachycardia: the clinical problem. In Josephson ME, editor: *Ventricular tachycardia: mechanisms and management,* Mt Kisco, NY, 1982, Futura.)

PHYSICAL SIGNS OF AV DISSOCIATION

The physical signs of VT are based on the presence of atrioventricular (AV) dissociation. The independent beating of the atria and ventricles is present in approximately 50% of VTs; the other half have some form of retrograde conduction to the atria (ventriculoatrial [VA] conduction). It should be noted that junctional tachycardia with aberration may also have AV dissociation when retrograde conduction from the junctional focus is not present. Although several cases of SVT with aberration and AV dissociation have been reported, AV dissociation remains a valid diagnostic clue.[10]

The following are physical signs of AV dissociation:
1. Irregular cannon "a" waves in the jugular pulse
2. Varying intensity of the first heart sound
3. Beat-to-beat changes in systolic blood pressure

Any one of these clues indicates AV dissociation. However, their absence does not rule out VT nor does it rule out AV dissociation. For example, in atrial fibrillation with VT there is AV dissociation without the usual physical or ECG signs.

The Jugular Pulse

During AV dissociation the atria and ventricles beat independently. This beating occasionally coincides so that the atria contract against closed AV valves and cause a reflux of blood up the jugular veins. Such irregular and unpredictable expansions in the pulsation of the jugular pulse are called *cannon a waves*.

The First Heart Sound

The first heart sound is caused by the closing of the AV valves. During sinus rhythm it has a fixed intensity because the position of the leaflets of the AV valves is the same for every ventricular systole. During AV dissociation this position differs from beat to beat, causing a varying intensity of the first heart sound. Other conditions in which there is varying intensity of the first heart sound are complete heart block, AV Wenckebach, and atrial fibrillation.

Systolic Blood Pressure

AV dissociation can be identified at the bedside by using the sphygmomanometer and cuff. During AV dissociation there are beat-to-beat changes in systolic blood pressure (changing Korotkoff sounds). These changes occur because the lapse of time between atrial and ventricular contraction is different with each cycle and results in varying ventricular filling times.

ECG SIGNS OF AV DISSOCIATION

AV dissociation is often missed on the surface ECG. In one study involving 150 patients with wide QRS tachycardia, AV dissociation was present in 67 patients (45%) but could be detected by the surface ECG in only 38 of those patients.[1] The greatest danger is that the clinician mistakes T waves for P waves—a mistake that leads to an incorrect diagnosis and possible lethal consequences.

Finding the Ps

In Figure 16-2 it is easy to recognize the ECG signs of AV dissociation because the ventricular rate is relatively slow (115 beats/min). Four of the P waves in this tracing are obvious and five are not. Note the distortion at the end of the third complex; there is a slur on the downstroke of the QRS complex and a pseudo S wave, both of which do not appear on the previous or following cycle. This is a partially hidden P wave; similar distortions are found in the sixth, ninth, and last beats.

Figure 16-3 provides a nice opportunity to track the sinus P waves through the new onset of VT in leads II and V_1. The little rounded nubbins following each ventricular complex are created by the s-ST-T combination but are often mistaken for P waves simply because they look like P waves. This is often the case in VT; somewhere in one or two leads can be found what looks like a P wave. To act on this "looks-like" urge is to place the patient in jeopardy. Because the independent P waves in a simultaneous lead II are clearly visible in Figure 16-3, the AV dissociation is obvious. This illustration also provides the opportunity to evaluate what P waves actually look like when they distort the ECG in less obvious leads. In the top strip of Figure 16-3, the four P waves that can be seen in V_1 during the tachycardia are marked with arrows. The first distorts the end of the T wave; the second distorts the nadir (lowest point) of the T wave; the third causes the T wave to flatten; and the last distorts the end of the T wave. Although themselves subtle, these P waves are easily seen by comparing one cycle with another and looking for distortions.

On viewing Figure 16-4, the first reaction may be to think that the P waves are the negative T waves following each QRS complex. However, by following the rule and looking for the distortions, the real P wave can be seen in front of the third complex. This distortion is not found in the previous or next cycles. Such a finding is diagnostic of VT. Other P waves are found by the same method. Note how the fourth P wave causes the R wave to be broader than it is in other QRS complexes.

ECG SIGNS OF VA CONDUCTION

During VT, some form of retrograde conduction to the atria occurs 50% of the time; the P′ waves are negative in leads II, III, and aV_F and positive in lead aV_R. However, to visualize this phenomenon on the ECG, VA conduction needs to be sufficiently long so that the P′ waves occur outside the QRS complex. VA conduction with a 1:1 ratio is

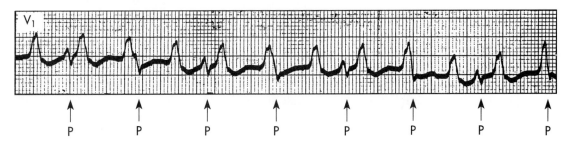

FIGURE 16-2 Ventricular tachycardia with AV dissociation. Note the independent sinus rhythm *(P)*.

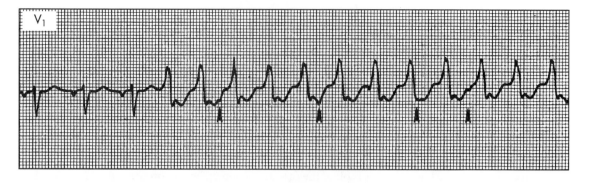

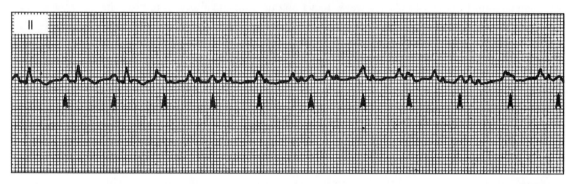

FIGURE 16-3 The onset of ventricular tachycardia with AV dissociation. The P waves that are obvious in lead II *(arrows)* can be seen in only four places in the concurrently recorded V₁ tracing *(arrows).* (From Wagner GS, Waugh RA, Ramo BW: *Cardiac arrhythmias,* New York, 1983, Churchill Livingstone.)

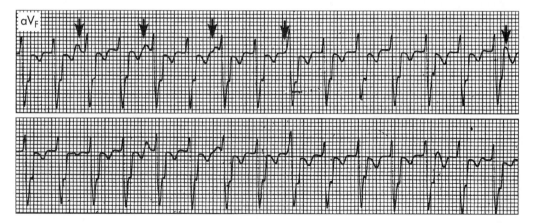

FIGURE 16-4 Ventricular tachycardia with AV dissociation. The P waves that can be seen are indicated with arrows. Notice that these waves are found because of the distortion they make in one cycle that is not found in another. The most subtle of these distortions occurs at the fourth arrow, where a hidden P wave causes an r wave to be slightly wider than those seen in the other cycles.

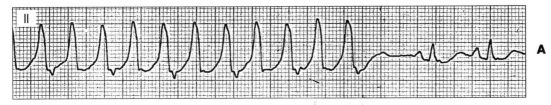

FIGURE 16-5 Ventricular tachycardia with 2:1 retrograde conduction. **A,** In lead II a negative P′ wave distorts every other T wave. (Figure 16-5 continued on p. 244.)

present in one fourth to one third of patients with VT at rates of less than 180 beats/min (without drugs). However, VA conduction is uncommon when the rate is more than 200 beats/min.[1]

Figure 16-5 illustrates VT with 2:1 retrograde conduction. In Figure 16-5, *A,* it is fairly easy to spot the negative P′ waves in every other T wave in lead II. In the 12-lead ECG shown in Figure 16-5, *B,* the 2:1 retrograde conduction can be seen only on lead aV_R, where a positive P′ wave is very prominent in every other T wave. A positive P′ in this lead indicates retrograde conduction. Strangely enough, the tracings shown in Figure 16-5 were originally published as an example of AV dissociation with the comment that the "AV dissociation is only recognizable to the expert eye in lead aV_R."[11] However, when there is VA conduction, the atria do not beat independently; they are under the control of the ventricles, and AV dissociation is *not* present.

Figure 16-6 illustrates VT with 5:4 retrograde Wenckebach conduction. The first clue for this diagnosis is the fact that two very visible P waves in front of the fourth and fifth beat show up repeatedly in front of every fourth and fifth beat (group beating). The fifth beat is not followed by a P wave; the T wave of that beat can be compared with other T waves to find those slight distortions that are P waves.

QRS CONFIGURATION

Two sets of rules help differentiate aberrancy from ectopy on the basis of QRS configuration. One set of rules applies to the V_1-positive wide complex tachycardia and uses leads V_1 and sometimes V_6. The other set of rules applies to the V_1-negative wide complex tachycardia* and uses leads V_1, V_2, and V_6. In applying the morphologic rules, it is important to understand that the clues specific for one type of tachycardia cannot be used for the other. For example, a little q wave in lead V_6 could mean either VT or SVT depending on the shape of the complex in V_1. If V_1 is upright, a little q in V_6 indicates SVT; VT is indicated if V_1 is negative.

WARNING: QRS patterns can be misleading if the entire clinical setting is not consid-

---

*In the medical literature the V_1-positive broad QRS complex is referred to as "right bundle branch block (RBBB)" or "RBBB-like" and the V_1-negative broad QRS complex as "left bundle branch block (LBBB)" or "LBBB-like." These terms do not imply the mechanism or precise QRS patterns; they imply merely the polarity of the QRS complex in V_1 (i.e., the RBBB pattern is positive in V_1 and the LBBB pattern is negative).

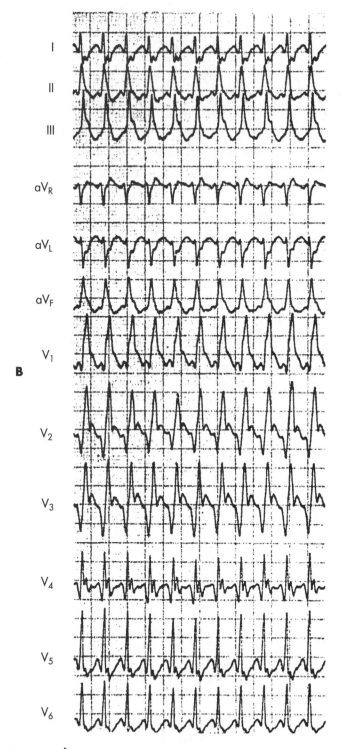

FIGURE 16-5, CONT'D   B, In the 12-lead ECG the retrograde P′ wave is fairly obvious in lead aV$_R$; it is the positive deflection that distorts every other T wave. (**B** from Brugada P, Brugada J, Mont L et al: A new approach to the differential diagnosis of a regular tachycardia with a wide QRS complex, *Circulation* 83:1649, 1991.)

ered. For example, SVT is morphologically identical to VT when an accessory pathway connects the atria and ventricle (Wolff-Parkinson-White syndrome) and when the patient is taking drugs that slow intraventricular conduction. Likewise, VT can be mistaken for SVT in cases of digitalis toxicity (fascicular VT), idiopathic VT, and bundle branch reentry VT. Thus an understanding of the clinical setting (e.g., drugs being taken, history of myocardial infarction, cardiomyopathy, presence or absence of heart disease) is critical. In such situations this information is not always available, which limits the value of the morphologic criteria.[1] On the other hand, the informed clinician who can evaluate the QRS configuration in light of the entire clinical spectrum often makes a stunning diagnosis and dramatically improves the quality of life for a patient. Chapter 17 addresses these important "other broads" (VTs that look like SVT and SVTs that look like VT).

V_1-Positive Broad QRS Tachycardia
ECG signs of supraventricular tachycardia

1. Triphasic pattern of RBBB (rSR′ in V_1 and qRs in V_6)
2. QRS complex <0.14 second
3. R:S ratio in V_6 >1 (R > S)

   NOTE: Certain types of VT may also have the triphasic pattern in V_1 and the relatively narrow QRS complex (i.e., fascicular VT, left ventricular idiopathic VT, and bundle branch reentry VT) (see Chapter 17).

ECG signs of ventricular tachycardia

1. Monophasic or diphasic complex (R, qR, or RS) in lead V_1[10,12,13]
2. The "rabbit ear" sign in V_1 (Rr′)
3. An R:S ratio in V_6 <1

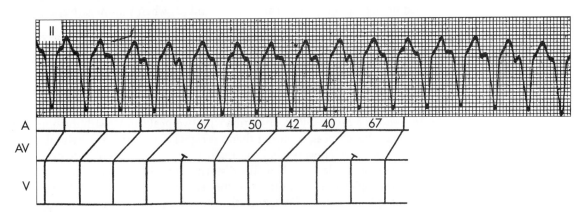

FIGURE 16-6 Ventricular tachycardia with 5:4 retrograde Wenckebach conduction. The laddergram helps identify the retrograde P′ waves. The P′ waves that are very apparent are the ones that produce pseudo r waves in the fifth, ninth, tenth, and fifteenth beats. These beats are not themselves followed by retrograde conduction and provide an opportunity to see what the T wave looks like when it is not distorted by a retrograde P′ wave.

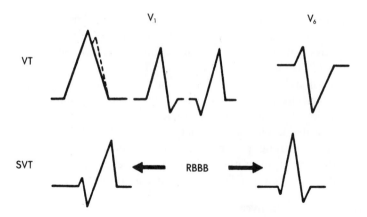

FIGURE 16-7 When V_1 is positive, ventricular ectopy is indicated in that lead by a monophasic or biphasic complex or by the rabbit ear clue (left peak taller than the right). RBBB aberration is indicated by triphasic patterns—rSR′ in V_1 and qRs in V_6. *VT,* Ventricular tachycardia; *SVT,* supraventricular tachycardia. (From Conover M: *Understanding electrocardiography,* ed 7, St Louis, 1996, Mosby.)

In 1970 Marriott[13] reported on the studies of Gozensky and Thorne,[14] describing the now widely accepted "rabbit ear clue" as an aid in distinguishing ventricular ectopy from aberration: When there are two positive peaks in V_1, ectopy is indicated if the left peak is taller. Gozensky and Thorne's findings were later confirmed by Wellens,[6] who found the taller left rabbit ear configuration only in patients with VT. Additional findings from that group demonstrated (1) when the right rabbit ear is the taller peak in V_1, it is not helpful in distinguishing ectopy from aberration; and (2) when V_1 is negative, a q or Q in V_6 indicates VT.

Figure 16-7 compares the patterns of RBBB in V_1 and V_6 with those of ventricular ectopy. The first two beats in Figure 16-8 are sinus rhythm with the triphasic pattern of RBBB in leads V_1 (rSR′) and V_6 (qRs) followed by an abrupt transition to a V_1-positive VT. Note the two positive peaks in V_1, with the left peak taller than the right. Also of note is the R:S ratio in V_6 of less than 1.

Figure 16-9 shows a broad QRS tachycardia with two peaks in V_1 with the opposite configuration (i.e., the left peak is shorter than the right). This sign is not helpful; clues must be sought elsewhere. However, in this case there is no need to look far—there are signs of AV dissociation in lead V_1. Note the distortion (a P wave) that occurs in front of the first QRS complex but not in front of the second. Other signs of VT in Figure 16-9 are the monophasic R in V_1, AV dissociation (best seen in aV_R), the excessive width of the QRS complex, and an R:S ratio in V_6 that is less than 1.

In Figure 16-9, the shape of the QRS complex in V_1 is what Moulton, Medcalf, and Lazzara[15] refer to as "ugly" and indicative of a dilated and globally hypokinetic left ven-

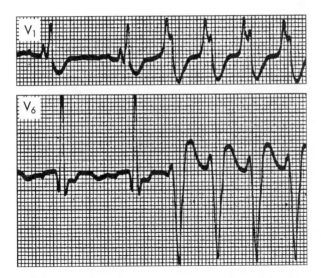

FIGURE 16-8 Sinus rhythm with RBBB (first two beats) followed by ventricular tachycardia with the rabbit ear clue (left peak taller than the right).

tricle in a nonspecifically diseased heart. A smoother, narrower beat reflects normal heart size and normal or near-normal systolic function despite the presence of underlying disease. "Ugliness" as described by these investigators is measured from the nadir of the notch to the peak of the R wave (Figure 16-10).

An rS pattern in V_6 favors VT. A left axis per se is one of the causes of an R:S ratio of less than 1. Therefore this pattern is more likely to be seen in the broad QRS tachycardias with left axis.

Axis

When V_1 is positive the only diagnostic axis for VT is that of -90 degrees to ± 180 degrees (sometimes also called "no man's land"; indeterminate, meaning extreme left or extreme right; or the northwest quadrant). Such an axis does not occur in SVT; it is an apical focus and therefore reliably distinguishes VT from SVT with aberration or accessory pathway conduction. In the V_1-positive broad QRS tachycardia, right or left axis deviation is supportive of VT but also can occur during SVT.

V_1-Negative Broad QRS Tachycardia
ECG signs of supraventricular tachycardia

1. Small, narrow r wave in V_1 and/or V_2 during LBBB aberration, if an r wave is present
2. Swift smooth S downstroke in V_1 and V_2, reflecting conduction in the His-Purkinje system
3. Early S nadir in V_1 and V_2, ≤ 0.06 second from the onset of the QRS complex

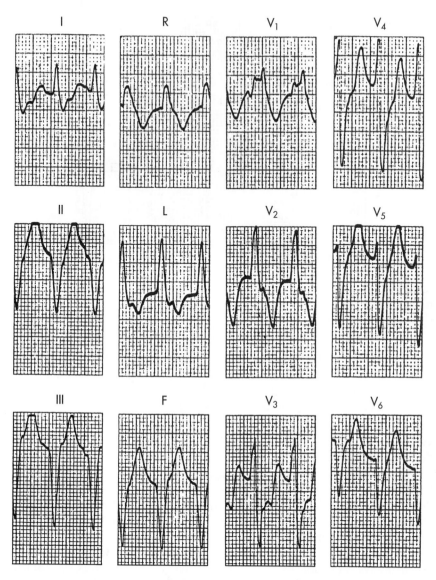

FIGURE 16-9 Ventricular tachycardia. The QRS pattern in V_1 is not helpful (left peak is shorter). The diagnosis is made because of the presence of AV dissociation (note the P wave in front of the first beat in V_1); another P wave may be distorting the initial peak of the QRS complex in the second beat. Supportive findings are the width of the QRS complex (0.16 second) and left axis deviation.

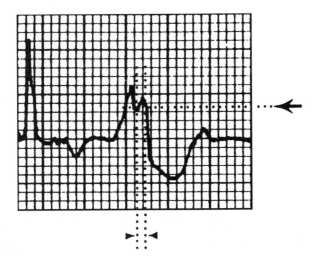

FIGURE 16-10 Method of measuring the notch in the ventricular ectopic beat. Draw a horizontal line at the level of the lowest point in the notch. Make vertical lines at the two peaks. A distance of at least 0.04 second indicates a dilated, globally hypokinetic left ventricle. (From Moulton KP, Medcalf T, Lazzara R: Premature ventricular complex morphology: a marker for left ventricular structure and function, *Circulation* 81:1245, 1990).

ECG signs of ventricular tachycardia

1. Wide R (V_1 and/or V_2); seen in more than 90% of VTs associated with inferior infarction and in only 25% of tachycardias associated with anterior infarction, in which a QS complex is more common[16]
2. Slurred S downstroke (V_1 and/or V_2); sensitivity of only 36% and usually occurs in anterior infarction
3. Delayed S nadir (V_1 and/or V_2); the distance from the onset of the QRS complex to the lowest point of the S wave (its nadir) is more than 0.06 second; seen in two thirds of patients having V_1-negative VT
4. Any Q in V_6; confirms VT, but *only* if the complex is mainly negative in V_1; this clue cannot be applied to the tachycardia that is positive in V_1

The wide R wave in V_1 and/or V_2 with an inferior axis as a sign of ventricular ectopy in normal hearts was first described in 1969 by Rosenbaum[17] and again in 1972 by Swanick, La Camera, and Marriott.[18] In 1988 Kindwall, Brown, and Josephson[19] published data supporting this finding plus the three more clues found in V_1, V_2, and V_6 for the V_1-negative broad QRS complex and important data regarding left axis deviation. The four clues discussed here have greatly improved the accuracy of using QRS patterns to identify VT.

The signs seen in leads V_1 and V_2 are diagrammatically illustrated in Figure 16-11. The absence of all four of the previously listed signs is highly suggestive of SVT. Even in the setting of preexisting BBB, the broad R and slurred or notched downstroke are characteristic of VT.[20,21] A diagnosis of SVT cannot be made if even one of the signs is present.

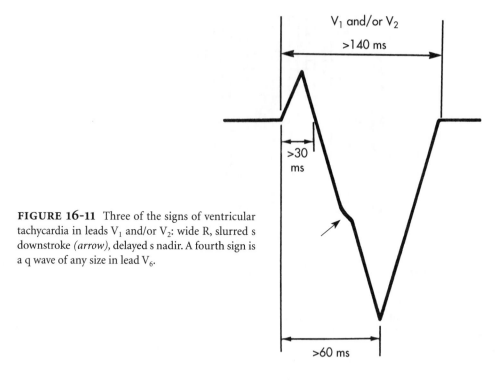

FIGURE 16-11 Three of the signs of ventricular tachycardia in leads V_1 and/or V_2: wide R, slurred s downstroke *(arrow)*, delayed s nadir. A fourth sign is a q wave of any size in lead V_6.

Table 16-1 lists the specificity, sensitivity, and predictive accuracy of each of these four findings. It is important to use both V_1 and V_2, especially when V_1 looks like SVT. The complex may have all of the signs of SVT in V_1, but in V_2 there will be a tell-tale sign of VT. Initial forces are often isoelectric in V_1, which leads to the misclassification of tracings. The criterion most susceptible to error is measurement of the distance to the nadir of the S wave because this point is sometimes so deep that it goes off the graph paper and cannot be seen and because of the inherent limitation in measuring intervals at the paper speed used clinically (25 mm/sec).[19]

Figure 16-12 compares the patterns of LBBB and V_1-negative VT. Atrial fibrillation with LBBB is seen in the top tracing and in the first half of the bottom tracing. Suddenly the rhythm becomes absolutely regular—this is the first sign of AV dissociation during atrial fibrillation. The broad r wave in lead MCL_1 identifies the VT.

Limitations[19]

1. LBBB in sinus tachycardia or atrial flutter with the same pattern as VT (e.g., broad R and slurred downstroke in V_1 and/or V_2). In such a case the sinus rhythm tracing without the tachycardia would expose the problem.
2. Antidromic circus movement tachycardia (using an accessory pathway in the antero-grade direction). This mechanism produces a tachycardia identical in shape to VT.
3. Antiarrhythmic drugs that slow conduction, possibly producing a QRS complex that fits the morphologic description for VT. These drugs may broaden the R wave and produce a delayed S nadir in V_1 or V_2, but a Q wave in V_6 would not be affected.

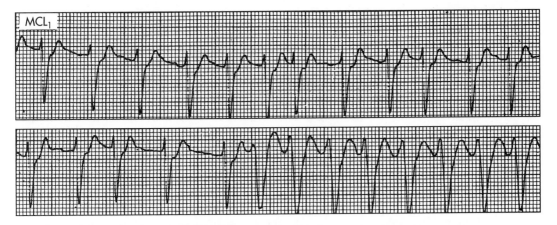

FIGURE 16-12 The pattern of atrial fibrillation and LBBB aberration is observed in the top tracing and in the first five beats of the bottom tracing. Note the narrow r wave and the swift clean downstroke to the S wave. A change suddenly occurs in the bottom strip; the R wave is much broader (a sign of ventricular tachycardia) and the rhythm becomes regular (a sign of AV dissociation in atrial fibrillation).

TABLE 16-1   ECG SIGNS OF VT WHEN MAINLY NEGATIVE IN V_1 (USING LEADS V_1, V_2, AND V_6)

CRITERIA	SPECIFICITY (%)	SENSITIVITY (%)	PREDICTIVE ACCURACY (%)
R >30 ms in V_1 or V_2	100	36	100
Any Q in V_6	96	55	98
>60 ms to S nadir in V_1 or V_2	96	63	98
Notched downstroke in S or QS in V_1 or V_2	96	36	97
Combined criteria	89	100	96

Modified from Kindwall E, Brown J, Josephson ME: Electrocardiographic criteria for ventricular tachycardia in wide complex left bundle branch block morphology tachycardia, *Am J Cardiol* 61:1279, 1988.

Axis

The two diagnostic QRS axes in the V_1-negative broad QRS tachycardia are "no man's land" and right axis deviation. Left axis deviation can occur with equal frequency in VT and SVT and therefore is of no help in the diagnosis.[19] A right axis when V_1 is negative is a diagnostic combination for VT. Akhtar, Shenasa, and Jazayeri et al[1] found that the combination of right axis and a V_1-negative complex (Figure 16-13) was seen only in VT (9 patients). This fact was first reported by Rosenbaum in 1969.[17]

Clinical Correlations of Axis[22]

- **Previous myocardial infarction.** When VT occurs in patients who have had a previous myocardial infarction, the QRS axis in the frontal plane is usually abnormal and often superior, that is, left or "no man's land" (negative complex in aV_F). This fact is especially true when V_1 is positive.
- **Idiopathic VT.** In the normal heart, VT can have a normal axis, but most commonly there is a marked left or right axis deviation (see Chapter 17). When V_1 looks like LBBB aberration (narrow r, smooth S), the axis is inferior (normal or right; aV_F positive). When V_1 looks like RBBB aberration (rSR′), the axis is superior (left or "no man's land"; aVF negative).
- **Preexisting BBB.** A markedly abnormal axis may occur in patients with preexisting BBB who have SVT.
- **Accessory pathways.** Marked left axis deviation (left of − 30 degrees) may be seen in SVT with conduction over a right-sided or posteroseptal accessory pathway; marked right axis deviation may be seen in SVT with conduction over a left lateral accessory pathway.
- **Class Ic drugs.** Patients taking class Ic drugs can have SVT with an axis to the left of − 30 degrees.

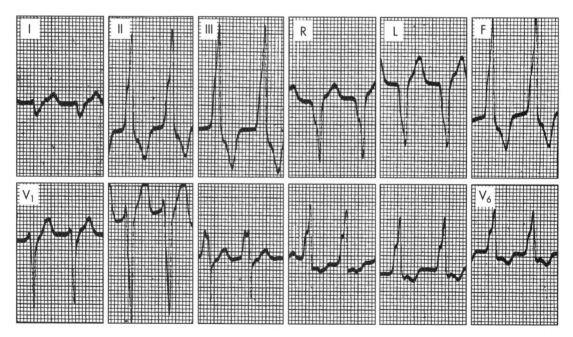

FIGURE 16-13 Ventricular tachycardia is identified by the broad r wave and the delayed S nadir in V_1 and V_2. The right axis deviation associated with this pattern is diagnostic of ventricular tachycardia.

QRS WIDTH

In the broad QRS tachycardia, a QRS complex of more than 0.14 second in duration is highly suggestive of VT. In a study of 100 cases of SVT with aberration, Wellens[22] showed a QRS complex width of ≤0.14 second to be present in all patients. He and his colleagues also examined 100 cases of VT and found that 59% had a QRS duration of more than 0.14 second. Akhtar, Shenasa, and Jazayeri et al[1] found "excellent" diagnostic accuracy for VT when they used a criterion for QRS duration of more than 0.14 second with a V_1-positive pattern and more than 0.16 second with a V_1-negative pattern.

CAPTURE BEATS AND FUSION BEATS

Capture beats and fusion beats occur during VT when a sinus impulse is conducted into the ventricle and either entirely captures the ventricle or collides with the ventricular ectopic impulse (fusion), which is discharged at approximately the same time. Either case results in a narrower beat. Figure 16-14 is an example of capture during VT. The capture beat is recognized because it ends a shorter cycle; the sinus P wave in front of it can usually be seen. Other signs of VT in this example are a broad r wave in leads V_1 and V_2 and a slurred S downstroke in V_2.

Figure 16-15 illustrates ventricular fusion during VT. A fusion beat or capture beat is strong evidence of VT but is not diagnostic. Fusion beats and capture beats are

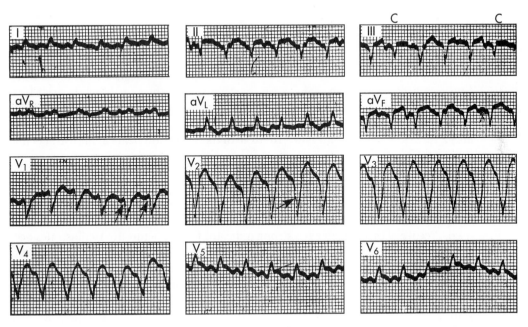

FIGURE 16-14 Capture *(C)* during ventricular tachycardia. The sinus P wave can be seen in front of the two captured beats in lead III. Note that capture is easily identified because it ends a shorter cycle. Leads V_1 and V_2 contain additional signs of ventricular tachycardia (broad r and delayed S nadir in both leads and slurred S downstroke in V_2 *[arrow]*).

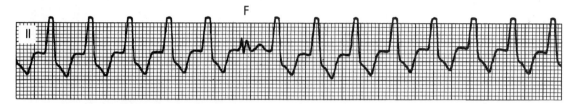

FIGURE 16-15 Ventricular fusion *(F)* during ventricular tachycardia.

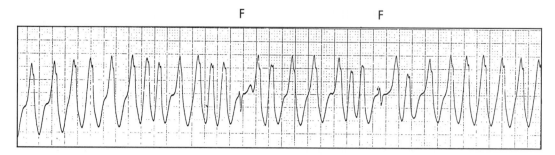

FIGURE 16-16 Two ventricular fusion beats *(F)* during atrial fibrillation with AV conduction down an accessory pathway (fast, broad, irregular rhythm). In this case, fusion occurs after two atrial impulses have entered the ventricles almost simultaneously via the AV node and the accessory pathway.

also seen in atrial fibrillation with conduction over an accessory pathway (a broad QRS tachycardia that is morphologically identical to VT). Two such fusion beats are shown in Figure 16-16. In the same clinical setting, capture beats are common when procainamide is given, in which case the accessory pathway is blocked or at least compromised (Figure 16-17). Fusion beats may also occur when an end-diastolic ventricular beat fires during sinus tachycardia with BBB. This phenomenon is probably a rare occurrence, but Figure 16-18 with its two fusion beats demonstrates that it is a possibility.

CONCORDANT PATTERN

When the precordial leads consist of complexes that are entirely negative or entirely positive during a broad QRS tachycardia, the term *precordial concordance* is used. Precordial concordance is a strong indicator for VT. Figure 16-19 illustrates negative precordial concordance, which reflects a focus in the anteroapical left ventricle. Negative precordial concordance is not possible in preexcited SVT because there is no accessory pathway location in which anterograde conduction would produce completely negative QRS complexes in the precordial leads, but it is sometimes seen with LBBB.

Positive precordial concordance results when ventricular activation originates in the posterobasal left ventricle. Thus such a pattern can result from both VT with a focus in that region (Figure 16-20) and from SVT with an accessory pathway in that region (Fig-

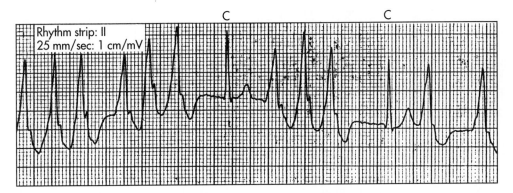

FIGURE 16-17 Two capture beats *(C)* during atrial fibrillation with AV conduction down an accessory pathway. The patient has just received procainamide, which is blocking the accessory pathway, slowing the ventricular rate, and allowing impulses to enter the ventricles via the AV node.

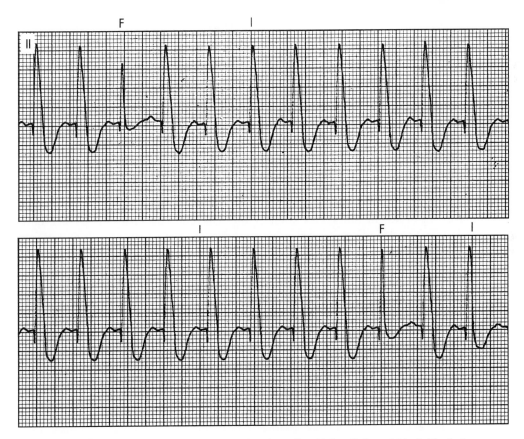

FIGURE 16-18 Two fusion beats *(F)* during sinus tachycardia with bundle branch block. The fusion is the result of a ventricular beat firing when the sinus impulse has entered the ventricles.

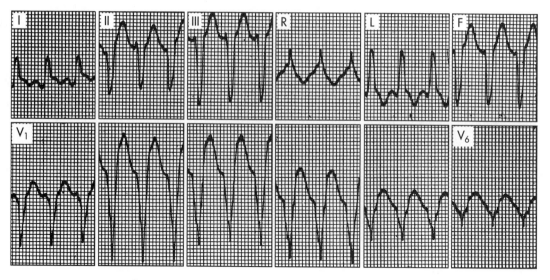

FIGURE 16-19 Negative precordial concordance, which is diagnostic of ventricular tachycardia from an apical focus. Note that the complexes across the precordial leads have no positive component.

ure 16-21). However, because positive precordial concordance caused by SVT is rare, the finding should raise the level of suspicion for VT. Other signs of VT are seen in this illustration: a monophasic R wave in V_1 and AV dissociation in aV_R.

OTHER FINDINGS

Swanick, La Camera, and Marriott[18] observed that two thirds of the examples of right ventricular ectopic beats under investigation had a negative QRS complex in lead I—a polarity not found in any of the examined examples of LBBB. This observation would reflect one of Rosenbaum's three findings[17] in right ventricular ectopy (right axis deviation), or it could indicate an axis in "no-man's-land," another strong indicator of ventricular ectopy.

In 1991 Brugada, Brugada, and Mont et al[11] pointed out that a duration of more than 100 ms from the onset of R to the nadir of the S wave in the precordial leads is an indication of VT. However, this criteria has limited usefulness because such a duration may also occur in SVT with the following conditions:[22]

- Conduction over an accessory pathway
- Administration of drugs that slow intraventricular conduction
- Preexisting BBB, most especially preexisting LBBB

Steurer et al[23] found the following criteria to be sensitive and highly specific for the differential diagnosis between VT in coronary artery disease and preexcited regular tachycardia. These criteria favor VT:

1. Presence of predominantly negative QRS complexes in the precordial leads V_4 to V_6
2. Presence of a QR complex in one or more of the precordial leads V_2 to V_6
3. AV relation different from 1:1 (more QRS complexes than P waves)

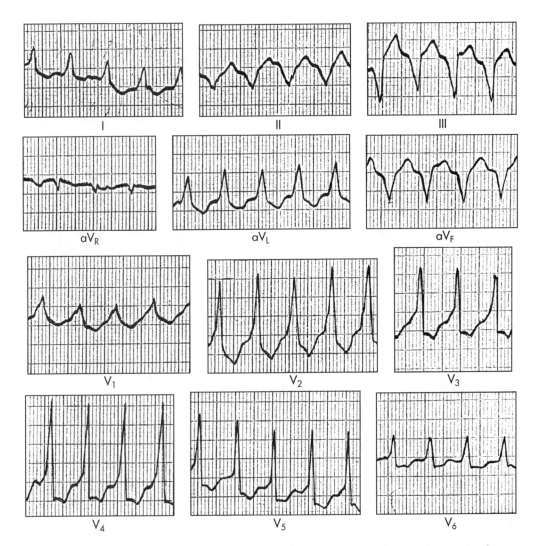

FIGURE 16-20 Positive precordial concordance, which is supportive but not diagnostic of ventricular tachycardia from the posterior base of the left ventricle. Note that the complexes across the precordial leads have no positive component. The other signs of ventricular tachycardia are a monophasic R wave in lead V_1 and AV dissociation. Note the negative P wave at the beginning of aV_R and again distorting the second T wave. (From Stein E: *The electrocardiogram,* Philadelphia, 1976, WB Saunders.)

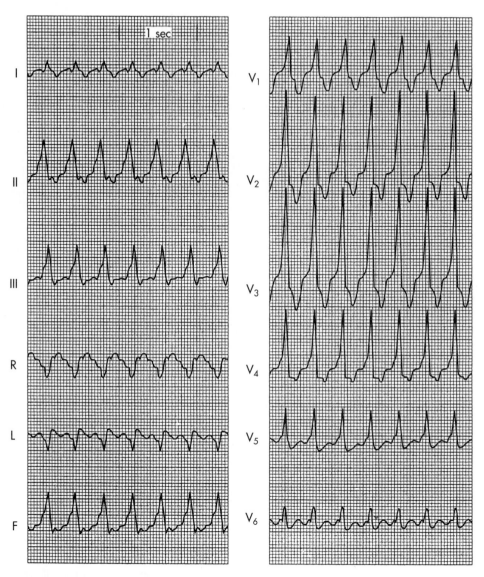

FIGURE 16-21 Positive precordial concordance caused by atrial flutter with 2:1 conduction over a posterior left ventricular accessory pathway. (From Wellens HJJ, Conover M: *The ECG in emergency decision making,* Philadelphia, 1992, WB Saunders.)

SUMMARY

When differentiating between aberrant ventricular conduction and ventricular ectopy it is important to keep the following points in mind:

1. VT is more common than SVT with aberration.
2. VT is commonly associated with structural heart disease and previous myocardial infarction.
3. When in doubt do not use verapamil; use procainamide.
4. A correct diagnosis can generally be made from the surface ECG when all criteria are applied.

The following are highly reliable ECG criteria for VT:

- AV dissociation
- Fusion beats
- Capture beats
- QRS duration >0.14 second in V_1-positive patterns
- QRS duration >0.16 second in V_1-negative patterns
- Precordial QRS concordance
- Axis of -90 degrees to ± 180 degrees
- Right axis deviation in V_1-negative broad QRS tachycardia
- QRS pattern in tachycardia that differs from that in sinus rhythm with BBB
- In V_1-negative patterns, a broad R, slurred S downstroke, and delayed S nadir in V_1 and/or V_2, or a Q wave in V_6
- In V_1-positive patterns, a monophasic R or biphasic complex (qR; RS) or a taller left "rabbit ear" in V_1

The following are highly reliable ECG criteria for SVT:

- QRS duration 0.14 second or less in V_1-positive patterns
- QRS duration 0.16 second or less in V_1-negative patterns
- QRS pattern in tachycardia same as that in sinus rhythm with BBB
- In V_1-negative patterns, a narrow r and clean S downstroke in V_1 and V_2
- In V_1-positive patterns, a triphasic pattern in V_1

REFERENCES

1. Akhtar M, Shenasa M, Jazayeri M et al: Wide QRS complex tachycardia: reappraisal of a common clinical problem, *Ann Intern Med* 109:905, 1988.
2. Wellens HJJ, Bär FW, Vanagt EJ et al: The differentiation between ventricular tachycardia and supraventricular tachycardia with aberrant conduction: the value of the 12-lead electrocardiogram. In Wellens HJJ, Kulbertus HE, editors: *What's new in electrocardiography?* The Hague, 1981, Martinus Nijhoff.
3. Buxton AE, Marchlinski FE, Doherty JU, Josephson ME: Hazards of intravenous verapamil for sustained ventricular tachycardia, *Am J Cardiol* 59:1107, 1987.
4. Wellens HJJ, Conover M: *The ECG in emergency decision making*, Philadelphia, 1992, WB Saunders.
5. Marchlinski FE, Buxton AE, Vassallo JA et al: Comparative electrophysiologic effects of intravenous and oral procainamide in patients with sustained ventricular arrhythmias, *J Am Coll Cardiol* 4:1247, 1984.
6. Wellens HJJ: The wide QRS tachycardia, *Ann Intern Med* 104:879, 1986.

7. Gorgels AP, van den Dool A, Hofs A et al: Procainamide is superior to lidocaine in terminating sustained ventricular tachycardia, *Circulation* 80(II-652):2590, 1989.

8. Wellens HJJ, Bär FWHM, Brugada P: Ventricular tachycardia: the clinical problem. In Josephson ME, editor: *Ventricular tachycardia: mechanisms and management,* Mount Kisco, NY, 1982, Futura.

9. Tchou P, Young P, Mahmud R et al: Useful clinical criteria for the diagnosis of ventricular tachycardia, *Am J Med* 84:53, 1988.

10. Wellens HJJ, Bär FWHM, Lie KI: The value of the electrocardiogram in the differential diagnosis of a tachycardia with a widened QRS complex, *Am J Med* 64:27, 1978.

11. Brugada P, Brugada J, Mont L et al: A new approach to the differential diagnosis of a regular tachycardia with a wide QRS complex, *Circulation* 83:1649, 1991.

12. Wellens HJJ, Bär FW, Vanagt EJ et al: Medical treatment of ventricular tachycardia: considerations in the selection of patients for surgical treatment, *Am J Cardiol* 49:186, 1982.

13. Marriott HJL: Differential diagnosis of supraventricular and ventricular tachycardia, *Geriatrics* 25:91, 1970.

14. Gozensky C, Thorne D: Rabbit ears: an aid in distinguishing ventricular ectopy from aberration, *Heart Lung* 3:634, 1975.

15. Moulton KP, Medcalf T, Lazzara R: Premature ventricular complex morphology: a marker for left ventricular structure and function, *Circulation* 81:1245, 1990.

16. Josephson ME, Wellens HJJ: Differential diagnosis of supraventricular tachycardia, *Cardiol Clin* 8:411, 1990.

17. Rosenbaum MB: Classification of ventricular extrasystoles according to form, *J Electrocardiol* 2:269, 1969.

18. Swanick EJ, La Camera F, Marriott HJL: Morphologic features of right ventricular ectopic beats, *Am J Cardiol* 30:888, 1972.

19. Kindwall E, Brown J, Josephson ME: Electrocardiographic criteria for ventricular tachycardia in wide complex left bundle branch block morphology tachycardia, *Am J Cardiol* 61:1279, 1988.

20. Josephson ME, Horowitz LN, Waxman HL, Cain ME: Sustained ventricular tachycardia: role of the 12-lead electrocardiogram in localizing site of origin, *Circulation* 64:257, 1978.

21. Miller JM, Marchlinski FE, Buxton AR, Josephson ME: Relationship between the 12-lead electrocardiogram during ventricular tachycardia and endocardial site of origin in patients with coronary artery disease, *Circulation* 77:759, 1988.

22. Wellens HJJ: Wide QRS tachycardia. In Willerson JT, Cohn JN, editors: *Cardiovascular medicine,* New York, 1995, Churchill Livingstone.

23. Steurer G, Gürsoy S, Frey B et al: The differential diagnosis on the electrocardiogram between ventricular tachycardia and preexcited tachycardia, *Clin Cardiol* 17:306, 1994.

CHAPTER 17

The Other Broads

Accessory pathways 261
Mahaim fibers 262
Supraventricular
tachycardias that look
like ventricular
tachycardia 262
Atrial fibrillation with an
accessory pathway 262
Atrial fibrillation with
multiple accessory
pathways 269
Atrial flutter with an
accessory pathway
269
Antidromic circus
movement tachycardia
269
Circus movement
tachycardia with two
accessory pathways
274
Broad QRS paroxysmal
supraventricular
tachycardia using
nodoventricular fibers
274
Ventricular tachycardias
that look like
supraventricular
tachycardia 276
Idiopathic ventricular
tachycardia 276
Idiopathic right ventric-
ular tachycardia 279
Idiopathic left ventricular
tachycardia 281
Bundle branch reentrant
ventricular tachycardia
282
Fascicular ventricular
tachycardia 286

THERE ARE EXCEPTIONS TO THE RULES FOR THE USE OF QRS PATTERNS IN DIFFER-entiating ventricular tachycardia (VT) from supraventricular tachycardia (SVT). Patients with Wolff-Parkinson-White (WPW) syndrome, concealed accessory pathways, or Mahaim fibers who develop SVT have a QRS pattern identical to that of VT. Conversely, certain types of VT have exactly the same QRS pattern as SVT with aberration.

ACCESSORY PATHWAYS

An accessory pathway is an extra muscle bundle composed of working myocardial tissue that forms a connection between the atria and ventricles outside the conduction system. Any supraventricular tachycardia that uses an accessory pathway or nodoven-tricular Mahaim fiber for AV conduction will have a broad QRS complex that is identical in shape to VT.

The most common locations of accessory pathways are the left free wall (50%) and posterior septum (30%). Right free wall pathways occur in 13% of patients; anterosep-tal locations are the least common (7%).[1] Surgical experience has demonstrated path-ways located at any depth between the valve annuli and the epicardium. Experience with radiofrequency ablation suggests that the majority of left-sided pathways are subepicardial (juxtaannular), whereas right-sided pathways tend to be more variable in depth, with some closer to the epicardium and others midway between the epicardium and endocardium.[2] They may be single or multiple, active or inactive, and may possess the capability to conduct both anterogradely and retrogradely or only retrogradely (con-cealed accessory pathway).[3]

In 60% to 70% of patients with an accessory pathway the diagnosis can be made from the surface ECG when the patient is in sinus rhythm (overt WPW syndrome). The remainder of cases (30% to 40%) are concealed or latent; the ECG during sinus rhythm does not have a delta wave as does the overt syndrome. In such cases the diagnosis can be made from rhythm strips obtained during the tachycardia. The concealed accessory pathway can conduct only retrogradely; thus the diagnosis is made during paroxysmal supraventricular tachycardia (PSVT). The latent accessory pathway is capable of both anterograde and retrograde conduction. Such patients may present with either PSVT or atrial fibrillation with a ventricular rhythm that is identical in pattern to VT with a fo-cus at the base of the heart (accessory pathway insertion).

High-risk patients are identified not from the size of the delta wave but from the duration of the refractory period of the accessory pathway in the anterograde direction. This duration varies considerably among patients and is influenced by sympathetic tone.[4] The following list contains the noninvasive ways of estimating the adequacy of the refractory period of the accessory pathway in the anterograde direction, which protects the patient from excessive ventricular rates should atrial fibrillation develop[5]:

1. Preexcitation is intermittent.
2. Preexcitation disappears (not just lessens) with exercise (secondary to the catecholamines).[6] Wellens[1] advises care in this interpretation in that sympathetic stimulation during exercise speeds up AV nodal conduction and may diminish the area of preexcitation. Concurrent multiple ECG leads should be recorded, with attention given to the ECG after exercise. In cases of exercise-induced block in the accessory pathway, a sudden marked change in the ECG occurs when conduction through this pathway is resumed.
3. The PR interval and QRS complex normalize following intravenous (IV) procainamide.[7]

NOTE: Before using procainamide for this purpose, one should become acquainted with the references that advise ruling out hypertrophic cardiomyopathy by echocardiogram.[8] Because procainamide prolongs the refractory period of both the accessory pathway and the His-Purkinje system, it is given in a setting in which complete heart block can be managed.[1]

Mahaim Fibers

Mahaim fibers are anomalous tracts between the lower AV node or His bundle and the ventricles. There are two main anatomic types of Mahaim fibers: *nodoventricular* fibers, which arise from the AV node itself and insert into the ventricle, and *fasciculoventricular* fibers, which arise from the His bundle or bundle branches. The nodoventricular fibers produce an SVT with a pattern identical to that of VT.

SUPRAVENTRICULAR TACHYCARDIAS THAT LOOK LIKE VENTRICULAR TACHYCARDIA
Atrial Fibrillation with an Accessory Pathway
ECG features

- **Rate.** Fast, usually more than 180 beats/min
- **QRS complex.** Broad; pattern is that of VT
- **Rhythm.** Irregular

Figure 17-1 is a 12-lead ECG from a patient with atrial fibrillation and AV conduction via an accessory pathway. Figure 17-2 demonstrates the consequences of gross mismanagement of this life-threatening arrhythmia. A 25-year-old man sustained a very rapid heart rate for 10 hours at home. At midnight he presented himself to the emergency room complaining of palpitations, a heaviness in his chest, and shortness of breath. His blood pressure was 95/60 mm Hg, and a 12-lead ECG revealed the broad, irregular, very rapid rhythm seen in Figure 17-2, *A*. He was incorrectly diagnosed as having atrial fibrillation with aberrant ventricular conduction and was given digitalis IV

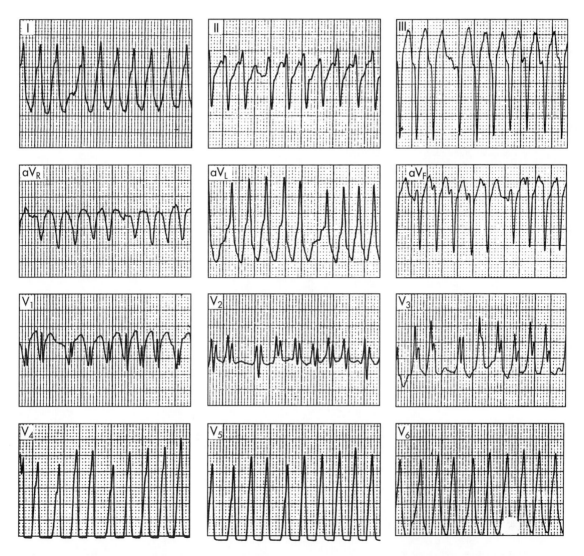

FIGURE 17-1 A typical ECG of atrial fibrillation with AV conduction over an accessory pathway. It is identified because it is more than 180 beats/min, the QRS complex is broad and like ventricular tachycardia, and the rhythm is irregular. The one feature that raises suspicion is its irregularity. Ventricular tachycardia is usually regular, except when polymorphic.

0.5 mg and 0.25 mg between 1:45 AM and 4 AM. At 6:30 AM he was in ventricular fibrillation and was successfully defibrillated. Later that day the mechanism was correctly identified by a cardiologist. Although these tracings are more than 25 years old, similar mismanagement is still seen in many emergency departments and intensive care units, which is especially regrettable because a safe transvenous cure with radiofrequency ablation is now available.

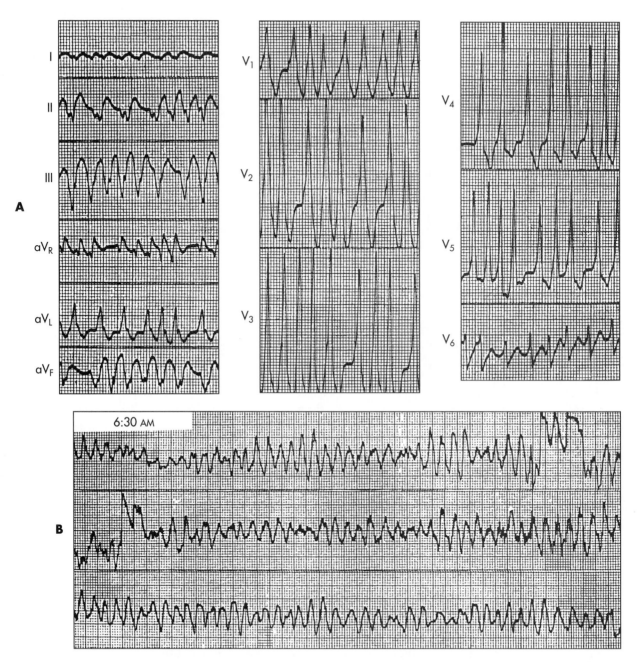

FIGURE 17-2 **A,** Atrial fibrillation with AV conduction down an accessory pathway. This is an emergency department ECG tracing from a 25-year-old man who was misdiagnosed and given digitalis. **B,** Ventricular fibrillation. This event occurred after 6 hours of mismanagement with digitalis and "observation" and 16 hours after the onset of atrial fibrillation. Procainamide should have been given intravenously in the emergency department to block conduction in the accessory pathway; if this did not work, the patient should have been cardioverted.

Differential diagnosis

Differentiating atrial fibrillation with an accessory pathway from atrial fibrillation with bundle branch block is not a diagnostic challenge. The differentiation is made on the basis of rate and QRS pattern. Atrial fibrillation with AV conduction over an accessory pathway is faster than 180 beats/min and is identical in shape to VT. Atrial fibrillation without an accessory pathway but with bundle branch block has a heart rate of approximately 140 to 150 beats/min, and the QRS pattern is that of bundle branch block (Figures 17-3 and 17-4).

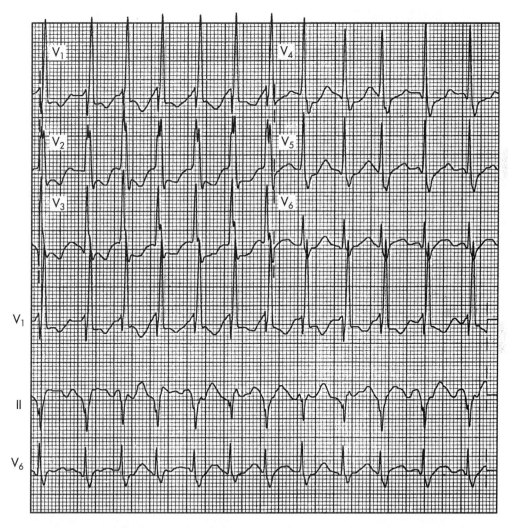

FIGURE 17-3 Atrial fibrillation with pathologic RBBB. The rate is 120 beats/min and the QRS duration is 0.12 second, with a triphasic rSR′ pattern in V_1 and qRS in V_6. This tracing is easily distinguishable from atrial fibrillation with an accessory pathway.

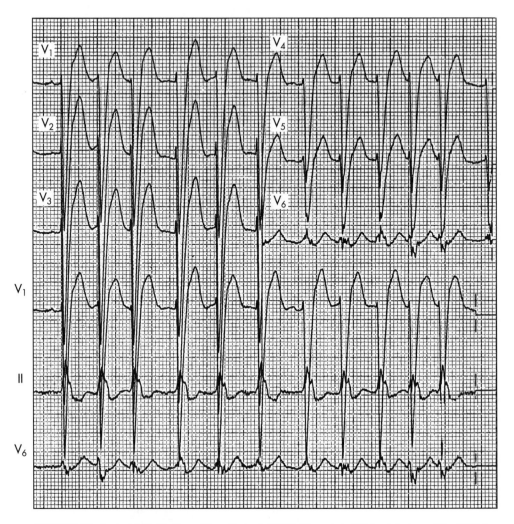

FIGURE 17-4 Atrial fibrillation with pathologic LBBB. The rate is 150 beats/min and the QRS duration is 0.13 second, with a sharp narrow r wave and a swift clean S downstroke in V_1 and V_2 (easily distinguishable from atrial fibrillation with an accessory pathway). (Compare with Figure 17-5.)

Incidence

Atrial fibrillation has been reported in 41 out of 157 patients with WPW syndrome.

Mechanism

When atrial fibrillation is not associated with an accessory pathway, the erratic electrical activity from the atria is slowed by the AV node in its passage to the ventricles, producing uncontrolled ventricular rates of 140 to 150 beats/min. In addition, because the impulse enters the ventricles through the normal AV nodal–His–Purkinje axis, the QRS complex is usually not as wide. However, a very rapid ventricular response with a broader QRS complex that is morphologically identical to VT results when there is an officiating accessory pathway (Figure 17-5). The mechanism of atrial fibrillation with conduction over an accessory pathway is diagrammatically illustrated in Figure 17-6 with the typical ECG tracing.

RATE. The following factors determine ventricular rate during atrial fibrillation[1]:
1. Refractory period duration of the accessory pathway in the anterograde direction
2. Refractory period of the AV node
3. Refractory period of the ventricle
4. Concealed anterograde and retrograde penetration into the accessory pathway and AV node[9]
5. Sympathetic stimulation shortens the refractory period of the accessory pathway and accelerates the rate.[10] It is important to terminate this tachycardia promptly and to reassure the patient in the meantime. A reflex sympathetic response to the fall in blood pressure is associated with the atrial fibrillation and the very rapid ventricular rate: anxiety adds to this response.

If the refractory period of the accessory pathway is short, the heart rate can exceed 300 beats/min. This life-threatening arrhythmia may deteriorate into ventricular fibrillation.

WIDTH. The QRS complex is broad (it looks like a VT) because ventricular activation is initiated outside of the normal conduction system. (Remember that this is not a reentry circuit. It is the accessory pathway that must be blocked, not the AV node.)

RHYTHM. The rhythm is irregular because of rapid stimulation from the fibrillating atria, concealed conduction into the accessory pathway and, perhaps, changing refractoriness of the accessory pathway. This type of irregularity is typical and distinguishes atrial fibrillation with conduction over an accessory pathway from VT, which is usually regular.

Emergency treatment

1. Obtain a 12-lead ECG during the tachycardia and one during sinus rhythm following conversion.
2. Administer procainamide 10 mg/kg body weight over 5 minutes. If procainamide does not slow the rhythm and block the accessory pathway (complexes become narrow as they pass down the AV node), proceed to step 3.
3. Cardioversion is, of course, the first-line emergency treatment for severe circulatory impairment.

WARNING: Calcium channel blockers and digitalis are absolutely contraindicated. Calcium channel blockers almost always cause the heart rate to increase, and digitalis causes such an increase in approximately 30% of cases. The drug of choice is procainamide; if this does not work, other drugs will not slow the rate either. Instead cardiovert and refer the patient for radiofrequency ablation.

Radiofrequency ablation involves the use of unmodulated, high-frequency alternating current flow through tissue to cause heat, cell desiccation, and coagulation necrosis for the purpose of destroying troublesome areas and pathways in the heart. The closed electrical circuit required for cardiac ablation is achieved by a radiofrequency generator, connecting leads, and unipolar or bipolar electrodes.

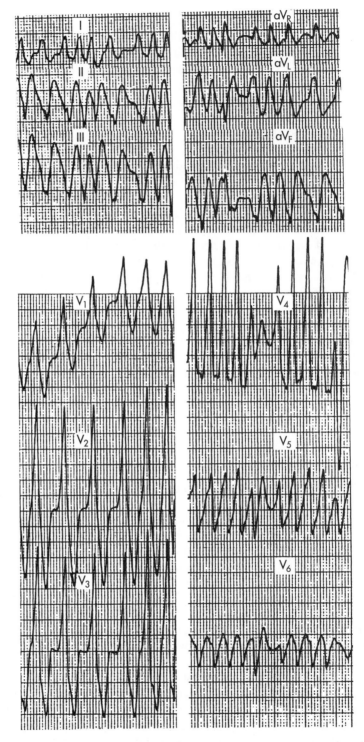

FIGURE 17-5 Atrial fibrillation with AV conduction down an accessory pathway. A comparison of this ECG with Figures 17-3 and 17-4 illustrates that it is not difficult to differentiate between atrial fibrillation with and without an accessory pathway (see text).

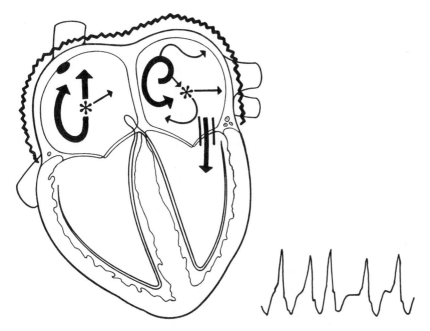

FIGURE 17-6 The mechanism of atrial fibrillation with AV conduction down an accessory pathway. A typical fast, broad, irregular tracing is shown. (From Conover M: *Understanding electrocardiography,* ed 7, St Louis, 1996, Mosby.)

Atrial Fibrillation with Multiple Accessory Pathways

When atrial fibrillation occurs in a patient with more than one accessory pathway, AV conduction via the extra connections plus the AV node results in an irregular rapid rhythm, fusion beats, and a polymorphous broad QRS tachycardia. Figure 17-7 illustrates the ECG during atrial fibrillation in a patient with both right-sided and left-sided accessory pathways.

Atrial Flutter with an Accessory Pathway

Figure 17-8 demonstrates the difficulty in determining the mechanism of a regular tachycardia with a wide QRS complex. The regularity of the rhythm, the monophasic R wave in V_1, and the precordial concordance would prompt an incorrect diagnosis of VT. Intracardiac recordings identified atrial flutter with 2:1 conduction over a left-sided accessory pathway. This difficulty would also be true in atrial tachycardia with 1:1 or 2:1 AV conduction over an accessory pathway and in antidromic circus movement tachycardia (CMT).[11] First-response treatment is directed toward slowing the heart rate and restoring sinus rhythm.

Antidromic Circus Movement Tachycardia

Antidromic CMT is a reentry circuit that uses the accessory pathway in the antero-grade direction (producing a broad QRS complex) and the AV node in the retrograde direction. Here again is a regular broad QRS paroxysmal supraventricular tachycardia

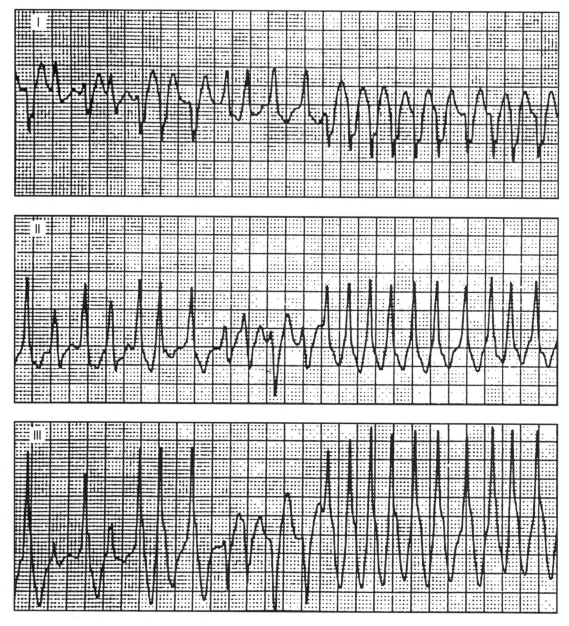

FIGURE 17-7 Atrial fibrillation with multiple accessory pathways. (From Yee R, Klein GJ, Sharma ADR et al: Tachycardia associated with accessory atrioventricular pathways. In Zipes DP, Jalife J, editors: *Cardiac electrophysiology,* Philadelphia, 1990, WB Saunders.)

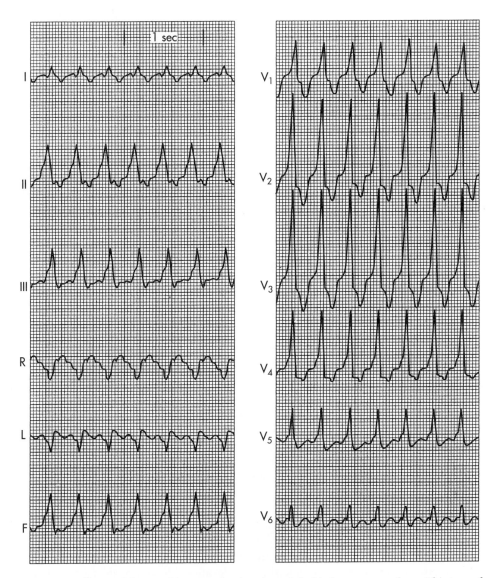

FIGURE 17-8 Atrial flutter with 2:1 conduction over a left-sided accessory pathway. This type of supraventricular tachycardia causes positive precordial concordance and an ECG identical to that of ventricular tachycardia. Intracardiac recordings are needed to make the diagnosis. (Courtesy Hein JJ Wellens, MD, The Netherlands.)

with the QRS pattern of VT (Figure 17-9). It is impossible to make the correct diagnosis without intracardiac recordings, although a strong suspicion exists when the delta wave during sinus rhythm is the same polarity as the tachycardia in all leads. Antidromic CMT indicates multiple accessory pathways in at least 50% of patients.[12] Electrophysiologic studies are necessary to rule out VT.

ECG features

- **Rate.** 150 to 250 beats/min.
- **QRS complex.** Broad; pattern is that of VT.
- **Rhythm.** Usually regular but may be slightly irregular because retrograde conduction times vary through the fascicles to the atria. Although this rhythm may help distinguish this broad QRS tachycardia from VT (which is regular 75% of the time), it may also be confused with atrial fibrillation with conduction over an accessory pathway, which also looks like VT but is irregular.
- **P waves.** Although P' waves are present following every QRS complex, they are usually not seen during antidromic CMT because of the width of the QRS complex.
- **Main diagnostic features.** A broad, regular QRS tachycardia morphologically identical to VT because of initial ventricular excitation outside of the conduction system. The diagnosis cannot be made from the ECG during the tachycardia, and electrophysiologic studies are necessary for confirmation. The ECG during sinus rhythm may be of some help and may create a high degree of suspicion if the delta force is identical to that of the initial forces of the tachycardia (see Figure 17-9).

Mechanism

The mechanism of antidromic CMT is schematically illustrated in Figure 17-10. Antidromic CMT begins like orthodromic CMT, with a critically timed atrial premature beat, ventricular premature beat, or a critical sinus rate. Note that anterograde conduction proceeds down the accessory pathway and lands within the ventricle outside of the conduction system. This path causes a relatively slow beginning to the broad QRS complex.

Emergency treatment

The treatment for antidromic and orthodromic CMT is the same; the problem lies in recognition. This tachycardia is identical in shape to that of VT. Treatment is as follows:

1. Perform a vagal maneuver. Both carotid sinus massage and gagging are strong vagal maneuvers. Others are squatting, leg elevation, blowing against a closed glottis, and cold water to the face. The vagal maneuver should be performed as soon as the tachycardia is recorded. The longer the wait, the more difficult to convert with a vagal maneuver because of the increasing dominance of the sympathetic nervous system.
2. Administer adenosine 6 mg IV, which may be increased to 12 mg and repeated at 1-minute intervals.
3. If adenosine is unsuccessful, administer procainamide 10 mg/kg IV over 5 minutes.
4. Pacing or cardioversion is rarely required to interrupt CMT. However, electrical cardioversion is used if vagal maneuvers and drugs do not terminate the tachycardia or if the patient is hemodynamically unstable at any time.

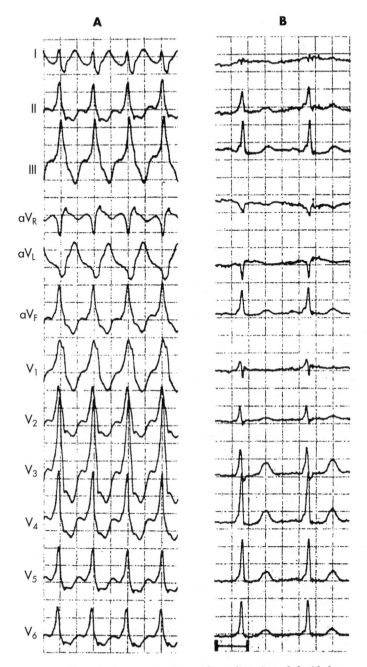

FIGURE 17-9 A, Antidromic circus movement tachycardia using a left-sided accessory pathway for AV conduction. This tracing is another example of a supraventricular tachycardia producing positive precordial concordance and an ECG that is identical to that of ventricular tachycardia. **B,** Sinus rhythm in the same patient. Note that the polarity of the delta waves is identical to that of the initial forces during the tachycardia. (Courtesy Hein JJ Wellens, MD, The Netherlands.)

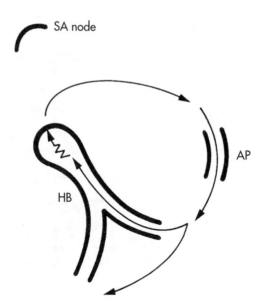

FIGURE 17-10 A schematic representation of the mechanism of antidromic circus movement tachycardia. The anterograde conduction down the accessory pathway *(AP)* produces an ECG identical to that of ventricular tachycardia. *HB,* His bundle.

Following resolution of the acute event, the patient is referred to a center experienced in treatment of the arrhythmias of WPW syndrome. Radiofrequency ablation is available as a cure.

Circus Movement Tachycardia with Two Accessory Pathways

CMT using two accessory pathways is another rare form of PSVT in which the QRS complexes are broad. Anterograde conduction is down one accessory pathway, and retrograde conduction is up another (Figure 17-11), producing a rhythm identical to both VT and the previously described antidromic CMT.

Broad QRS Paroxysmal Supraventricular Tachycardia Using Nodoventricular Fibers

When a supraventricular impulse is conducted in an anterograde direction down the extra fiber and not down the AV node, it may return in a retrograde direction to the atria via the bundle branch(es), His bundle, and AV node (Figure 17-12). The resulting reciprocating SVT has a broad QRS complex because the ventricles are activated outside the conduction system. If the extra fiber inserts into the right ventricle, the QRS complex resembles left bundle branch block (LBBB) (Figure 17-13). Thus there is usually an rS in V_1 and an RS in V_2 with left axis deviation.

ECG during sinus rhythm

The PR interval and QRS duration during sinus rhythm depend on the origin, insertion, length, and conduction time of the Mahaim fiber. Nodoventricular fibers may

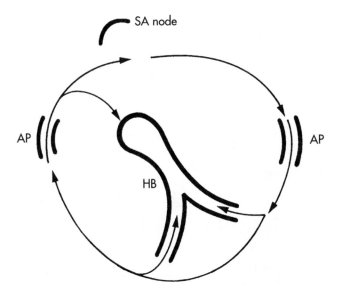

FIGURE 17-11 A schematic representation of the mechanism of circus movement tachycardia using two accessory pathways. The ECG is identical to that of ventricular tachycardia. *AP,* Accessory pathway; *HB,* His bundle.

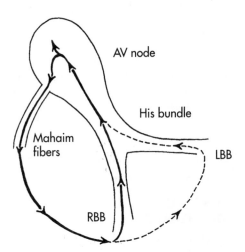

FIGURE 17-12 Schematic representation of a reentry circuit using a nodoventricular (Mahaim) fiber. The nodoventricular fiber may insert into either the right ventricle or the right bundle branch *(RBB)*. The retrograde return circuit can conceivably be completed by either the RBB or the left bundle branch *(LBB)*. This is a relatively rare mechanism in which a supraventricular tachycardia (using the AV node and a short circuit to the ventricle) can produce an ECG identical to that of ventricular tachycardia. (From Gallagher JJ, Smith WM, Kasell JH et al: Role of Mahaim fibers in cardiac arrhythmias in man, *Circulation* 64:176, 1981.)

A   **B**

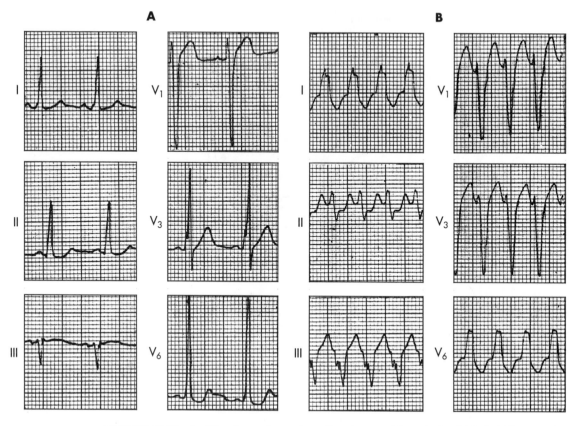

FIGURE 17-13 An AV reciprocating tachycardia using a nodoventricular (Mahaim) fiber running from the AV node to the posteroinferior part of the right ventricle to produce an ECG identical to that of ventricular tachycardia. **A,** The sinus rhythm. During tachycardia (**B**) the ventricle is activated exclusively by way of the nodoventricular fiber. (Courtesy Hein JJ Wellens, MD, The Netherlands.)

be manifested by either a short or a normal PR interval. There may or may not be a delta wave, and the QRS complex is often a fusion beat that results from conduction over the extra fiber and over the normal pathway.

VENTRICULAR TACHYCARDIAS THAT LOOK LIKE SUPRAVENTRICULAR TACHYCARDIA

When VTs have a focus close to or within the conduction system or use the intraventricular conduction system for a reentry circuit, the QRS pattern is that of SVT with aberration. Three types of VT look like SVT: idiopathic, fascicular, and bundle branch reentry.

Idiopathic Ventricular Tachycardia

Idiopathic VT is diagnosed when the only abnormality is the arrhythmia as determined by current diagnostic techniques. Identifiable underlying etiologies are ruled out by echocardiography, signal averaging during sinus rhythm, magnetic resonance imaging, and cardiac catheterization with angiography. Of 706 patients with VT who were studied in the electrophysiology laboratory at one institution, 75 were found to have idiopathic VT.[13] General localization of the focus area of the VT is possible from the surface 12-lead electrocardiogram. Accurate localization of the focus site is accomplished by activation mapping and pace mapping.[14]

Idiopathic VT is usually of monomorphic configuration and can be classified according to its site of origin as either right monomorphic (70%) or left monomorphic VT. Several physiopathologic types of monomorphic VT can be individualized according to their mode of presentation, relationship to adrenergic stress, or response to various drugs. Different sensitivities to adenosine and isoproterenol between right and left ventricular idiopathic VT suggest different underlying mechanisms for both types of VT.[15]

The most common form of idiopathic VT is repetitive monomorphic VT, which typically occurs at rest and is characterized by frequent ventricular ectopy and salvos of nonsustained VT with intervening sinus rhythm.[16]

ECG warning of the onset

There is a significant change in autonomic influence on the heart during the last few minutes before the onset of idiopathic VT. This change seems to result mainly from impaired vagal efferent cardiac activity rather than from enhanced sympathetic input to the heart.[17] Although there is no significant change in the QT or QTc interval, the high frequency component of heart rate variability is significantly decreased. The relationship between QT interval and heart rate variability (QT/RR relationship) is also significantly altered in patients with idiopathic VT as compared with normal subjects. A transient, inappropriate shortening of ventricular repolarization may play an important role in the pathogenesis of idiopathic VT.[18-20]

Prognosis

The long-term prognosis for monomorphic idiopathic VT is usually good. Sudden cardiac death is rare as opposed to the very high mortality associated with postischemic recurrent VT. Frequent episodes of this arrhythmia may result in cardiomyopathy and render the decision for radiofrequency ablation of the focus more imperative. Idiopathic polymorphic VT is a much rarer type of arrhythmia and has a less favorable prognosis. Idiopathic ventricular fibrillation may represent an underestimated cause of sudden cardiac death in ostensibly healthy patients.[21-24]

Symptoms

The symptoms of idiopathic VT are palpitations or episodes of syncope.[25]

Pediatrics

It is uncommon for a previously healthy child to present to the emergency department with hemodynamically stable VT.[26] The clinical characteristics and long-term prognosis of 163 children with ventricular arrhythmias without underlying heart disease were studied (46 children had VT). It was concluded that ventricular arrhythmias in children without underlying disease often disappeared, and the prognosis was generally favorable. However, appropriate treatment and follow-up were required in children with sustained VT, symptomatic VT, or VT with a high rate.[27]

In a study of six consecutive children it was found that radiofrequency catheter ablation is a safe and effective treatment for right ventricular outflow tachycardia during childhood and adolescence.[28] However, the late effects of radiofrequency energy application in the human ventricle remain undetermined. Animal studies suggest that the lesions resulting from radiofrequency energy application enlarge over time and that its use in very young children may carry a higher long-term risk.[28,29]

History

Paroxysmal VT occurring in young healthy hearts was first described by Gallavardin in 1922[30] and was known as "right ventricular outflow tract tachycardia." This condition was described again in 1953.[31] In 1979, Zipes, Foster, Troup, and Pedersen[32] described the ECG characteristics of idiopathic VT with a focus in the left ventricle (i.e., QRS duration <0.12 second and an RBBB-like pattern with left axis deviation). This tachycardia could be induced by exercise, atrial or ventricular pacing, and atrial or ventricular premature beats. In 1980 Wellens, Farré, and Bär[33] reported that this type of VT may be terminated by verapamil; this observation was confirmed in a later series.[34] The focus is thought to be in the posterior fascicle of the left bundle branch (LBB).[33,35,36]

Emergency treatment

Zipes and colleagues[32] recommend that idiopathic VT be managed like other VTs. Unless the physician is an expert electrophysiologist, verapamil is contraindicated for all wide QRS tachycardias. Adenosine can also be used and is effective for some of the right ventricular outflow tract VTs.[37]

Long-term treatment

Map-guided transcatheter radiofrequency ablation of idiopathic VT is safe and effective.[13,24,33,35,36,38-44] Figure 17-14 shows ablation sites in the right ventricular outflow tract. The efficacy of the procedure depends on the site of origin of the VT, with the efficacy greater for those originating from the outflow tract of the right ventricle than for those from other locations.[45] However, radiofrequency ablation therapy was also found to be effective and safe in 20 consecutive patients with idiopathic left VT and was considered to be the primary therapeutic modality for these patients.[44]

Pacing is performed in the right ventricular outflow tract. The complexes are analyzed with respect to the R:S ratio and fine notching in each lead until the paced complexes match the spontaneous QRS patterns during tachycardia. This site becomes the site of ablation.[46]

Unfortunately, in patients with VT associated with organic heart disease the success rate is lower, the recurrence is higher, and the procedure can be applied only to patients who can tolerate the relatively long episodes of induced VT necessary for mapping and successful ablation. For patients who lose consciousness during tachycardia or present with prehospital cardiac arrest, transcatheter radiofrequency ablation is inappropriate as definitive treatment and does not obviate the need for other therapies such as cardioverter-defibrillator implantation or antiarrhythmic drug therapy.[47]

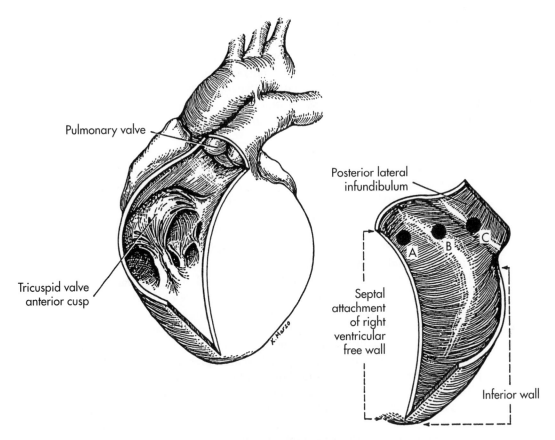

FIGURE 17-14 Ablation sites in the right ventricular outflow tract. The heart is represented in an angulated left anterior oblique projection. The right ventricle is opened, with the endocardial surface of the free wall depicted on the segment to the right. *A, B,* and *C* mark the sites in the right ventricular outflow tract that, during pace mapping, produced QRS complexes identical to those of ventricular tachycardia. (From Wilbur DJ, Baerman J, Olshansky B et al: Adenosine-sensitive ventricular tachycardia, *Circulation* 87:126, 1993.)

Complications following radiofrequency ablation

Radiofrequency arrhythmogenicity in the ablation of supraventricular tachycardia seems to be restricted to infrequent short runs of VT in the first week after the procedure.[48] There are few such reports following the procedure for idiopathic VT. One case of ventricular fibrillation is reported.[49]

Idiopathic Right Ventricular Tachycardia
ECG recognition

- LBBB pattern
- Inferior axis (normal or right)

- QRS duration 0.13 to 0.16 second
- Response to adenosine and verapamil[15]

Figure 17-15 is an example of idiopathic right VT with the focus in the right ventricular outflow tract compared with a normal sinus rhythm in the same patient. The relative narrowness of the QRS and the QRS pattern in V_1, V_2 (not shown), and V_6 cause this VT to be misdiagnosed as SVT with LBBB aberration. Note the swift clean S downstroke in V_1 and the absence of a q wave in V_6 during the tachycardia.

Mechanism

The study by Ng, Wen, and Yeh et al[50] strongly supports the view that idiopathic VT of right ventricular outflow tract origin may be a heterogenous group with triggered activity as the predominant mechanism, whereas idiopathic VT of left ventricular inferoapical origin is a reentry mechanism.

Location of the foci; value of lead I and the precordial leads

Idiopathic right ventricular adenosine-sensitive tachycardia appears to arise from relatively discrete sites that are predominantly located in the free wall of the pulmonary infundibulum (see Figure 17-14). The localized nature of this tachycardia renders it amenable to long-term cure by catheter ablation techniques.[37]

Pace mapping used to locate the site for ablation of idiopathic right ventricular outflow tract VT is difficult and time-consuming. One study has described an ECG-guided approach using lead I and R wave progression in precordial leads to find an identical pace map. The most common site of origin of idiopathic right ventricular outflow tract VT is on the middle to anterior and superior aspect of the septum of the outflow tract. The polarity of the QRS complex in lead I indicates anterior (monophasic Q) or posterior (monophasic R). Precordial R wave transition assists in identifying superior and inferior positioning of the catheter tip. The R wave transition occurs later as the pacing catheter is moved from the posterior superior aspect of the septum to the anterior inferior septal location.[51]

Differential diagnosis

Although the majority of cases of VTs with an LBBB pattern are attributable to acquired structural heart disease (including ischemia, prior infarction, or dilated cardiomyopathy), the consideration of specific right ventricular processes is essential to proper evaluation and treatment. The approach to older patients or those with evidence of heart disease begins with an evaluation for coronary artery disease and an assessment of biventricular function. Careful evaluation for bundle branch reentry should be performed during electrophysiologic study, especially when there is underlying conduction system disease.

Younger patients without overt heart disease or those with isolated right ventricular disease receive a complete, noninvasive evaluation of right and left ventricular size and function. An abnormal signal-averaged ECG or identification of intracardiac late potentials suggests right ventricular dysplasia or cardiomyopathy, whereas responsiveness to adenosine and the absence of detectable heart disease support the diagnosis of idiopathic right VT.

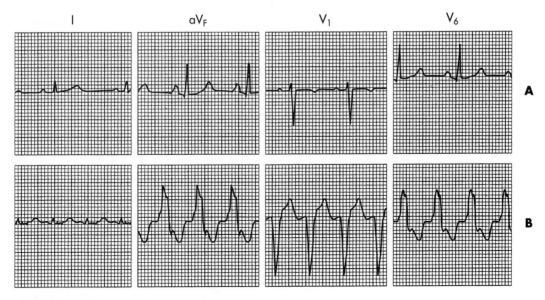

FIGURE 17-15 A, Sinus rhythm in leads I, aVF, V$_1$, and V$_6$. **B,** Idiopathic right ventricular tachycardia in the same patient. The focus is in the right ventricular outflow tract. Note that the QRS pattern is identical to that of supraventricular tachycardia with LBBB aberration. The typical features of ventricular tachycardia from this focus are the LBBB pattern and an inferior axis (aV$_F$ positive). (From Bhadha K, Marchlinski FE, Iskandrian AS: Ventricular tachycardia in patients without structural heart disease, *Am Heart J* 126:1194, 1993.)

Newer techniques, including magnetic resonance imaging, show promise in identifying subtle right ventricular disease not otherwise detectable even in the setting of presumed idiopathic right VT. Following the surgical repair of selected congenital heart defects (particularly tetralogy of Fallot), symptoms of recurrent palpitations, near syncope, syncope, or aborted sudden death may be attributable to recurrent VT; diagnostic electrophysiologic study should be considered for these patients. Finally, SVTs with an LBBB pattern, particularly cases associated with right-sided or septal accessory pathways, should always be considered in the differential diagnosis.[52]

Idiopathic Left Ventricular Tachycardia

Idiopathic left ventricular tachycardia is a distinct clinical syndrome that demonstrates a characteristic response to verapamil and inducibility from the atrium in patients without structural heart disease.[53]

ECG recognition

- Right bundle branch block (RBBB) pattern
- Superior axis, usually left (right in a minority of cases)[54]
- QRS duration 0.13 to 0.16 second
- Response to verapamil
- Inducibility from the atrium[53,55]

Both the relative narrowness of the QRS complex and the QRS pattern itself cause idiopathic left VT to be misdiagnosed as SVT with RBBB aberration. Figure 17-16 illustrates idiopathic left VT. The QRS duration is 0.14 second, and the pattern in V_1 is not helpful. There is typically a left axis deviation.

Mechanism

Idiopathic left VT with the RBBB pattern and left-axis deviation has been shown to be a result of reentry. The slow conduction zone of this VT shows tachycardia-dependent conduction delay, and the mechanism of this slow conduction involves mainly calcium channel–dependent conduction and partly depressed sodium channel–dependent conduction.[22,50,56,57] In six patients with idiopathic left VT, Aizawa, Chinushi, and Kitazawa et al[58] estimated the spatial orientation of the reentrant circuit from the results of transient entrainment of the tachycardia with rapid pacing at different sites. The entrance to the area of slow conduction was toward the outflow tract; the exit was at the apicoposterior area of the left interventricular septum.[58]

Location of the foci

As identified by successful radiofrequency catheter ablation, the tachycardia originates from different areas of the left ventricular septum—from the base to the mid-apical region.[59]

Pathology

A false tendon in the left ventricle has been described in a patient with idiopathic left VT in whom surgical resection of the false tendon resulted in a cure. A false tendon extending from the posteroinferior left ventricle to the septum is a consistent finding in patients with idiopathic left VT; there is speculation that this false tendon is the anatomic substrate for this unique arrhythmia. The mechanism by which the false tendon precipitates tachycardia is speculative, but possibilities include conduction through the false tendon or the production of stretch in the Purkinje fiber network on the interventricular septum.[53] In addition, echocardiographic findings demonstrate the entire spectrum of involvement of the right side of the heart in patients with apparent idiopathic VT; these findings can give insight into the clinical history, arrhythmia inducibility, and prognosis.[60]

Bundle Branch Reentrant Ventricular Tachycardia

Sustained bundle branch reentrant VT (BBR-VT) is a highly malignant form of monomorphic VT that commonly presents as syncope, palpitations, or sudden cardiac death. It is associated with severe myocardial disease or with significant disease of the intraventricular conduction system. There is a higher incidence of this condition in patients with idiopathic cardiomyopathy compared with those with ischemic heart disease.[61] It is important to recognize BBR-VT because it can be cured with radiofrequency ablation.[62]

ECG recognition

- QRS complex during sinus rhythm: incomplete LBBB consistent with His-Purkinje system disease
- QRS complex during VT: the most common form of BBR-VT is an LBBB pattern (present in 98% of patients)[63]

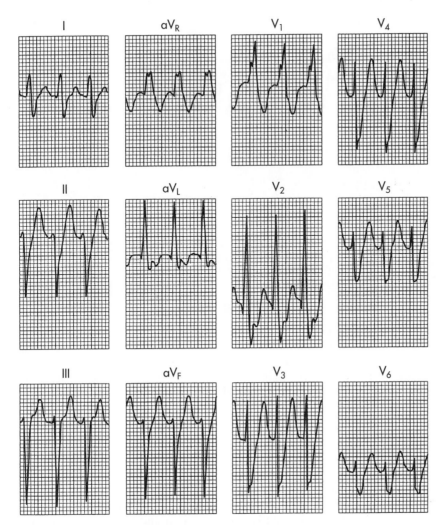

FIGURE 17-16 Idiopathic left ventricular tachycardia. The QRS complex is relatively narrow and the pattern in V_1 is not helpful. The typical features of ventricular tachycardia from this focus are an RBBB pattern and a superior axis, usually left (aV_F negative). (Courtesy Ara Tilkian, MD, Van Nuys, Calif.)

Figure 17-17 illustrates BBR-VT with anterograde conduction down the right bundle branch (RBB). Note that the negative complex in lead V_1 has none of the signs of VT described on p. 249. This phenomenon occurs because the mechanism is being sustained by a reentry loop that uses the His-Purkinje system. Figure 17-18 illustrates a less common form of BBR-VT in which the ventricles are activated with anterograde conduction down the LBB, resulting in an RBBB pattern.

When a patient is not in VT, he or she is either in atrial fibrillation or sinus rhythm, in which case the QRS contour reflects a nonspecific intraventricular conduction delay or an LBBB pattern. If there is sinus rhythm the PR is prolonged.[62] In rare cases of interfascicular reentry the QRS pattern during sinus rhythm and VT are the same—RBBB with right axis deviation.[64]

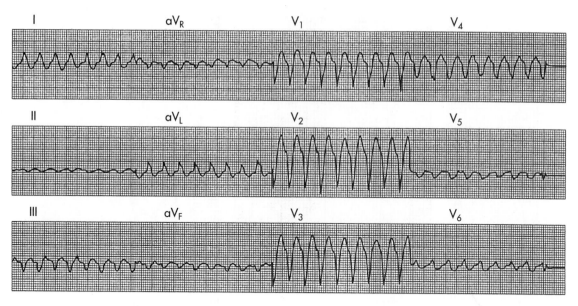

FIGURE 17-17 A bundle branch reentrant ventricular tachycardia with an LBBB pattern and left axis deviation at a rate of 215 beats/min. Because ventricular activation occurs by way of the RBB, the QRS complex is relatively narrow, and its configuration suggests supraventricular tachycardia with LBBB aberrant ventricular conduction. (From Blanck Z, Sra J, Dhala A et al: Bundle branch reentry: mechanisms, diagnosis, and treatment. In Zipes DP, Jalife J, editors: *Cardiac electrophysiology from cell to bedside,* ed 2, Philadelphia, 1995, WB Saunders.)

Mechanism

BUNDLE BRANCH REENTRANT VENTRICULAR TACHYCARDIA. The mechanisms of the two forms of BBR-VT are illustrated in Figure 17-19. BBR-VT is a well-defined macroreentry circuit in which the His bundle, right and left bundle branches, and transseptal ventricular muscle conduction are the obligatory components.[65,66] An absolute prerequisite for such a reentry loop is conduction delay in the His-Purkinje system.[63] Note the slow conduction depicted within the LBB. The mechanism usually consists of anterograde conduction over the RBB and retrograde conduction over the LBB; rarely does the circuit proceed in the opposite direction. Thus an LBBB pattern is most common during the tachycardia. Because the mechanism of this tachycardia uses the His-Purkinje system, the resultant QRS pattern is that of *SVT with aberration.*

INTERFASCICULAR REENTRANT VENTRICULAR TACHYCARDIA. Interfascicular reentrant VT is a rare form of BBR-VT that uses the anterior fascicle of the left bundle anterogradely and the posterior fascicle retrogradely. This path produces identical QRS patterns during sinus rhythm and VT—RBBB with right axis deviation.[66] The RBB does not participate in the reentry circuit. A cure is accomplished by catheter ablation of anterior fascicular conduction.[64]

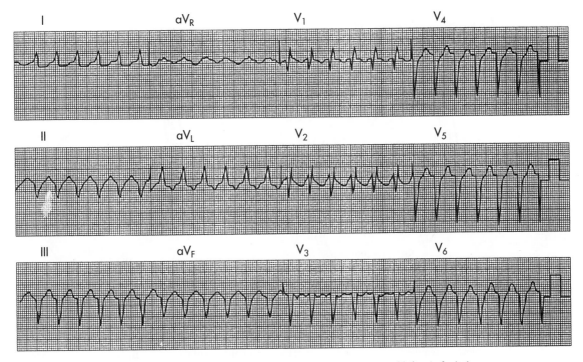

FIGURE 17-18 A bundle branch reentrant tachycardia with an RBBB pattern and left axis deviation at a rate of 150 beats/min. Because ventricular activation occurs by way of the LBB, the QRS complex is relatively narrow; its configuration suggests SVT with RBBB aberrant ventricular conduction. (From Blanck Z, Sra J, Dhala A et al: Bundle branch reentry: mechanisms, diagnosis, and treatment. In Zipes DP, Jalife J, editors: *Cardiac electrophysiology from cell to bedside*, ed 2, Philadelphia, 1995, WB Saunders.)

Pathophysiology

BBR-VT usually occurs in individuals with significant structural heart disease, usually in the form of dilated ischemic or idiopathic cardiomyopathy.[63,66,67] The critical prerequisite for the development of this arrhythmia is conduction delay in the His-Purkinje system, which manifests as a nonspecific conduction delay or LBBB in the surface ECG and a prolonged His-ventricular (HV) interval in the intracardiac recordings.[63] BBR-VT may also occur in the setting of dilated ventricles secondary to coronary or significant valvular heart disease.[68] Three cases of BBR-VT have been reported in patients with conduction abnormalities on the surface ECG that are suggestive of His-Purkinje system disease but no manifestation of myocardial or valvular dysfunction.[69]

Clinical presentation

- Syncope and sudden death (70%)[63,66]
- Sustained palpitations during wide complex tachycardia

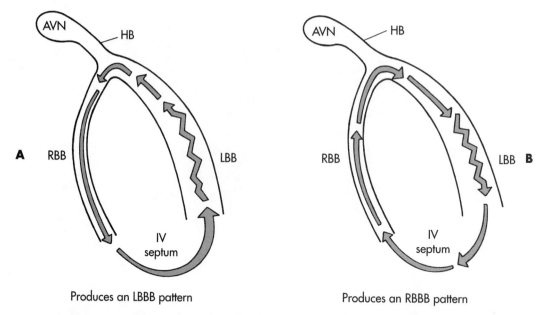

FIGURE 17-19 The mechanism of bundle branch reentry ventricular tachycardia. **A,** The most common form of BBR-VT, with anterograde conduction in the RBB to produce an LBBB pattern. Note the required delay of conduction in the ascending limb of the circuit. **B,** The least common form of BBR-VT, with anterograde conduction in the LBB to produce an RBBB pattern. *AVN,* Atrioventricular node; *HB,* His bundle.

Long-term treatment

Transcatheter ablation of the RBB with the use of radiofrequency current is the treatment of choice for BBR-VT because it effectively eliminates this condition.[63,70-72] Because of the availability of such a cure, the recognition of BBR-VT through electrophysiologic studies avoids therapy with the automatic implantable defibrillator or antiarrhythmic drugs.[66] After ablation, long-term follow-up of 48 patients did not document bundle branch reentry, but congestive heart failure was a common cause of death.[63,73]

Prognosis

The prognosis for BBR-VT is generally poor. Some patients with a combination of BBR-VT and dilated cardiomyopathy may be considered for cardiac transplantation.[68]

Fascicular Ventricular Tachycardia

Fascicular VT was discussed in Chapter 13 and is illustrated again here for completeness and because it is often misdiagnosed. The QRS pattern in this life-threatening arrhythmia is identical to that of SVT with RBBB aberration.

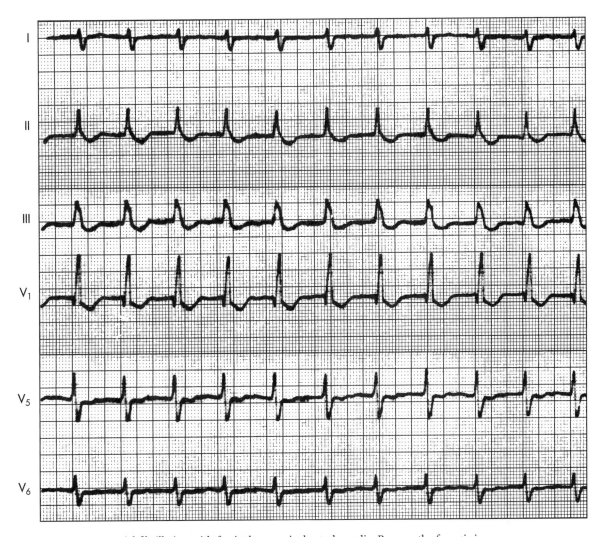

FIGURE 17-20 Atrial fibrillation with fascicular ventricular tachycardia. Because the focus is in the posterior fascicle of the LBB, the ECG is identical to that of supraventricular tachycardia with RBBB aberration. (Courtesy Hein JJ Wellens, MD, The Netherlands.)

The QRS width is approximately 0.12 second, and the rate is between 90 and 160 beats/min. At this point of toxicity the patient is usually symptomatic. If left untreated the mortality is 100%. Digitalis-specific Fab fragments (Digibind) is lifesaving in this clinical setting.

Figure 17-20 illustrates fascicular VT in a patient with atrial fibrillation. Note the typical ECG features mentioned and the digitalis effect of a scooped-down ST segment.

SUMMARY

The guidelines for recognizing ventricular tachycardia by QRS patterns are aptly applied most of the time. However, an informed clinician is also aware of the clinical situations in which such guidelines serve only to misguide. The supraventricular tachycardias that look like ventricular tachycardia are those that use accessory pathways for anterograde conduction. In such cases the QRS pattern is identical to that of ventricular tachycardia. These arrhythmias are atrial tachycardia, atrial flutter, atrial fibrillation, antidromic circus movement tachycardia, and circus movements using more than one accessory pathway. Correct identification is essential not only for correct emergency response but also because there is a cure.

The ventricular tachycardias that look like supraventricular tachycardia are a mixed group. They appear in patients without any indication of heart disease (idiopathic ventricular tachycardia), in patients with dilated cardiomyopathy (bundle branch reentry ventricular tachycardia), and in patients with digitalis toxicity (fascicular ventricular tachycardia). The correct identification of these mechanisms is imperative for their cure and management.

REFERENCES

1. Wellens HJJ: Pre-excitation. In Willlerson JT, Cohn JN, editors: *Cardiovascular medicine,* New York, 1995, Churchill Livingstone.
2. Cox JL, Ferguson TB Jr: Surgery for the Wolff-Parkinson-White syndrome: the endocardial approach, *Semin Thorac Cardiovasc Surg* 1:34, 1989.
3. Wellens HJJ, Brugada P, Penn DC et al: Pre-excitation syndromes. In Zipes DP, Jalife J, editors: *Cardiac electrophysiology,* Philadelphia, 1990, WB Saunders.
4. Wellens HJJ, Brugada P: Value of programmed stimulation of the heart in patients with Wolff-Parkinson-White syndrome. In Josephson ME, Wellens HJJ, editors: *Tachycardias: mechanisms, diagnosis, treatment,* Philadelphia, 1984, Lea & Febiger.
5. Wellens HJJ: Wolff-Parkinson-White syndrome. Part I. *Mod Concepts Cardiovasc Dis* 52:53, 1983.
6. Levy S, Bronstet JP, Clemency J: Syndrome de Wolff-Parkinson-White, *Arch Mal Coeur* 72:634, 1979.
7. Wellens HJJ, Braat SH, Brugada P et al: Use of procainamide in patients with the Wolff-Parkinson-White syndrome to disclose a short refractory period of the accessory pathway, *Am J Cardiol* 50:921, 1982.
8. Wellens HJJ et al: Death after ajmaline administration, *Am J Cardiol* 50:1087, 1982.
9. Josephson ME, Wellens HJJ: Differential diagnosis of supraventricular tachycardia, *Cardiol Clin* 8:411, 1990.
10. Wellens HJJ, Brugada P, Roy D et al: Effect of isoproterenol on the antegrade refractory period of the accessory pathway in patients with Wolff-Parkinson-White syndrome, *Am J Cardiol* 50:180, 1982.
11. Wellens HJJ, Bär FW, Vanagt EJ et al: The differentiation between ventricular tachycardia and supraventricular tachycardia with aberrant conduction: the value of the 12-lead electrocardiogram. In Wellens HJJ, Kulbertus HE, editors: *What's new in electrocardiography,* Boston, 1981, Martinus Nijhoff.
12. Wellens HJJ, Josephson ME: *Diagnosis of difficult arrhythmias,* Miami, 1987, Medtronic.
13. Wellens HJJ, Rodriquez LM, Smeets JL: Ventricular tachycardia in structurally normal hearts. In Zipes DP, Jalife J, editors: *Cardiac electrophysiology from cell to bedside,* Philadelphia 1995, WB Saunders.

14. Lokhandwala YY, Smeets JL, Rodriguez LM et al: Idiopathic ventricular tachycardia: characterization and radiofrequency ablation, *Indian Heart J* 46:281, 1994.

15. Lee SH, Chen SA, Tai CT et al: Electropharmacologic characteristics and radiofrequency catheter ablation of sustained ventricular tachycardia in patients without structural heart disease, *Cardiology* 87:33, 1996.

16. Lerman BB, Stein K, Engelstein ED et al: Mechanism of repetitive monomorphic ventricular tachycardia, *Circulation* 92:421, 1995.

17. Fei L, Statters DJ, Hnatkova K et al: Change of autonomic influence on the heart immediately before the onset of spontaneous idiopathic ventricular tachycardia, *J Am Coll Cardiol* 24:1515, 1994.

18. Fei L, Gill JS, Katritsis D, Camm AJ: Abnormal autonomic modulation of QT interval in patients with idiopathic ventricular tachycardia associated with clinically normal hearts, *Br Heart J* 69:311, 1993.

19. Fei L, Camm AJ: Shortening of the QT interval immediately preceding the onset of idiopathic spontaneous ventricular tachycardia, *Am Heart J* 130:915, 1995.

20. Gill JS, Baszko A, Xia R et al: Dynamics of the QT interval in patients with exercise-induced ventricular tachycardia in normal and abnormal hearts, *Am Heart J* 126:1357, 1993.

21. Belhassen B, Viskin S: Idiopathic ventricular tachycardia and fibrillation, *J Cardiovasc Electrophysiol* 4:356, 1993.

22. Ohe T: Idiopathic verapamil-sensitive sustained left ventricular tachycardia, *Clin Cardiol* 16:139, 1993.

23. Ohe T, Aihara N, Kamakura S et al: Long-term outcome of verapamil-sensitive sustained left ventricular tachycardia in patients without structural heart disease, *J Am Coll Cardiol* 25:54, 1995.

24. Bhadha K, Marchlinski FE, Iskandrian AS: Ventricular tachycardia in patients without structural heart disease, *Am Heart J* 126:1194, 1993.

25. Buston AE, Waxman HL, Marchlinski FE et al: Right ventricular tachycardia: clinical and electrophysiological characteristics, *Circulation* 68:917, 1983.

26. Suner S, Simon HK, Feit LR, Linakis JG: Child with idiopathic ventricular tachycardia of prolonged duration, *Ann Emerg Med* 25:706, 1995.

27. Tsuji A, Nagashima M, Hasegawa S et al: Long-term follow-up of idiopathic ventricular arrhythmias in otherwise normal children, *Jpn Circ J* 59:654, 1995.

28. O'Connor BK, Case CL, Sokoloski MC et al: Radiofrequency catheter ablation of right ventricular outflow tachycardia in children and adolescents, *J Am Coll Cardiol* 27:869, 1996.

29. Saul JP, Hulse JE, Papagiannis J et al: Late enlargement of radiofrequency lesions in infant lambs: implications for ablation procedures in small children, *Circulation* 90:492, 1994.

30. Gallavardin L: Extrasystolie ventriculaire a paroxysmes tachycardiques prolonges, *Arch Mal Coeur* 15:298, 1922.

31. Froment R, Gallavardin L, Cahen P: Paroxysmal ventricular tachycardia: a clinical classification, *Br Heart J* 15:172, 1953.

32. Zipes DP, Foster PR, Troup PJ, Pedersen DH: Atrial induction of ventricular tachycardia: reentry versus triggered automaticity, *Am J Cardiol* 44:1, 1979.

33. Wellens HJJ, Farré J, Bar FW: The significance of the slow response in ventricular arrhythmias. In Zipes D, Bailey J, Elmarrar V, editors: *The slow inward current,* The Hague, 1980, Martinus Nijhoff.

34. Belhassen B, Rotmensch HH, Laniado S: Response of recurrent sustained ventricular tachycardia to verapamil, *Br Heart J* 16:679, 1981.

35. Nakagawa H, Beckman KJ, McClelland JH et al: Radiofrequency catheter ablation of idiopathic left ventricular tachycardia guided by a Purkinje potential, *Circulation* 88:2607, 1993.

36. Wellens HJJ, Smeets JLRM: Idiopathic left ventricular tachycardia: cure by radiofrequency ablation (editorial), *Circulation* 88:2978, 1993.

37. Wilber LDJ, Baerman J, Olshansky B et al: Adenosine-sensitive ventricular tachycardia: clinical characteristics and response to catheter ablation, *Circulation* 87:126, 1993.

38. Aizawa Y, Chinushi M, Naitoh N et al: Catheter ablation with radiofrequency current of ventricular tachycardia originating from the right ventricle, *Am Heart J* 125:1269, 1993.

39. Klein SL, Shih HT, Hackett K et al: Radiofrequency catheter ablation of ventricular tachycardia in patients without structural heart disease, *Circulation* 85:1666, 1992.

40. Smeets JLRM, Rodriquez LM, Metzger J et al: Can ventricular tachycardia in the absence of structural heart disease be cured by radiofrequency catheter ablation? *Eur Heart J* 14(suppl):256, 1993.

41. Yoshifusa A, Chinushe M, Naitoh N et al: Catheter ablation with radiofrequency current of ventricular tachycardia originating from the right ventricle, *Am Heart J* 125:1269, 1993.

42. Morady F, Kadish AH, DiCarlo L et al: Long-term results of catheter ablation of idiopathic right ventricular tachycardia, *Circulation* 82:2093, 1990.

43. Breithardt G, Borggrefe M, Wichter T: Catheter ablation of idiopathic right ventricular tachycardia (editorial), *Circulation* 82:2273, 1990.

44. Wen MS, Yeh SJ, Wang CC et al: Radiofrequency ablation therapy in idiopathic left ventricular tachycardia with no obvious structural heart disease, *Circulation* 89:1690, 1994.

45. Calkins H, Kalbfleisch SJ, el-Atassi R et al: Relation between efficacy of radiofrequency catheter ablation and site of origin of idiopathic ventricular tachycardia, *Am J Cardiol* 71:827, 1993.

46. Coggins DL, Lee RJ, Sweeney J et al: Radiofrequency catheter ablation as a cure for idiopathic tachycardia of both left and right ventricular origin, *J Am Coll Cardiol* 23:1333, 1994.

47. Garan H: A perspective on the ESVEM trial and current knowledge: catheter ablation for ventricular tachyarrhythmias, *Prog Cardiovasc Dis* 38:457, 1996.

48. Chiang CE, Chen SA, Wang DC et al: Arrhythmogenicity of catheter ablation in supraventricular tachycardia, *Am Heart J* 125:388, 1993.

49. Lacroix D, Kacet S, Lekieffre J: Ventricular fibrillation after successful radiofrequency catheter ablation of idiopathic right ventricular tachycardia, *Am Heart J* 128:1044, 1994.

50. Ng KS, Wen MS, Yeh SJ et al: The effects of adenosine on idiopathic ventricular tachycardia, *Am J Cardiol* 74:195, 1994.

51. Movsowitz C, Schwartzman D, Callans DJ et al: Idiopathic right ventricular outflow tract tachycardia: narrowing the anatomic location for successful ablation, *Am Heart J* 131:930, 1996.

52. Nibley C, Wharton JM: Ventricular tachycardias with left bundle branch block morphology, *Pacing Clin Electrophysiol* 18:334, 1995.

53. Thakur RK, Klein GJ, Sivaram CA et al: Anatomic substrate for idiopathic left ventricular tachycardia, *Circulation* 93:497, 1996.

54. Gaita F, Giustetto C, Leclercq JF et al: Idiopathic verapamil-responsive left ventricular tachycardia: clinical characteristics and long-term follow-up of 33 patients, *Eur Heart J* 15:1252, 1994.

55. Zardini M, Thakur RK, Klein GJ, Yee R: Catheter ablation of idiopathic left ventricular tachycardia, *Pacing Clin Electrophysiol* 18:1255, 1995.

56. Okumura K, Yamabe H, Tsuchiya T et al: Characteristics of slow conduction zone demonstrated during entrainment of idiopathic ventricular tachycardia of left ventricular origin, *Am J Cardiol* 77:379, 1996.

57. Kottkamp H, Chen X, Hindricks G et al: Radiofrequency catheter ablation of idiopathic left ventricular tachycardia: further evidence for microreentry as the underlying mechanism, *J Cardiovasc Electrophysiol* 5:268, 1994.

58. Aizawa Y, Chinushi M, Kitazawa H et al: Spatial orientation of the reentrant circuit of idiopathic left ventricular tachycardia, *Am J Cardiol* 76:316, 1995.

59. Sreeram N, Smeets JL, Wellens HJ: Radiofrequency catheter ablation of idiopathic left ventricular tachycardia in young adults, *Int J Cardiol* 42:288, 1993.

60. Orlov MV, Brodsky MA, Allen BJ et al: Spectrum of right heart involvement in patients with ventricular tachycardia unrelated to coronary artery disease or left ventricular dysfunction, *Am Heart J* 126:1348, 1993.

61. Scheinman MM: The role of catheter ablation in the management of patients with ventricular tachycardia. In Podrid PJ, Kowey PR, editors: *Cardiac arrhythmia: mechanisms, diagnosis, and management,* Baltimore, 1995, Williams & Wilkins.

62. Blanck Z, Sra J, Dhala A et al: Bundle branch reentry: mechanisms, diagnosis, and treatment. In Zipes DP, Jalife J, editors: *Cardiac electrophysiology from cell to bedside,* ed 2, Philadelphia, 1995, WB Saunders.

63. Blanck Z, Akhtar M: Ventricular tachycardia due to sustained bundle branch reentry: diagnostic and therapeutic considerations, *Clin Cardiol* 16:619, 1993.

64. Crijns HJ, Smeets JL, Rodriguez LM et al: Cure of interfascicular reentrant ventricular tachycardia by ablation of the anterior fascicle of the left bundle branch, *J Cardiovasc Electrophysiol* 6:486, 1995.

65. Akhtar M, Damato AN, Batsford WP et al: Demonstration of reentry within the His-Purkinje system in man, *Circulation* 50:1150, 1974.

66. Blanck Z, Dhala A, Deshpande S et al: Bundle branch reentrant ventricular tachycardia: cumulative experience in 48 patients, *J Cardiovasc Electrophysiol* 4:253, 1993.

67. Caceres J, Jazayeri M, McKinnie J et al: Sustained bundle branch reentry as a mechanism of clinical tachycardia, *Circulation* 79:256, 1989.

68. Akhtar M: Clinical spectrum of ventricular tachycardia, *Circulation* 82:1561, 1990.

69. Blanck Z, Jazayeri M, Dhala A et al: Bundle branch reentry: a mechanism of ventricular tachycardia in the absence of myocardial or valvular dysfunction, *J Am Coll Cardiol* 22:1718, 1993.

70. Tchou P, Jazayeri M, Denker S, Dongas J: Transcatheter electrical ablation of the right bundle branch: a method of treating macroreentrant ventricular tachycardia due to bundle branch reentry, *Circulation* 78:246, 1988.

71. Langberg JJ, Desai J, Dullet N, Scheinman MM: Treatment of macroreentrant ventricular tachycardia with radiofrequency ablation of the right bundle branch, *Am J Cardiol* 62:220, 1989.

72. Gallay P: Ventricular tachycardia caused by bundle branch reentry, *Arch Mal Coeur Vaiss* 85:77, 1992.

73. Blanck Z, Deshpande S, Jazayeri MR, Akhtar M: Catheter ablation of the left bundle branch for the treatment of sustained bundle branch reentrant ventricular tachycardia, *J Cardiovasc Electrophysiol* 6:40, 1995.

CHAPTER 18

Polymorphic Ventricular Tachycardia

Classification 293
Acquired long QT
  syndrome 294
Congenital long QT
  syndrome 300
Polymorphic ventricular
  tachycardia (without QT
  prolongation) 303

POLYMORPHIC VENTRICULAR TACHYCARDIA (VT) HAS A CONTINUOUSLY CHANG-ING QRS complex pattern and is viewed as having a more ominous prognosis than that of sustained monomorphic VT. The majority of polymorphic VT episodes terminate spontaneously, although prolonged rapid events (≤200 beats/min) are associated with hemodynamic collapse and usually degenerate into ventricular fibrillation.

Recognition of this life-threatening arrhythmia is important because it is not treated like other VTs. This condition can be exacerbated by the administration of class Ia drugs, some class Ic drugs, and sotalol, but it responds to intravenous (IV) magnesium and, possibly, class Ib drugs.[1,2]

CLASSIFICATION

Polymorphic VT occurs in two clinical settings: long QT syndrome (LQTS) and normal QT. The LQTS setting is divided into (1) *acquired* (iatrogenic) and (2) *congenital* (idiopathic). In both types of LQTS prolonged repolarization and abnormal TU waves result in a rapid polymorphic VT with a distinctive, twisting configuration known as *torsade de pointes (TdP)*. In contrast, when polymorphic VT occurs against a background of normal QT intervals, the resultant VT is simply called polymorphic.

Torsade de pointes is a French expression that means "twisting of the points," which is descriptive of the typical undulating pattern in which the QRS peaks first appear to be up and then down. The singular form, *torsade de pointes,* refers to one episode. The plural form, *torsades de pointes,* refers to more than one episode or to a prolonged attack.[3]

The normal QT type of polymorphic VT has a pattern similar to that of TdP. However, unlike TdP it is not related to sinus bradycardia, preceding pauses, or electrolyte abnormalities.[4] It is important to distinguish between LQTS and normal QT because they have different mechanisms and treatments. Standard antiarrhythmic drugs are given for normal QT polymorphic VT.[2]

ACQUIRED LONG QT SYNDROME

Acquired LQTS often begins with the critical combination of hypokalemia and a potassium channel blocker, which causes the QT to lengthen and early afterdepolarizations (see p. 53) to appear on the action potential recording, resulting in TdP.

ECG Warning Signs

- Progressive lengthening of the QT interval
- T wave alternans or bizarre T wave aberration following a postextrasystolic pause in idiopathic TdP[5]
- Development of prominent U waves in the sinus beats
- Significant heart rate increase in the last minute before the arrhythmic events[6]
- Long-short sequences and salvos of VT[6]
- The shorter the short intervals and the longer the postextrasystolic pauses, the greater the probability of TdP[6]

ECG Recognition of the Tachycardia Itself

- Initiation is pause-dependent (long-short preceding cycles)
- An undulating pattern of the QRS complex appears to twist around the isoelectric line (Figure 18-1)
- Heart rate >170 beats/min

QT prolongation

The QT interval is an indirect measure of the time between ventricular depolarization and repolarization. The uncertainty regarding the true range of the normal QT interval is compounded by the fact that this interval varies with heart rate, gender, and time of day (circadian variability).

The QT interval is usually more than 0.50 second in the sinus beats preceding the tachycardia; this sign is the hallmark of TdP and is an important way to differentiate it from ischemia-related polymorphic VT.[7] The precise degree of QT prolongation that predicts TdP is not known. In quinidine-induced TdP the QT intervals have exceeded 0.60 second. Oberg and Bauman[8] found that in 7 out of 9 episodes of TdP the peak QT

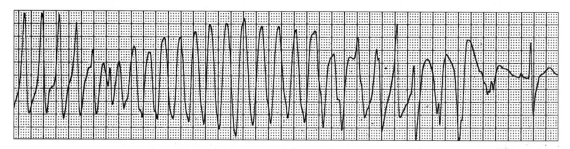

FIGURE 18-1 Torsade de pointes. Note the typical undulating spindle appearance of the pattern in this Holter recording.

prolongation occurred 6.5 to 43 hours before the attack. In all cases the QT was either greater than 0.50 second or prolonged by more than 33%. They found that it is important to watch for a relative change in the QT interval.

The corrected QT interval

Because the QT interval lengthens with bradycardia and shortens with tachycardia, it is corrected for heart rate (QTc) using a formula introduced by Bazett in 1920 (QTc = QT ÷ square root of the RR interval).[9] Since then several other formulas have been proposed, but none of them can be applied universally.[10] Bazett's formula is still in use but has a disadvantage in that it overcorrects at high heart rates. A heart rate of 60 beats/min is the only one in which the QTc is the same as the measured normal QT (i.e., 0.39 second). Some computer readouts provide the QTc, in which case it is only necessary to know the normal (0.39 ± 0.4 second) to evaluate QT prolongation. It should be noted that, according to one study, the uncorrected QT interval may be a better predictor of pause-induced TdP than the QTc interval.[11]

Individual QTc measurements are highly variable. Studies by Molnar, Zhang, and Weiss et al[12] showed that even with 460 ms selected as the upper limit of normal, 23% of their normal subjects exceeded that limit (6% women and 42% men). In their study QTc intervals of >500 ms were not uncommon. Therefore they have suggested that the upper limits now used for the QTc interval (440 ms) may be too low and should be increased. Continuous measurement of QTc intervals over 24 hours in healthy subjects placed the average maximum QTc interval at 495 ± 21 ms, with the average range between minimum and maximum QTc interval at 95 ± 20 ms. Women consistently had longer QTc intervals than men and also had a wider range between minimum and maximum. One study showed that QT prolongation was more than three times as likely in elderly women as in elderly men.[13]

Long-short sequence

The long-short sequence is a hallmark of TdP.[14] Figure 18-2 illustrates the sequence of long-short that initiates the paroxysms of TdP.[15] The long cycle causes the beat that follows it to have an even more prolonged QT interval and dispersion of refractoriness.[16] Waldo's group found characteristic long-short ventricular cycle lengths as the initiating sequence in 41 out of 44 episodes of TdP.[17] For example, in Figure 18-3 there is a long-short sequence that results in TdP against a background of sinus tachycardia and a long QT interval. A ventricular ectopic beat ends the pause and is itself followed by a short cycle of 520 ms. (long-short). The tachycardia typically arises after the peak of the T wave in the cycle following the pause.

The *cascade phenomenon* consists of at least three consecutive long-short sequences, with the ventricular arrhythmias preceding an episode of TdP becoming increasingly more complex.[6] The escalating sequence of events is described as follows:

1. A premature beat is followed by a pause.
2. The pause is followed by a sinus beat with marked TU changes.
3. A ventricular beat originates from the TU changes and is itself followed by a pause and more bizarre TU changes from which progressively longer and faster runs of TdP originate.

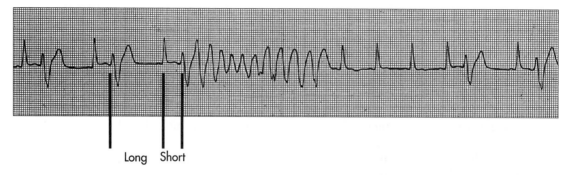

Long   Short

FIGURE 18-2 Note the long-short prelude of this episode of torsade de pointes.

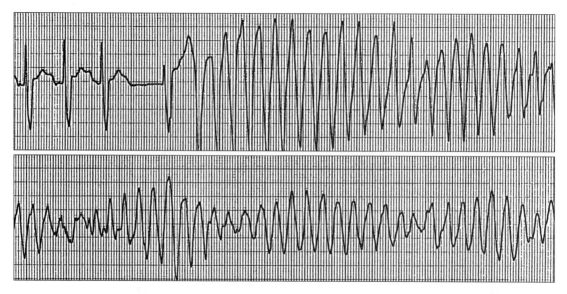

FIGURE 18-3 The onset of torsade de pointes. In the top tracing, note a prolonged QTU, the short-long-short sequence, and the typical undulating pattern of torsade de pointes.

Potassium Channel Blockers and Torsades de Pointes

Drugs such as quinidine suppress a range of potassium currents, including the rapidly activating delayed potassium rectifier current (I_{Kr}). Drugs that block I_{Kr} markedly prolong the QT interval and produce TdP in some patients. For some of these drugs the development of TdP is related to high dosages and/or high plasma concentrations; with other drugs this is not the case. Characteristic features of quinidine-related TdP are low quinidine plasma concentrations, the absence of marked QRS prolongation, hypokalemia (potassium less than 4 mEq/L), and slowing of the heart rate just before the initiation of TdP.[18]

Hypokalemia

Hypokalemia and bradyarrhythmias are important risk factors for the development of TdP. Studies suggest that the level of extracellular potassium is a major factor in modulating the physiology of I_{Kr} and its response to blocking drugs. Action potential durations are shorter at higher extracellular concentrations of potassium and longer at lower levels. At low levels of extracellular potassium there is an increase in sensitivity to drug block of potassium channels so that even a modest degree of hypokalemia is critical during TdP.[19]

Erythromycin

Daleau, Lessart, Groleau, and Turgeon[20] demonstrated in guinea pig ventricular myocytes that erythromycin blocks an outward, time-dependent potassium current that has characteristics similar to those of I_{Kr}. Torsades de pointes induction by injectable erythromycin lactobionate is rare, but QT prolongation is common. Some patients may be at risk for suffering TdP because of this agent, particularly if heart disease or other factors that may further delay ventricular repolarization are present.[8]

Antihistamines

It is now well known that nonsedating H_1-selective antihistamines such as astemizole (Hismanal)[21-23] and terfenadine (Seldane)[24-32] can cause TdP in certain individuals. The modulation of histamine receptors in cardiac tissue can have a profound effect on AV conduction and arrhythmogenesis. Studies suggest that the mechanism of action of nonsedating antihistamines causing TdP is potassium channel blockade; a significant blockade of the channel for inward potassium rectifier current (I_{K1}) was demonstrated.[32] It should also be noted that terfenadine metabolism is prevented by the antifungal agent itraconazole (Sporanox), which increases the risk of TdP already present with terfenadine.[33]

Antihistamines are prescribed for the treatment of allergies, urticarial diseases, and symptoms associated with upper respiratory infections. They act by blocking the H_1 histamine receptors present in skin, pulmonary, gastrointestinal, neural, and cardiac tissues. Astemizole and terfenadine are second-generation H_1-receptor antagonists that differ from first-generation antihistamines because they have a preferential affinity for the peripheral H_1 receptors (vs the brain and cholinergic receptors). Their proarrhythmic effects (TdP) have typically been seen only with overdose, liver disease, or concomitant administration of a medication that interferes with hepatic cytochrome P-450 enzymatic metabolism (e.g., cimetidine [Tagamet], macrolide antibiotics [the erythromycins], ketoconazole [Nizoral]).[34]

Summary of mechanisms

In summary, the concatenation of events leading to acquired LQTS may begin with hypokalemia and a potassium channel blocker (e.g., quinidine), which leads to the prolongation of action potential duration, the development of early afterdepolarizations, and critically slow conduction that contributes to the development of reentry.[7,35-38] The early afterdepolarizations initiate the tachycardia; reentry sustains it.[37,38] Reentrant waves normally rotate around a stationary spiral core. However, if action potential duration is prolonged in excess of the perimeter of this stationary unexcited spiral core, the core becomes unstable and drifts, resulting in polymorphic VT. One of two things may then happen: the wave front fragments may annihilate one another, producing nonsustained TdP, or multiple spiral wavelets may arise, causing fibrillation and sudden cardiac death.[39]

Common Clinical Causes

In a study involving 65 patients with 74 episodes of TdP the most common cause was therapy with diuretics (30 episodes); second place was shared by D-1-sotalol and hypokalemia of less than 3.6 mM (23 episodes each); quinidine was the third most common cause (18 episodes).[40] One study has shown that quinidine and disopyramide, although both class Ia drugs, have significantly different effects on repolarization after a pause, which may account for the greater frequency of TdP with quinidine.[41]

Clinical Characteristics

1. An important clinical characteristic of the class Ia antiarrhythmic drug–induced TdP is that it appears to occur early in the drug course, permitting in-hospital detection and treatment.
2. TdP is more common in women. Women represent almost half of the cases of TdP even though they constitute the minority of patients receiving antiarrhythmic drugs for ventricular arrhythmias.[42,43]
3. TdP that results from electrolyte disturbances and drugs tends to recur with high frequency until the underlying cause is corrected, which usually takes from several hours to several days.

Latent Long QT Syndrome

The identification of patients at risk for developing TdP involves computing the QTc during rest and after a stress test. Kadish et al[44] have shown that although patients may have a normal QTc interval during rest, they are at risk for developing TdP if they demonstrate a prolonged QTc with exercise and are given type Ia antiarrhythmic agents. In this study, 10 out of 11 patients with newly documented drug-related TdP had an abnormal repolarization response to exercise compared with 11 control patients. The patients who developed TdP when drug-free had a normal QTc at rest but a long QTc with exercise (although the uncorrected QT actually shortened with exercise).

Symptoms

With TdP, the patient is often unaware of palpitations. However, if the attack is prolonged there are episodes of dizziness, syncope and, rarely, sudden death, probably from a deterioration of TdP into ventricular fibrillation.[2] When syncope is the presenting symptom, patients are sometimes misdiagnosed as epileptic.[45] The term *quinidine syncope* was used to describe these symptoms before knowledge of the mechanism and ECG identification of TdP.

Emergency Treatment

Treatment of the acquired form of TdP is primarily directed at identifying and withdrawing the offending agent. Emergency therapy using maneuvers and agents that favorably modulate transmembrane ion currents can be lifesaving. The following measures are taken for the emergency treatment of TdP:[40,46]

1. The patient is monitored continuously, and it is ascertained that the condition is truly a long QT (QTU) duration in the basic rhythm.
2. All agents that may be potentially responsible for TdP and QT prolongation are immediately discontinued.
3. IV potassium is given to correct this electrolyte abnormality. Blood samples are drawn for later evaluation and confirmation of deficiencies and drug levels.
4. IV magnesium is regarded as the treatment of choice for TdP and is even suggested for normomagnesemia.[47,48]
5. If IV magnesium is unsuccessful, overdrive ventricular pacing or isoproterenol may be necessary as a way to increase the basic heart rate and thus shorten the QT interval. Temporary ventricular or atrial pacing suppresses the VT, and it may remain abated after pacing is discontinued.[49]
6. Direct current cardioversion is usually transiently effective in terminating TdP. Repeated cardioversions may be necessary when the arrhythmia is caused by high doses of class Ia agents.

Possible Outcomes

- Slowing and then spontaneous conversion
- Conversion and then a new attack
- Ventricular standstill
- Ventricular fibrillation

Patients with idiopathic LQTS who are at increased risk for sudden death are those with a family member who died suddenly at an early age and those who have had syncope.

Contraindications for Magnesium

The continued use of magnesium is contraindicated in the following situations:

- Renal failure
- Disappearance of deep tendon reflex
- Rise in serum Mg above 5 mEq/L
- Drop in systolic blood pressure below 80 mm Hg
- Drop in pulse below 60 beats/min

Advantages of Magnesium for Torsades de Pointes

Studies have shown that the prompt suppression of TdP arrhythmia in both acquired and congenital LQTS can be achieved with IV magnesium.[50] Magnesium has the advantage of safety and simplicity of administration. If the diagnosis of TdP is uncertain, magnesium will not aggravate the VT that is not TdP, as would isoproterenol.

Magnesium plays an essential role in maintaining the cellular resting membrane potential. It is a necessary intracellular ingredient for the phosphorylation of ATP and sodium in the sodium pump.[51,52]

Isoproterenol or cardiac pacing is sometimes used to shorten the QT interval by a rate increase. Although effective, both have disadvantages. Isoproterenol is contraindicated in patients with hypertension or ischemic heart disease; cardiac pacing requires skilled personnel and fluoroscopy.

Prevention

The following steps should be taken after initiating drugs to prolong the QT interval:[50]
1. Monitor the QT interval.
2. Modify the dosage of the drug if the QT interval reaches 0.56 to 0.60 second.
3. Discontinue the drug and hospitalize the patient immediately if the patient complains of lightheadedness or syncope or if there is increased frequency and complexity of ventricular premature beats (VPBs).

CONGENITAL LONG QT SYNDROME

The congenital LQTS is an inherited disease characterized by prolonged repolarization resulting in QT, T, and U wave abnormalities. There is a high incidence of sudden death in some affected families but not in others.[53]

Three forms of congenital LQTS have been named. Two are hereditary, one with and one without accompanying deafness, and one is sporadic. Although uncommon, congenital LQTS is a potentially treatable cause of sudden cardiac death.

Chromosomal Defects

Exciting new molecular genetic findings in LQTS have opened new areas of research. Mutations in three genes that encode the cardiac ion channel protein have been identified and account for >90% of cases. The currents that pass through ion channels determine cardiac repolarization.

In families linked to chromosome 3, mutations in *SCN5A* cause LQTS. This gene encodes the human cardiac sodium channel; defects result in defective sodium channel inactivation. In families linked to chromosome 7, mutations in *HERG* cause LQTS. This gene encodes the delayed rectifier potassium channel; defects result in decreased outward potassium current. In families linked to chromosome 11, mutations in *KVLQT1* cause LQTS. This newly cloned gene appears to encode a potassium channel; such defects decrease net outward current during repolarization, which accounts for long QT intervals.[53]

ECG Recognition

The following ECG characteristics of congenital LQTS are illustrated in Figure 18-4:
- **QTc.** Prolonged (>0.46 second); may be in the normal–to–upper normal range (0.41 to 0.45 second);[54] borderline QT prolongation is more sensitive but less specific
- **QT dispersion.** Normal: 46 ± 18 ms; LQTS: 33 ± 21 ms

The difference between the longest and shortest QT intervals on the 12-lead ECG is increased in LQTS. Figure 18-5 demonstrates QT alternans:
- **T wave.** Alternans (varies from beat to beat and with sympathetic activation);[55] often notched or biphasic[5,53,56,57]
- **U waves.** Prominent in some patients; exaggerated in sinus bradycardia or after pauses (Figure 18-6); may display alternans; marked prolongation of the QT interval can represent a very prominent U wave
- **Sinus rate.** Bradycardia and decreased heart rate with exercise in some individuals
- **Initiation:** Long-short sequence may be seen at onset of congenital LQTS (as in acquired TdP);[14] cascade phenomenon has also been described in pause-dependent TdP

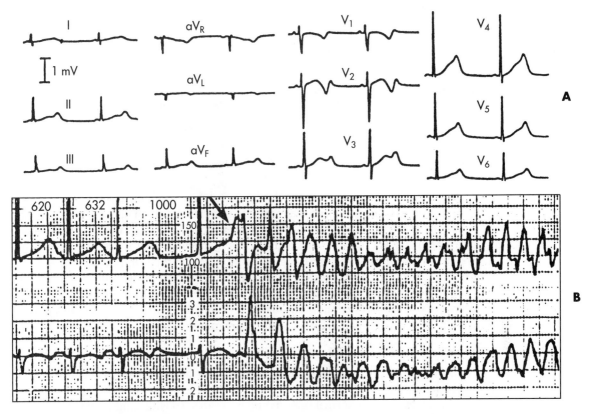

FIGURE 18-4 ECG recordings from an 11-year-old girl with congenital LQTS and recurrent syncope. **A,** A 12-lead rest ECG demonstrates biphasic and notched T waves. **B,** Holter recording during a syncopal episode triggered by sudden arousal from sleep and accompanied seizures. The RR intervals during sinus rhythm are shown in milliseconds. The sinus complex after the longest RR interval shows marked augmentation of TU wave amplitude *(arrow)* and is immediately followed by torsade de pointes. (From Viskin S, Alla SR, Barron HV et al: Mode of onset of torsades de pointes in congenital long QT syndrome, *J Am Coll Cardiol* 28:1262, 1996.)

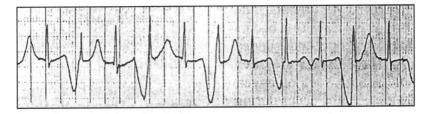

FIGURE 18-5 QT alternans. The QT interval on alternate beats is as long as the RR interval. (From Roden DM, Lazzara R, Rosen M et al: Multiple mechanisms in the long QT syndrome: current knowledge, gaps, and future directions, *Circulation* 94:1996, 1996.)

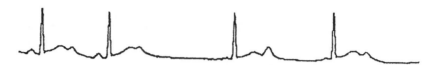

FIGURE 18-6 Pause-dependent lability of a prominent U wave. (From Roden DM, Lazzara R, Rosen M et al: Multiple mechanisms in the long QT syndrome: current knowledge, gaps, and future directions, *Circulation* 94:1996, 1996.)

Abnormal T Waves

Abnormal T wave patterns may also be useful in identifying asymptomatic family members, which may be an especially valuable diagnostic tool in light of the limitations of QT measurements and correction for heart rate. Nador, Beria, and De Ferrari et al[56] have noted biphasic, bifid, or notched T waves (particularly in the precordial leads) associated with abnormal echocardiographic findings, syncope, and cardiac arrest.[5] Figure 18-7 illustrates three grades of T wave humps collected from a study of 13 families with congenital LQTS.[58] Grade I, although subtle, demonstrates a distinct bulge in the downslope of the T wave that is unusual when compared with the usually brisk normal T descent. In grades II and III the T humps are more distinct.

The Corrected QT Interval

In the diagnosis of nonsymptomatic members of a family with congenital LQTS, measurement of the QTc interval may not be diagnostic. There may be an overlap in the range of QTc values between normal subjects and those affected with congenital LQTS.[54]

Treatment

The present treatment for congenital LQTS is antiadrenergic therapy (β-blocking agents, left cervicothoracic sympathetic ganglionectomy) because an increase in sympathetic stimulation can precipitate TdP in these patients. The efficacy of permanent pacing and a β-blocker has also been reported, with the main goal being the prevention of the pauses that precede TdP.[14]

One study based on the fact that I_{Kr} is activated by an increase in potassium (which shortened the duration of repolarization) found potassium to be effective in the treatment of congenital LQTS.[59]

Screening

1. Congenital TdP can be screened with stress testing and the Valsalva maneuver because such maneuvers can prolong the QT interval, produce T wave alternans, and cause TdP in afflicted patients. In contrast, acquired TdP is usually manifested during bradycardia or long pauses in the ventricular rhythm.
2. When an individual is found to have symptoms of TdP, all family members should have ECG monitoring. During ECG monitoring they are subjected to various stresses (e.g., auditory stimuli, psychologic stress, cold pressor stimulation, and exercise).

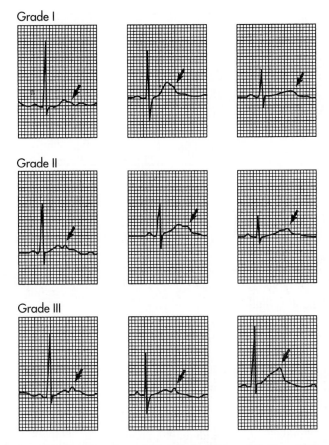

FIGURE 18-7 A grading for T-wave humps in patients with congenital long QT syndrome. In grade I there is a slight bulge on the downslope of the T wave. The distortions in grades II and III are more obvious. (From Lehmann HM, Suzuki F, Fromm BS et al: T wave "humps" as a potential electrocardiographic marker of the long QT syndrome, *J Am Coll Cardiol* 24:746, 1994.)

POLYMORPHIC VENTRICULAR TACHYCARDIA (WITHOUT QT PROLONGATION)

Most of the patients with polymorphic VT without QT prolongation have coronary artery disease. Akhtar[60] describes two subgroups: one associated with chronic coronary artery disease and the other with acute myocardial ischemia caused by critical coronary artery stenosis.

Chronic Coronary Artery Disease

Figure 18-8 shows a polymorphic VT without QT prolongation in a patient with stable coronary artery disease and prior myocardial damage but no evidence of acute ischemia. Treatment options are similar to those for sustained monomorphic VT in association with chronic coronary artery disease.[60]

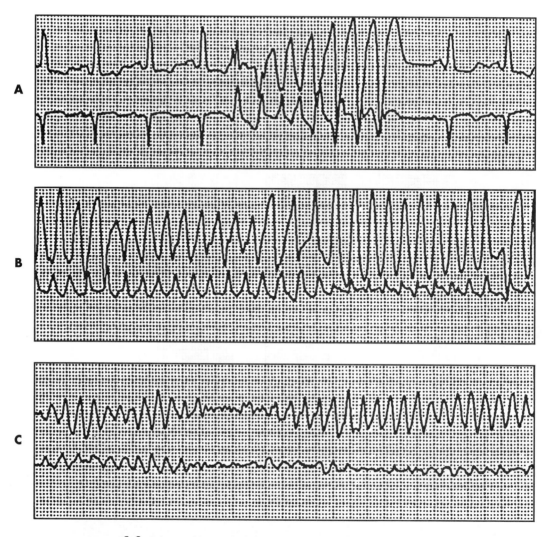

FIGURE 18-8 Polymorphic ventricular tachycardia with a normal QT interval in a patient with chronic coronary artery disease. **A,** Spontaneous episode of polymorphic ventricular tachycardia. **B,** Sustained episode leading to ventricular fibrillation. **C,** Patient had coronary artery disease but continued to have such episodes after myocardial revascularization and beta blockade. Class I agents readily controlled this arrhythmia. (From Akhtar M: Clinical spectrum of ventricular tachycardia, *Circulation* 82:1561, 1990.)

Acute Myocardial Ischemia

Figure 18-9 shows a polymorphic VT in a patient with acute ischemia caused by an occluding bypass graft. This type of VT is often but not always accompanied or preceded by angina or ischemic ECG changes, and it responds well to β-blockers and myocardial revascularization.

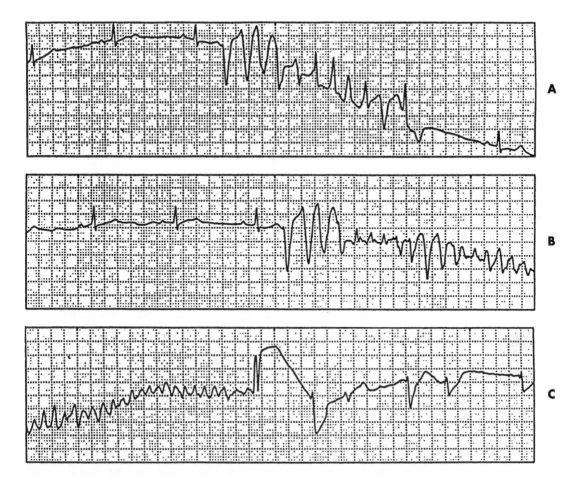

FIGURE 18-9 Polymorphic ventricular tachycardia with a normal QT interval in a patient with acute myocardial ischemia. **A,** Nonsustained polymorphic ventricular tachycardia. **B** and **C,** Another episode that leads to rapid degeneration into ventricular fibrillation. (From Akhtar M: Clinical spectrum of ventricular tachycardia, *Circulation* 82:1561, 1990.)

Figures 18-10 and 18-11 are tracings from patients who had symptoms of angina and/or ST segment deviation immediately before the initiation of the polymorphic VT. Wolfe, Nibley, and Bhandari et al[4] found the following in patients with post–myocardial infarction polymorphic VT:

1. Although the QT interval and the QTc were normal or mildly prolonged, the arrhythmia failed to respond to class I antiarrhythmics.
2. IV amiodarone appeared to be effective in suppressing the VT.
3. The tachycardia was associated with symptoms or ECG evidence of recurrent ischemia.

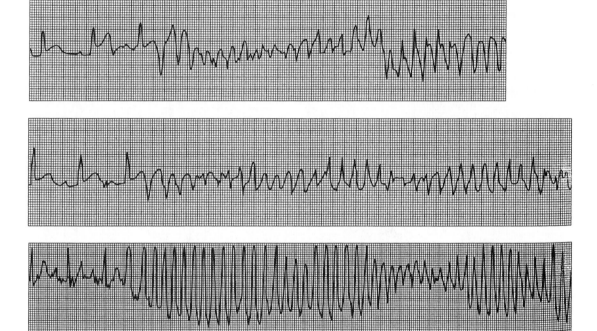

FIGURE 18-10 Recording of three episodes of polymorphic ventricular tachycardia in a patient on day five after an acute inferior myocardial infarction. The first two episodes were preceded by ST segment elevation on the ECG. Note the normal QT interval and the absence of bradycardia or a sinus pause immediately before the initiation of polymorphic ventricular tachycardia. (From Wolfe CL, Nibley C, Bhandari A et al: Polymorphous ventricular tachycardia associated with acute myocardial infarction, *Circulation* 84:1543, 1991.)

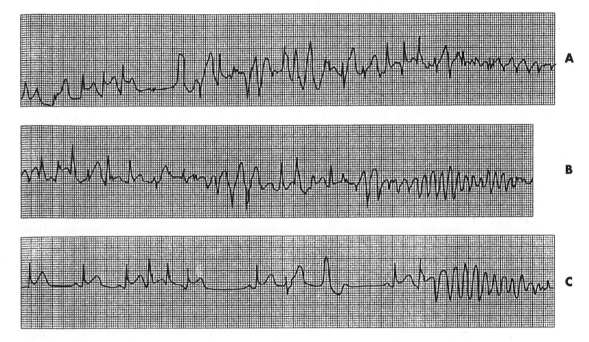

FIGURE 18-11 Recordings from recurrent episodes of polymorphic ventricular tachycardia in a patient who had received IV tissue-type plasminogen activator for treatment of an acute anterior myocardial infarction. All three tracings show ST-segment elevation before the onset of the tachycardia. **A** and **C,** Tracings are continuous. A pause immediately precedes the onset of the tachycardia. **B,** An episode of ventricular tachycardia that is not preceded by a sinus pause. (From Wolfe CL, Nibley C, Bhandari A et al: Polymorphous ventricular tachycardia associated with acute myocardial infarction, *Circulation* 84:1543, 1991.)

SUMMARY

Polymorphic VT has a continuously changing QRS complex pattern and is classified according to whether the baseline QT (or QTU) interval is normal or prolonged. The term *torsade de pointes* (TdP) is reserved exclusively for the type of polymorphic VT associated with a prolonged QT interval.

Polymorphic VT with a normal QT interval is usually associated with coronary artery disease or acute myocardial infarction. It has a pattern similar to that of TdP, but unlike TdP it is not related to sinus bradycardia, preceding pauses, or electrolyte abnormalities.[4] It is important to distinguish between prolonged and normal QT intervals because the polymorphic VTs associated with them have different mechanisms and treatments.

REFERENCES

1. Arstall MA, Hii JT, Lehman RG, Horowitz JD: Sotalol-induced torsade de pointes: management with magnesium infusion, *Postgrad Med J* 68:289, 1992.
2. Zipes DP: Specific arrhythmias: diagnosis and treatment. In Braunwald E, editor: *Heart disease*, ed 4, Philadelphia 1992, WB Saunders.
3. Coumel P, Leclercq JF, Dessertenne F: Torsades de pointes. In Josephson ME, Wellens HJJ, editors: *Tachycardias: mechanisms, diagnosis, treatment*, Philadelphia, 1984, Lea & Febiger.
4. Wolfe CL, Nibley C, Bhandari A et al: Polymorphous ventricular tachycardia associated with acute myocardial infarction, *Circulation* 84:1543, 1991.
5. Malfatto G, Beria G, Sala S et al: Quantitative analysis of T wave abnormalities and their prognostic implications in the idiopathic long QT syndrome, *J Am Coll Cardiol* 23:296, 1994.
6. Locati EH, Maison-Blanche P, Dejode P et al: Spontaneous sequences of onset of torsade de pointes in patients with acquired prolonged repolarization: quantitative analysis of Holter recordings, *J Am Coll Cardiol* 25:1564, 1995.
7. Roden DM: Torsade de pointes, *Clin Cardiol* 16:683, 1993.
8. Oberg KC, Bauman JL: QT interval prolongation and torsades de pointes due to erythromycin lactobionate, *Pharmacotherapy* 15:687, 1995.
9. Bazett HC: An analysis of the time relations of electrocardiograms, *Heart,* p 353, 1920.
10. Puddu PE, Jouve R, Mariotti S et al: Evaluation of 10 QT prediction formulas in 881 middle-aged men from the Seven Countries Study: emphasis on the Cubic Root Fridericia's Equation, *J Electrocardiol* 21:219, 1988.
11. Keren A, Tzivoni D, Gavish D et al: Etiology, warning signs and therapy of torsade de pointes: a study of 10 patients, *Circulation* 64:1167, 1981.
12. Molnar J, Zhang F, Weiss J et al: Diurnal pattern of QTc interval: how long is prolonged? Possible relation to circadian triggers of cardiovascular events, *J Am Coll Cardiol* 27:76, 1996.
13. Rautaharju PM, Manolio TA, Psaty BM et al: Correlates of QT prolongation in older adults (the cardiovascular health study), *Am J Cardiol* 73:999, 1974.
14. Viskin S, Alla SR, Barron HV et al: Mode of onset of torsade de pointes in congenital long QT syndrome, *J Am Coll Cardiol* 28:1262, 1996.
15. Cranefield PF, Aronson RS: Torsade de pointes and other pause-induced ventricular tachycardias: the short-long-short sequence and early afterdepolarizations, *Pacing Clin Electrophysiol* 11(6 pt 1):6708, 1988.
16. El-Sherif N, Gough WB, Restivo M: Reentrant ventricular arrhythmias in the late myocardial infarction period: mechanism by which a short-long-short cardiac sequence facilitates the induction of reentry, *Circulation* 83:268, 1991.
17. Clark M et al: Torsade de pointes: serum drug levels and ECG warning signs, *Circulation* 66:282, 1982 (abstract).

18. Roden DM, Thompson KA, Hoffman BF, Woosley RL: Clinical features and basic mechanisms of quinidine-induced arrhythmias, *J Am Coll Cardiol* 8(1 suppl A):73A, 1986.

19. Yang T, Roden DM: Extracellular potassium modulation of drug block of I_Kr: implications for torsade de pointes and reverse use–dependence, *Circulation* 93:1996.

20. Daleau P, Lessart E, Groleau MF, Turgeon J: Erythromycin blocks the rapid component of the delayed rectifier potassium current and lengthens repolarization of guinea pig ventricular myocytes, *Circulation* 91:3010, 1995.

21. Vorperian VR, Zhou Z, Mohammad S et al: Torsade de pointes with an antihistamine metabolite: potassium channel blockade with desmethylastemizole, *J Am Coll Cardiol* 28:1556, 1996.

22. Saviuc P, Danel V, Dixmerias F: Prolonged QT interval and torsade de pointes following astemizole overdose, *J Toxicol Clin Toxicol* 31:121, 1993.

23. Katyal VK, Jagdish Choudhary D, Choudhary D: Occurrence of torsade de pointes with use of astemizole, *Indian Heart J* 46:181, 1994.

24. Pinney SP, Koller BS, Franz MR, Woosley RL: Terfenadine increases the QT interval in isolated guinea pig heart, *J Cardiovasc Pharmacol* 25:30, 1995.

25. Koh KK, Rim MS, Yoon J, Kim SS: Torsade de pointes induced by terfenadine in a patient with long QT syndrome, *J Electrocardiol* 27:343, 1994.

26. Smith SJ: Cardiovascular toxicity of antihistamines, *Otolaryngol Head Neck Surg* 111:348, 1994.

27. Tran HT: Torsades de pointes induced by nonantiarrhythmic drugs, *Conn Med* 58:291, 1994.

28. Rao KA, Adlakha A, Verma-Ansil B et al: Torsades de pointes ventricular tachycardia associated with overdose of astemizole, *Mayo Clin Proc* 69:589, 1994.

29. Botstein P: Is QT interval prolongation harmful? A regulatory perspective, Office of Drug Evaluation I, Food and Drug Administration, Rockville, Md 20857, *Am J Cardiol* 72:50B, 1993.

30. Hasan RA, Zureikat GY, Nolan BM: Torsade de pointes associated with astemizole overdose treated with magnesium sulfate, *Pediatr Emerg Care* 9:23, 1993.

31. Sakemi H, VanNatta B: Torsade de pointes induced by astemizole in a patient with prolongation of the QT interval, *Am Heart J* 125:1436, 1993.

32. Berul CI, Morad M: Regulation of potassium channels by nonsedating antihistamines, *Circulation* 91:2220, 1995.

33. Pohjola-Sintonen S, Viitasalo M, Toivonen L, Neuvonen P: Itraconazole prevents terfenadine metabolism and increases risk of torsades de pointes ventricular tachycardia, *Eur J Clin Pharmacol* 45:191, 1993.

34. Honig PK, Wortham DC, Zamani K et al: Terfenadine-ketoconazole interaction, *JAMA* 269:1513, 1993.

35. Jackman WM, Szabo B, Friday KJ et al: Ventricular tachyarrhythmias related to early afterdepolarizations and triggered firing: relationship to QT interval prolongation and potential therapeutic role for calcium channel blocking agents, *J Cardiovasc Electrophys* 1:170, 1990.

36. El-Sherif N, Craelius W, Boutjdir M, Gough WB: Early afterdepolarizations and arrhythmogenesis, *J Cardiovasc Electrophysiol* 1:145, 1990.

37. Pertsov AM, Davidenko JM, Salomonsz R et al: Spiral waves of excitation underlie reentrant activity in isolated cardiac muscle, *Circ Res* 72:631, 1993.

38. Schwartz PJ, Locati EH, Napolitano C, Priori SG: The long QT syndrome. In Zipes DP, Jalife J, editors: *Cellular electrophysiology from cell to bedside,* Philadelphia, 1992, WB Saunders.

39. Starmer CF, Romashko DN, Reddy RS et al: Proarrhythmic response to potassium channel blockade: numerical studies of polymorphic tachyarrhythmias, *Circulation* 92:595, 1996.

40. Haverkamp W, Shenasa M, Borggrefe M, Breithardt G: Torsades de pointes. In Zipes DP, Jalife J, editors: *Cardiac electrophysiology from cell to bedside,* Philadelphia, 1995, WB Saunders.

41. Bursill JA, Qyse KR, Campbell TJ: Quinidine but not disopyramide prolongs cardiac Purkinje fiber action potentials after a pause, *J Cardiovasc Pharmacol* 23:833, 1994.

42. Makkar RR, Fromm BS, Steinman RT et al: Female gender as a risk factor for torsades de pointes associated with cardiovascular drugs, *JAMA* 270:2590, 1993.

43. Kawasaki R, Machado C, Reinoehl J et al: Increased propensity of women to develop torsades de pointes during complete heart block, *J Cardiovasc Electrophysiol* 6:1032, 1995.

44. Kadish AH, Weisman HF, Veltri EP et al: Paradoxical effects of exercise on the QT interval in patients with polymorphic ventricular tachycardia receiving type Ia antiarrhythmic agents, *Circulation* 81:14, 1990.

45. Gospe SM Jr, Choy M: Hereditary long Q-T syndrome presenting as epilepsy: electroencephalography laboratory diagnosis, *Ann Neurol* 25:514, 1989.

46. Wellens HJJ, Conover M: *The ECG in emergency decision making*, Philadelphia, 1991, WB Saunders.

47. Banai S, Tzivoni D: Drug therapy for torsade de pointes, *J Cardiovasc Electrophysiol* 4:206, 1993.

48. Iseri LT, Chung P, Tobis J: Magnesium therapy for intractable ventricular tachyarrhythmias in normomagnesemic patients, *West J Med* 138:823, 1983.

49. Jackman WM, Friday KJ, Clark M et al: The long QT syndromes: a critical review, new clinical observations and unifying hypothesis, *Prog Cardiovasc Dis* 31:115, 1988.

50. Keren A, Tzivoni D: Torsades de pointes: prevention and therapy, *Cardiovasc Drugs Ther* 5:509, 1991.

51. Tzivoni D, Keren A: Suppression of ventricular arrhythmias by magnesium, *Am J Cardiol* 65:1397, 1990.

52. Gadsby DC: The Na/K pump of cardiac myocytes. In Zipes DP, Jalife J, editors: *Cardiac electrophysiology*, Philadelphia, 1990, WB Saunders.

53. Roden DM, Lazzara R, Rosen M et al: Multiple mechanisms in the long QT syndrome: current knowledge, gaps, and future directions, *Circulation* 94:1996, 1996.

54. Vincent GM, Timothy KW, Leppert M, Keating M: The spectrum of symptoms and QT intervals in carriers of the gene for the long QT syndrome, *N Engl J Med* 327:846, 1992.

55. Schwartz PJ, Malliani A: Electrical alternation of the T wave: clinical and experimental evidence of its relationship with the sympathetic nervous system and with the long QT syndrome, *Am Heart J* 89:45, 1975.

56. Nador F, Beria G, De Ferrari GM et al: Unsuspected echocardiographic abnormality in the long QT syndrome: diagnostic, prognostic, and pathogenetic implications, *Circulation* 84:1530, 1991.

57. Schwartz PJ, Moss AJ, Vincent GM, Grampton RS: Diagnostic criteria for the long QT syndrome: an update, *Circulation* 88:782, 1993.

58. Lehmann HM, Suzuki F, Fromm BS et al: T wave "humps" as a potential electrocardiographic marker of the long QT syndrome, *J Am Coll Cardiol* 24:746, 1994.

59. Compton SJ, Lux RL, Ramsey MR et al: Genetically defined therapy of inherited long-QT syndrome: correction of abnormal repolarization by potassium, *Circulation* 94:1018, 1996.

60. Akhtar M: Clinical spectrum of ventricular tachycardia, *Circulation* 82:1561, 1990.

The PR interval 311
Nonconducted beats 311
Type I and type II block
   312
Anatomy versus
   behavior 312
Wenckebach periodicity
   and RP/PR reciprocity
   314
2:1 AV block 316
"Skipped" P waves 317
High-grade (or advanced)
   AV block 318
Complete AV block 319
Ventricular asystole 320
Need to reclassify 320
Remedial measures 326

CHAPTER **19**

AV Block

EVERYONE AT ALL CONVERSANT WITH THE TERMINOLOGY OF CARDIOLOGY IS FAMILIAR with the conventional division of AV block into first, second, and third degrees. Few, however, appreciate what confusion, misunderstanding, and mismanagement this oversimplified classification has created. The situation has been compounded by deficient definitions and multiple misconceptions. It is with these unfortunate aspects of the subject that much of this chapter is concerned.

THE PR INTERVAL

The normal PR interval, measured from the beginning of the P wave to the beginning of the QRS complex, ranges between 0.12 and 0.20 second. This is not to say that somewhat longer and shorter intervals necessarily indicate abnormality; in a study of normal youths between the ages of 15 and 23 years, 1.3% had PR intervals longer than 0.20 second, and the same percentage had intervals shorter than 0.12 second.[1] It may well be that these exceptions to the general rule represent merely the extremities of a normal bell curve.

The term *first-degree AV block* is generally applied when all atrial impulses that should be conducted to the ventricles are so conducted, but with a PR interval of greater than 0.20 second.

NONCONDUCTED BEATS

The term *second-degree AV block* is applied when one or more (but not all) atrial impulses that should be conducted fail to reach the ventricles. This term thus covers a great variety of conduction patterns of markedly variable significance.

When an atrial impulse fails to reach the ventricles, it is often referred to as a "dropped" beat. The use of this term has been criticized, but it is difficult to find an adequate and appropriate substitute; it at least has the blessing of traditional use since Lewis.[2] *Faute de mieux,* we shall use it!

When an atrial impulse fails to reach the ventricles and a beat is "dropped," the individual circumstances must be considered. If the atrial impulse arrives at the AV junction early in the cycle when the junction is still normally refractory, it is not conducted but neither is it blocked; *block* implies a *pathologic* failure of conduction. One of the determinants of the prematurity with which an atrial impulse arrives at the junction is the atrial rate; when the rate is exceedingly fast, as in atrial flutter, it is only proper that every other impulse should not be conducted. One of the normal functions of the AV node is to protect the ventricles from excessively rapid and therefore ineffective beating when the atria have gone berserk. Therefore 2:1 conduction resulting from normal refractoriness should not be called 2:1 block, which immediately places it in an abnormal category.

Before assessing the significance of a dropped beat, the atrial rate and its inseparable partner the RP interval must always be considered. The failure of an atrial impulse to reach the ventricles can have a quite different significance if its P wave lands after the end of the T wave than if it is perched on the first part of the ST segment.

TYPE I AND TYPE II BLOCK

In 1899 Wenckebach,[3] without benefit of electrocardiograph and by simple observation of the pulses in the neck, described the form of AV block that bears his name, in which the AV conduction time progressively lengthens until a beat is dropped (Figure 19-1).

Seven years later Wenckebach[4] in Vienna and Hay[5] in Scotland both described a second form of AV block in which there was no progressive lengthening of conduction time before conduction failed (Figure 19-2).

In 1924 Mobitz[6] correlated these earlier clinical findings with those in the electrocardiogram and suggested that the first type be called "type I" (1899) and the second type "type II" (1906). They have since been commonly referred to as Mobitz type I and Mobitz type II block but are just as appropriately called Wenckebach type I and Wenckebach type II.[7,8] In later years His bundle recordings have repeatedly demonstrated that type I block is usually a manifestation of AV nodal block, whereas type II is always infranodal block and is usually a manifestation of bilateral bundle branch block (BBB).[9-12]

As useful as this classification has proved to be and as widely as the terms *type I* and *type II* are used, most authorities fail to explain fully how they are using them, and the simple division into two types is beset with ambiguities.

If the terms are confined only to the basic patterns of block originally described, the terms are too restrictive and their usefulness is decreased. For example, if a patient has an atrial rate of 80 beats/min with 3:2 Wenckebach periods, it is generally accepted as classical type I block. If the atrial rate increases to 100 beats/min with the result that the conduction ratio changes to 2:1, it is still the same type of block (i.e., type I); however, there is no longer the progressive increase in conduction times (PR intervals) before each dropped beat, which is characteristic of the classical Wenckebach. Thus if only examples with increasing PR intervals are included, important samples of type I block are excluded.

ANATOMY VERSUS BEHAVIOR

Two ingredients blend to produce both type I and type II block: pathophysiologic behavior and the anatomic level of the block. Unfortunately, there is an irreconcilable dichotomy between anatomy and behavior. Most authorities, correctly following traditional usage, use the terms *type I* and *type II* as behavioral descriptions.[13-16] Yet there is little doubt that the anatomic level of the lesion is clinically more important than its physiologic behavior. For example, in the presence of contralateral bundle branch block, Wenckebach periodicity in a bundle branch is behaviorally type I but clinically and prognostically more appropriately considered type II.[8,17] Consequently, a division into nodal and infranodal, or proximal and distal, has much to commend it.[17]

It would be ideal if we could infallibly distinguish between AV nodal block (and call it type I) and infranodal block (and call it type II) from the clinical tracing. Unfortunately we cannot; in many situations intracardiac recordings—the only sure way of accurately lo-

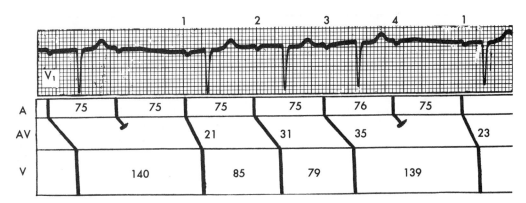

FIGURE 19-1 Typical 4:3 Wenckebach period. Of the four atrial impulses *(1, 2, 3, 4)*, only three reach the ventricles. Characteristic features include the following: the first PR is slightly prolonged (0.21 second); the larger PR increment is between the first and second PR (from 0.21 to 0.31 second); as the increment decreases, the ventricular cycle shortens (from 0.85 to 0.79 second); the longest cycle (of the dropped beat—1.39 second) is less than twice the shortest ventricular cycle (0.79 second); and there is no bundle branch block.

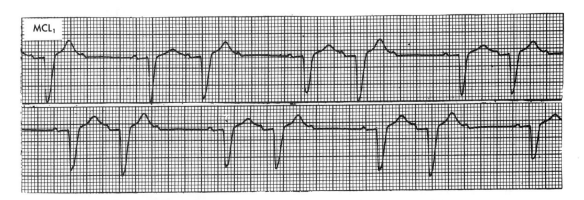

FIGURE 19-2 Typical example of type II 3:2 AV block. Characteristic features include the following: consecutive atrial impulses are conducted with the same PR interval (0.18 second) immediately before the dropped beat, the PR after the dropped beat is the same as the PR before it, the PR is of normal duration, and there is a bundle branch block.

calizing the level of the block—are neither available nor desirable. However, with a knowledge of the attributes of both types of block, aided at times by the result of carotid sinus massage and/or atropine administration[18] and exercise and catecholamines,[19] we can usually make an intelligent and correct guess (Table 19-1). Table 19-2 lists the three noninvasive means of differentiating AV nodal from infranodal block.

Important exceptions to the usual findings are as follows:
1. Many Wenckebach periods are atypical and fail to show all the classical features depicted in Figure 19-1.[20]

TABLE 19-1   ESTABLISHED CHARACTERISTICS OF TYPE I AND TYPE II BLOCK

	TYPE I	TYPE II
Clinical	Usually acute	Usually chronic
	Inferior infarction	Anteroseptal infarction
	Rheumatic fever	Lenegre's disease
	Digitalis	Lev's disease
	Propranolol	Cardiomyopathy
Anatomic	Usually AV nodal, sometimes His bundle	Always subnodal, usually bundle branches
Electrophysiologic	Relative refractory period	No relative refractory period
	Decremental conduction	All-or-none conduction
Electrocardiographic	RP/PR reciprocity	Stable PR
	Prolonged PR	Normal PR
	Normal QRS duration	Bundle branch block

TABLE 19-2   NONINVASIVE ASSESSMENT OF BLOCK LEVEL

	TYPE I (NODAL)	TYPE II (INFRANODAL)
Atropine	Improves	Worsens
Exercise and catecholamines	Improves	Worsens
Carotid sinus massage	Worsens	Improves

2. Rarely, the classical Wenckebach period can develop in the His bundle, and then the ECG is indistinguishable from the nodal Wenckebach period.
3. The all-or-none conduction that characterizes the bundle branches may be found in the His bundle, and then type II block may be encountered with a narrow QRS complex.[8,21-24] This combination occurs almost exclusively in elderly women.[8]
4. In the presence of existing BBB, progressive lengthening of the PR interval before a dropped beat is caused in perhaps 25% of cases by progressive delay in the contralateral bundle branch.[17,25,26]

Despite such significant exceptions, "in most instances, the differentiation can be made easily and reliably from the surface ECG."[15] What it all boils down to is that when we say type I, we mean "probably nodal and usually benign"; when we say type II, we mean "certainly infranodal and definitely malignant." Genuine type II block is an unequivocal indication for an artificial pacemaker, whereas type I block seldom is.

WENCKEBACH PERIODICITY AND RP/PR RECIPROCITY

Although it may well prove to be an oversimplification, it is a convenient and practical concept to think of type I *behavior* as caused by an abnormally long relative refractory period (RRP) and type II as the result of little or no RRP.[16] In the prolonged RRP the rate of conduction depends on the moment of impulse arrival—the earlier it

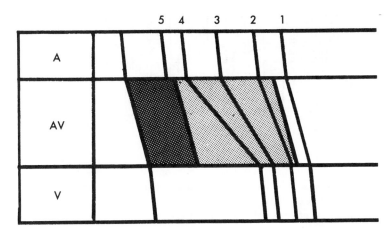

FIGURE 19-3 Diagrammatic behavior of AV conduction during type I AV block. Dark stippling in the AV junction represents the absolute refractory period (ARP); light stippling represents the relative refractory period (RRP). If an atrial impulse *(1)* arrives at the AV node after the RRP is over, it is conducted normally. If it arrives a little earlier *(2)*, there will be some delay in AV conduction. As the atrial impulse arrives earlier and earlier *(3* and *4)*, conduction time becomes longer and longer. Finally, the impulse arrives during the ARP *(5)* and is not conducted.

arrives at the AV node, the longer it takes to penetrate; the later it arrives, the shorter the penetration time (Figure 19-3).

It becomes obvious that the Wenckebach type of conduction develops because each successive impulse arrives earlier and earlier in the RRP of the AV node until, at last, one arrives during the absolute refractory period (ARP) and fails to get through.

A clinically practical concept results from translating this earlier and earlier arrival into terms of the surface tracing. Other things being equal, the earlier the impulse sets out from the SA node, the earlier it reaches the AV node. The RP interval (measured from the beginning of the QRS complex to beginning of the next P wave) gives us an approximate—and in practice highly satisfactory—indication of the relative earliness of arrival at the AV node. In terms of the clinical tracing, the shorter the RP, the longer the PR; the longer the RP, the shorter the PR. We can think and talk of "RP/PR reciprocity" and "RP-dependent" PR intervals. If such reciprocity in the clinical tracing can be demonstrated, some part of the AV junction is exhibiting Wenckebach (type I) behavior.

In Figure 19-4 the reciprocal relationship between RP and its associated PR is nicely demonstrated. After the first three beats, which are conducted normally with a PR of 0.17 second complementing an RP of 0.48 second, the last four beats are conducted with progressively shortening PR intervals (exactly the converse of what happens in a Wenckebach sequence) because they complement progressively lengthening RP intervals (again, exactly the opposite of what happens in a Wenckebach sequence).

In the classical Wenckebach period (see Figure 19-1) the dropped beat fails to penetrate the diseased stratum of the AV node, which therefore enjoys a relatively long rest (RP interval = 1.13 second) with consequent optimal AV conduction (PR = 0.21 sec-

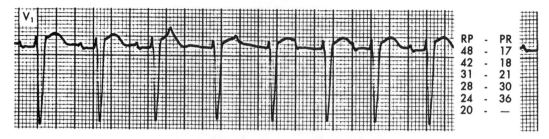

FIGURE 19-4 Illustration of the reciprocal relationship between the RP interval and its complementing PR (see table at end of tracing). The last four conducted beats demonstrate the converse of what happens in Wenckebach conduction. As the RP gets longer with each successive beat, its complementary PR gets progressively shorter, whereas in Wenckebach conduction the PR progressively lengthens in response to a progressively shortening RP.

ond). Suddenly the RP dramatically shortens from 1.13 to 0.52 second, and consequently the PR in dramatically lengthens from 0.21 to 0.31 second. This phenomenon explains why the second PR in the Wenckebach sequence almost always shows the largest increment over the preceding PR—it follows the most dramatic shortening of the RP (i.e., it arrives much earlier in the RRP of the sick AV node).

On the other hand, if there is virtually no RRP, it follows that beats are conducted with the same facility (i.e., with the same PR interval) whether early or late in diastole, provided they arrive after the ARP is finished (see Figure 19-2). The PR is the same regardless of the preceding RP, and RP/PR reciprocity is lacking.

It follows from all this information that when *consecutive* atrial impulses are conducted, type I block is characterized by progressive lengthening of the PR before conduction fails altogether, whereas type II block has constant PR intervals when *consecutive* impulses are conducted before the dropped beat.

2:1 AV BLOCK

What about when only alternate beats are conducted, with a resulting 2:1 ratio? With this ratio in both type I (Figure 19-5) and type II (Figure 19-6), the PR interval is, of course, constant in the beats that are conducted. This is true for type II because all PRs are constant in this type of block; it is also true of type I block because, provided the atrial rhythm is regular, the RP intervals will be constant and therefore so will the PRs (recall that in type I block the PR is RP-dependent). This fact has been the source of much misunderstanding, with consequent misdiagnosis and mistreatment.

Although a block no longer qualifies as the Wenckebach phenomenon when the classic form of Wenckebach conduction alternates with 2:1 conduction (see Figure 19-5), the type of block has not changed. Sometimes changes in atrial rate produce changes in conduction ratios, and sometimes the conduction ratios change spontaneously. In these cases there can be no doubt that the type of block is unchanged. When the conduction ratio in Wenckebach periods changes from 5:4 to 4:3 or from 4:3 to 3:2, there is no doubt that the type of block is unchanged. Why, when it goes one stage further and becomes 2:1, should there be an immediate flurry to change the type and its prognostic significance?

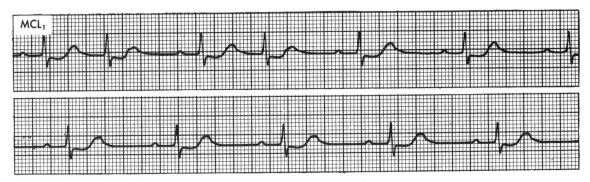

FIGURE 19-5 From a patient with acute true posterior infarction. Note the prominent initial R wave with reciprocal ST depression. Strips are continuous; atrial rate throughout is 103 beats/min. At the beginning of the top strip there are two 3:2 Wenckebach periods; through the bottom strip the conduction ratio changes to 2:1. Note that the PR interval is prolonged during the 2:1 conduction (0.25 second).

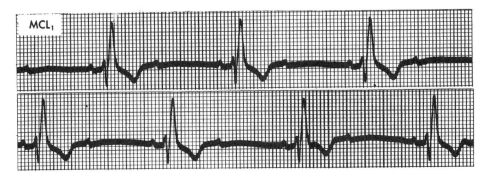

FIGURE 19-6 Strips are continuous and show 2:1 AV block with right bundle branch block. The atrial rate is 82 beats/min, and the combination of a normal PR interval (0.15 second) with bundle branch block makes it likely that this is type II AV block.

Figures 19-5 and 19-6 illustrate two other features that are highly characteristic of the two types of second-degree AV block and that can be of assistance in differentiating types when only 2:1 conduction is present. The prolonged PR and the absence of BBB are typical of pure type I block, whereas the normal PR and the presence of BBB are characteristic of type II.

"SKIPPED" P WAVES

Another point that is not well appreciated and leads to faulty diagnosis is that the atrial impulse that is conducted to the ventricles is not always represented by the P wave that immediately precedes the QRS complex. In Figure 19-7 the group beating and the other "footprints" clearly identify a Wenckebach period.

Moreover, the increasing PR intervals in each group of beats are evident. However, in

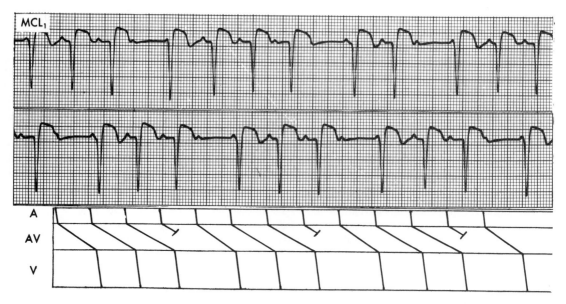

FIGURE 19-7 Strips are continuous. Sinus tachycardia (rate = 125 beats/min) with 3:2, 4:3, and 5:4 Wenckebach periods. Note that the PR intervals are longer than the PP intervals.

each group the first and second PR intervals are clearly too short for conduction, and therefore conduction must come from the preceding P wave (see the laddergram in Figure 19-7).

Furthermore, these rather long PR intervals, which reach 0.69 second, bring to mind the commonly asked question: How long can a PR be and still represent conduction? There is no established answer, but at least it can be said that a PR of 0.60 second is not uncommon, one of 0.70 second is sometimes seen, and one of 0.80 to 0.90 second is rare. Reports of PR intervals of more than 1 second have been published, but the validity of some of these reports is doubtful.

HIGH-GRADE (OR ADVANCED) AV BLOCK

High-grade AV block represents a stage between the occasionally, or even alternately, dropped beats and complete block. High-grade block may be diagnosed when, *at a reasonable atrial rate* (e.g., 135 beats/min or less), at least two consecutive atrial impulses fail to be conducted. This failure of conduction must happen *because of the existing block itself*, not because an escaping junctional or ventricular pacemaker anticipates and prevents conduction. Figure 19-8 presents two examples of high-grade AV block. One is probably type I because of the inferior infarction and absence of BBB, and the other type II because there is both BBB and a normal PR interval in the conducted beats.

The two conditions italicized in the previous paragraph are necessary ingredients in the definition. For example, if the fluttering atria are beating at a frantic rate of 300 beats/min, it would be absurd to call 4:1 block (in which three consecutive impulses are not conducted) "high-grade" because a 4:1 ratio, producing a ventricular rate of 75, is

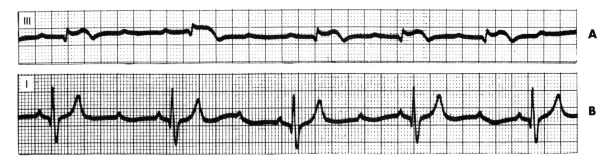

FIGURE 19-8 High-grade (advanced) AV block. **A,** From a patient with acute inferior infarction, sinus tachycardia, and 3:1 and 2:1 AV block—presumably type I. **B,** From a 47-year-old patient with no history of heart disease, initially seen with Adams-Stokes attacks. There is sinus tachycardia (rate = 122 beats/min) with 3:1 AV block. In this clinical context the normal PR (0.16 second) with right bundle branch block makes this likely to be type II block caused by sclerodegenerative disease of the conduction system.

exactly what both the therapist and the patient desire. As discussed later in this chapter, the ventricular escape rate, quite apart from the block, can be a major determinant of nonconduction and a cause of overdiagnosis.

COMPLETE AV BLOCK

The AV block should be called complete when (and only when) the opportunity for conduction is optimal and yet none occurs. The key word here is *opportunity* because it is obvious that if there is no opportunity to do something, one cannot be blamed for not doing it. If there is less than optimal opportunity for the AV conduction system to conduct, it cannot be regarded as a failure if it does not conduct. On the other hand, if it has every conceivable opportunity to conduct and invariably fails, it may well be blamed as a total failure. What then determines the presence or absence of an opportunity for conduction? The several factors involved are listed on p. 326.

To make the diagnosis of complete block, there should be no conduction as recognized by the changing P-to-R relationship in the presence of a regular ventricular rhythm. That absence of conduction must be in the presence of a slow enough ventricular rate (less than 45 beats/min, although some clinicians[27,28] require a ventricular rate of less than 40 beats/min), with P waves fully deployed across the RR intervals landing at every conceivable RP interval. Only then is the opportunity for conduction optimal and the diagnosis of complete block justified. These features require repeated emphasis because there is probably no entity in cardiology that is so often overdiagnosed and then overtreated.

Figure 19-9 illustrates complete AV block: the ventricular rate is less than 45 beats/min, the ventricular rhythm is absolutely regular, and the P-to-R relationship is constantly changing as the P waves march resolutely through all phases of the ventricular cycle. Every possible chance for conduction is afforded but none occurs; therefore the diagnosis of the ultimate in block (complete) is warranted.

Acute complete block is usually caused by a lesion in the AV node such as in acute inferior infarction and less often in severe digitalis intoxication. In acute anterior infarc-

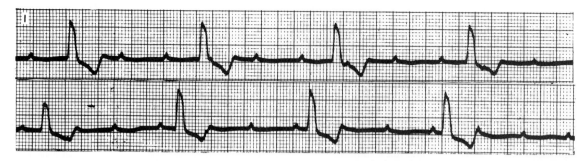

FIGURE 19-9 Complete AV block. Strips are continuous. In the presence of sinus tachycardia (rate = 108 beats/min) there is an independent idioventricular rhythm (rate = 36 beats/min). Note that the ventricular rhythm is absolutely regular, whereas the P-to-R relationship constantly changes.

tion complete block is more devastating and is almost always caused by a simultaneous block in both bundle branches. Approximately 90% of chronic complete block is caused by bilateral BBB, with the remaining 10% caused by block at the level of the His bundle.

VENTRICULAR ASYSTOLE

As a rule an escaping pacemaker, junctional or ventricular, comes to the rescue when AV conduction fails. However, if the failure of conduction is associated with reluctant subsidiary pacemakers, ventricular asystole results. This sinister situation, if unrelieved, is obviously and rapidly fatal. The most common context for this occurrence is as an ominous and usually fatal climax of type II block; that is, it develops spontaneously against a background of existing BBB, presumably because the other bundle branch is suddenly blocked (Figure 19-10, *A*).

Ventricular asystole is not always so sinister. If it develops as a result of a vagal storm such as with vomiting (Figure 19-10, *C*), the level of block is in the AV node and the disturbance may be relatively mild and transient. A third mechanism of asystole (Figure 19-10, *B*) is tentatively assumed to be caused by a phase 4 phenomenon because the block and consequent asystole develop only after a lengthening of the atrial cycle, which suggests that the AV node may have spontaneously depolarized to an unresponsive level.

NEED TO RECLASSIFY

The diagnosis and management of the AV blocks are in a state of confusion for several reasons, which are discussed in the following sections.

Definitions are Wanting

Most authors do not seem to realize that there is any uncertainty in the current situation. In fact, in more than 50 articles that deal with the subject of complete AV block and have been published in English since the advent of coronary care in 1962, not a single author considered it necessary to define AV block—presumably because it is tacitly but erroneously assumed that the term is uniformly used by and means the same to all. How far this is from the truth will become apparent.

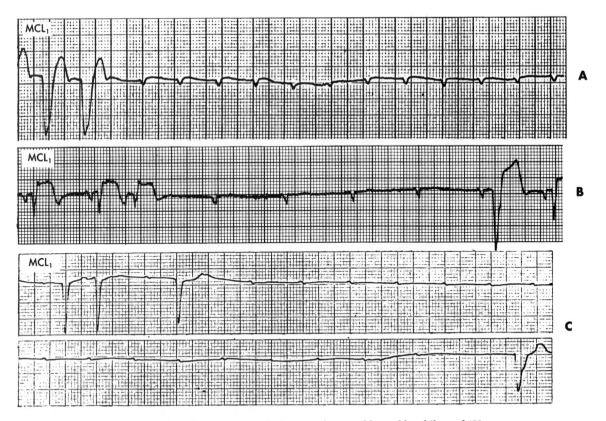

FIGURE 19-10 Three examples of transient ventricular asystole caused by sudden failure of AV conduction in the absence of an escaping pacemaker. **A,** *Spontaneous* asystole in the presence of left bundle branch block, probably representing end-stage type II block. **B,** From a patient with acute anteroseptal infarction. Asystole is precipitated by an atrial premature beat (as were many repeated periods of asystole); the atrial premature beat lengthens the ensuing sinus cycle, which suggests that the failure of conduction might be caused by a *phase 4 phenomenon.* **C,** Strips are continuous. *Vagal* asystole, precipitated by vomiting, in a patient with acute inferior infarction.

Not only is complete block almost never defined, but on the rare occasions in which it is, the definition is usually found wanting. Much the same is true of the usage and definition of other important categories of block such as "type II block" and "high-grade block."

Nondegrees of Block

The second source of inconsistency resides in the usage of "degrees." This word, by definition, should indicate a measure of the severity of the AV conduction disturbance. However, this is not necessarily the case (Figure 19-11). By any criterion Figure 19-11, *A,* is an example of 2:1 AV block, a ratio that some regard as "high-grade" block (see the following discussion).[8,29,30] Figure 19-11, *B,* shows no sign of any block. In fact, the patient in strip *B* has worse block than the patient in strip *A* because patient *B* develops 2:1 block when the atrial rate accelerates to only 84 beats/min (Figure 19-11, *D*); patient *A*

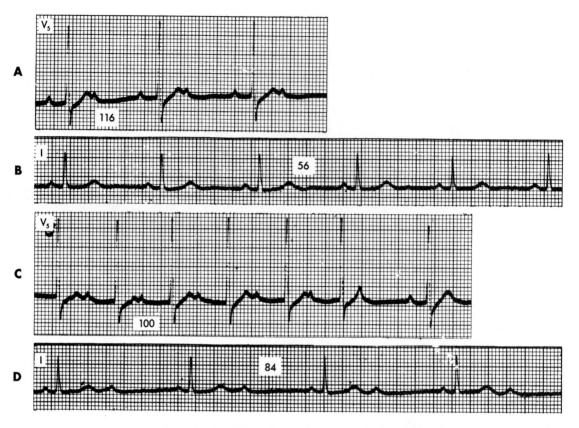

FIGURE 19-11 Strips **A** and **C** are from one patient; strips **B** and **D** are from a second patient. The first patient has 2:1 block at an atrial rate of 116 beats/min (**A**) but can conduct 1:1 at an atrial rate of 100 beats/min (**C**). In contrast, the second patient conducts normally at 56 beats/min (**B**) but develops 2:1 block at a rate of only 84 beats/min (**D**).

is able to conduct 1:1 even at a rate of 100 beats/min (Figure 19-11, *C*). A patient who develops 2:1 conduction at a rate of 84 beats/min has worse block than one who can conduct every beat at a rate of 100 beats/min.

In evaluating the severity of AV block, *rate* is far more important than *ratio*. Unfortunately, however, the definitions of "degrees" have for decades been partially predicated on ratios to the neglect of rate. Indeed, when the conduction ratio changes with an increase in rate, it may be described by some as a change for the worse in the degree of block rather than be recognized for what it is: a change in *rate* with a secondary and consequent change in the conduction *ratio*, not in the degree of block.[31]

This point is well illustrated in Figure 19-12, in which each conducted beat is followed by an identical prolonged refractory period (shaded area); that is, the degree of severity of block is the same throughout the diagram. At the beginning of the strip the atrial cycle length is 100 (rate = 60 beats/min), but after three beats the atrial cycle short-

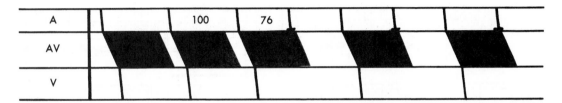

FIGURE 19-12 Diagram illustrating the effect of atrial rate on the AV conduction ratio. Note that the abnormally long refractory period is identical throughout (i.e., there is no worsening of the block). However, if the atrial cycle shortens from 100 (rate = 60 beats/min) to 76 (rate = 79 beats/min), the conduction ratio changes from 1:1 to 2:1.

ens to 76 (rate = 79 beats/min) and 2:1 conduction develops. Nevertheless, it is obvious that the severity (i.e., degree) of block has not changed. The primary change is the atrial rate, and the secondary change is the conduction ratio. From this it is clear that the seriousness of any AV block should not be assessed from the conduction ratio alone without taking the associated rate into consideration.

Misconceptions are Rife

The third circumstance that fosters confusion is the prevalence of certain important misconceptions, some of which have been hinted at earlier in this chapter.

First, some authorities regard 2:1 AV block as high-grade or advanced.[8,29,30] The absurdity of using the conduction ratio as an index of severity is obvious after the realization that 2:1 block can be anything from a disaster to a boon. At an atrial rate of 70 beats/min, 2:1 block may be a disaster; at an atrial rate of 130 beats/min, 2:1 block may prove a blessing. Clearly the ratio alone, when used in ignorance of the prevailing atrial and ventricular rate, cannot provide even an approximate idea of the severity of the block.

A second, commonly encountered misapprehension is that all 2:1 block is type II block. This misunderstanding results from the fact that the PR intervals are constant and that it is not necessary to look far to find defective definitions of type II block such as "AV block with constant PR intervals"[32] and "constant PR intervals for conducted sinus beats irrespective of the ratio of atrial to ventricular depolarizations."[33] Faulty definitions such as these very often omit the key word *consecutive*, which was carefully emphasized earlier in this chapter. The constant PR criterion can be applied only when **consecutive** atrial impulses are conducted with identical PR intervals immediately before the beat is dropped. Another common (and appropriate) way of stating the constant PR rule is to say that the PR after the dropped beat is the same as the PR before it. In the classical example of type II block in Figure 19-2 the two consecutive PRs before the dropped beat are identical, and the PR immediately before the dropped beat is the same the returning PR after it. What these variations of the rule are stating is simply that the PR is independent of the RP. It is the same after a short RP (before the dropped beat) as after a long RP (after the dropped beat) and, of course, the hallmark of type I block is RP/PR reciprocity.[34] Notice again the additional characteristic—but not invariable—features of type II block: the normal PR and the BBB.

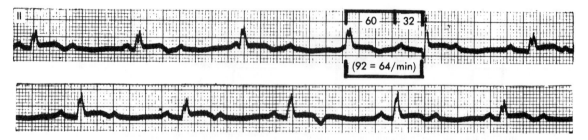

FIGURE 19-13   Strips are continuous. From a patient with acute inferior myocardial infarction. Some (undetermined) degree of AV block (presumably type I) combined with an atrial rate of 88 beats/min and a ventricular escape rate of 47 beats/min precludes conduction except for the one capture beat (fifth beat in the top strip) and two or three possible fusion beats in the bottom strip. The capture beat reveals that the patient is capable of conducting 1:1, with prolonged PR, at an atrial rate of 64 beats/min (see text).

In the acute setting of myocardial infarction, type I 2:1 block is, in fact, 20 or 30 times more common than type II 2:1 block. It is important to remember this point when temporary pacemakers are being brandished.

A third misconception is that when AV block is evident and most of the atrial impulses are not conducted, the block is "high-grade" or "advanced." Figure 19-13 illustrates AV block in which there are 21 atrial impulses, only one of which is completely conducted (there are possibly one or two fusion beats); yet, with so little conduction, the block is comparatively mild.

The way to avoid the error of overdiagnosis in such cases is to focus on the conducted beat rather than on the numerous nonconducted ones because the beat that *is* conducted tells far more about the patient's conduction capability than do all the nonconducted beats combined. It shows quite specifically the patient's current requirements for conduction. Concentrate on the solitary capture beat (fifth beat in top strip). When the RP interval reaches a length of 0.60 second, the patient is able to conduct with a PR interval of 0.32 second. Thus it can be deduced that at that time the patient had a 1:1 conduction capability if the atrial cycle equaled the cycle of the capture beat (i.e., cycle length = 0.92 second = 64 beats/min). Furthermore, a person capable of conducting every beat at a rate of 64 beats/min but who has a prolonged PR interval certainly does not have an advanced degree of AV block. Add to this reasoning the fact that the patient has an inferior wall infarction and that the capture beat manifests no BBB and it is clear that the block is almost certainly in the AV node.

A fourth misconception is that when AV block is clearly present and *none* of the atrial impulses is conducted, the block is necessarily complete. In a tracing like that in Figure 19-14, *A,* there is an obvious block because P waves are seen in situations in which conduction should but does not occur. In fact, there is no AV conduction because the junctional rhythm is absolutely regular. Thus there is AV block and complete AV dissociation, but this is by no means the same as complete AV block.[13] These tracings should be diagnosed as "*some* (undetermined) degree of AV block that, combined with an accelerated junctional rhythm, produces complete AV dissociation." Yet on a questionnaire mailed to

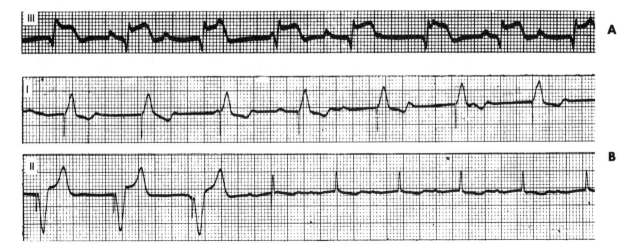

FIGURE 19-14   A, Block/acceleration dissociation. Some (undetermined) degree of AV block (presumably type I) combined with an accelerated junctional rhythm at a rate of 68 beats/min produces complete AV dissociation. **B,** Illustration of how mild a degree of AV block, when combined with an accelerated ventricular rate, can produce complete dissociation. In lead I there is obvious AV block, the paced rhythm has a rate of 62 beats/min, and there is complete AV dissociation. However, in lead II a few seconds later an atrial impulse (represented by a P wave landing at a critical RP interval) captures the ventricles and reveals the mildness of the underlying conduction disturbance.

directors of cardiology departments and coronary care units that asked how such an arrhythmia should be described, more than half of 550 respondents called it complete AV block.[35] Published examples of this same interpretative error are abundant.

The argument here is that, although it is not definite that the block is not complete, there is a real possibility that it is relatively mild. Therefore it is a mistake to assume the worst, label it the ultimate in block, and run the attendant risks of overdiagnosis, especially because it is known that patients with acute myocardial infarction who show this arrhythmia as their worst manifestation of block usually have an excellent prognosis.

Figure 19-14, *B*, shows how mild such a block may be. In lead I there is a paced ventricular rhythm of 62 beats/min. The P wave emerges from the QRS complex and marches backward across the RR interval without effecting capture—complete dissociation. However, after the third beat in lead II, the P wave happens to land at exactly the correct RP interval, and the atrial impulse captures the ventricles with a long PR interval. Once capture occurs, the atria remain in control for the rest of the strip with gradually lengthening PR intervals; this indicates that, at the prevailing atrial rate, the underlying block is far from being complete and is a mild form of type I block. The fundamental truth so poorly appreciated is that the *combination of quite mild block with a ventricular rate in the 50s or 60s can produce periods of complete AV dissociation.* The absence of conduction is not necessarily the same as block. Langendorf and Pick[36] demonstrated years ago that complete AV dissociation could be produced in a patient with only first-degree AV block by pacing the ventricle two or three beats faster than the sinus rate.

Therefore when faced with a sample of AV block in which all or a significant majority of beats are not conducted, it is important to mentally rehearse the many influences that determine AV conduction and to assess the relative contribution of each:

1. State of AV junction and bundle branches
   a. Physiologic refractoriness
   b. Pathologic refractoriness
   c. Concealed conduction
2. Autonomic influences
3. Atrial rate
4. R/P relationships
5. Ventricular rate
6. Level of ventricular pacemaker

Dysrhythmia (such as that in Figure 19-14, *A*) caused by the conspiracy of an undetermined degree of block with a subsidiary pacemaker beating at a rate faster than usual clearly requires a separate designation. Marriott[35] has therefore suggested the term *block/acceleration dissociation*.

REMEDIAL MEASURES

To introduce some semblance of order into the current chaos, three modifications commend themselves: (1) disturbances of AV conduction must be classified into many more categories than the long-standing oversimplification into three misleading "degrees"; (2) "degrees" of AV block as presently defined (or not defined!) should be abandoned or at least deemphasized because they have caused more confusion than they have contributed precision; and (3) in view of the major role they play in determining the frequency and ratio of AV conduction, both atrial and ventricular rates must be included in all definitions and diagnostic categorizations of block.

With the above considerations in mind, the AV blocks should be divided into more meaningful categories—meaningful from the viewpoint of placing the site of the lesion, assessing the prognosis, and deciding on the appropriate management. This division can, as has been emphasized, usually be performed from the surface tracing together with an informed appraisal of the clinical setting. As a short step in the right direction, the disturbances of AV conduction should be categorized and considered under at least the following number of subdivisions:

1. Prolonged PR interval
2. Block/acceleration dissociation
3. Occasional "dropped" beats
   a. Type I (Wenckebach periodicity)
   b. Type II
4. 2:1 AV block
   a. Type I
   b. Type II
5. High-grade block
   a. Type I
   b. Type II

6. Complete block
   a. Junctional escape
   b. Ventricular escape
7. Transient ventricular asystole
   a. Spontaneous
   b. Phase 4 (?)
   c. Vagal

REFERENCES

1. Van Hemel MM, Robles de Medina EO: Electrocardiographic findings in 781 males between the ages of 15 and 23 years. I. Arrhythmias and conduction disorders, *Excerpta Medica Cardiovasc Dis Cardiovasc Surg* 23:981, 1975 (abstract).
2. Lewis T: *The mechanism and graphic registration of the heart beat,* London, 1925, Shaw & Sons.
3. Wenckebach KF: Zur Analyse des unregelmässigen Pulses. II. Ueber den regelmässig intermittirenden Puls, *Z Klin Med* 37:475, 1899.
4. Wenckebach KF: Beiträge zur Kenntnis der Menschlichen Herztätigkeit, *Arch Anat Physiol,* p 297, 1906.
5. Hay J: Bradycardia and cardiac arrhythmia produced by depression of certain functions of the heart, *Lancet* 1:139, 1906.
6. Mobitz W: Ueber die unvollständige Stäorung der Erregungsüberleitung zwischen Vorhof und Kamme des menschlichen Herzens, *Z Ges Exp Med* 41:180, 1924.
7. Knoebel SB, Parsons MN, Fisch C: The role of transvenous pacing in acute myocardial infarction, *Heart Lung* 1:56, 1972.
8. Narula OS: *His bundle electrocardiography and clinical electrophysiology,* Philadelphia, 1975, FA Davis.
9. Damato AN, Lau SH: Clinical value of the electrogram of the conducting system, *Prog Cardiovasc Dis* 12:119, 1970.
10. Rosen KM: The contribution of His bundle recording to the understanding of cardiac conduction in man, *Circulation* 43:961, 1971.
11. Rosen KM, Gunnar RM, Rahimtoola SH: Site and type of second degree AV block, *Chest* 61:99, 1972.
12. Haft JI, Weinstock M, DeGuia R: Electrophysiologic studies in Mobitz type II second degree heart block, *Am J Cardiol* 27:682, 1971.
13. Langendorf R, Pick A: Atrioventricular block, type II (Mobitz)—its nature and clinical significance, *Circulation* 38:819, 1968.
14. Barold SS, Friedberg HD: Second degree atrioventricular block: a matter of definition, *Am J Cardiol* 33:311, 1974.
15. Zipe DP: Second-degree atrioventricular block, *Circulation* 60:465, 1979.
16. Pick A, Langendorf R: *Interpretation of complex arrhythmias,* Philadelphia, 1979, Lea & Febiger.
17. Del Negro AA, Fletcher RD: Indications for and use of artificial cardiac pacemakers, *Curr Probl Cardiol* 3(7):9, 1978.
18. Mangiardi LM, Bonamini R, Conte M et al: Bedside evaluation of atrioventricular block with narrow QRS complexes: usefulness of carotid sinus massage and atropine administration, *Am J Cardiol* 49:1136, 1982.
19. Bar FW, Den Bulk K, Wellens HJJ: Atrioventricular dissociation. In MacFarlane PW, Veitch Lawrie T: *Comprehensive electrocardiology,* New York, 1989, Pergamon Press.

20. Denes P, Levy L, Pick A, Rosen KM: The incidence of typical and atypical AV Wenckebach periodicity, *Am Heart J* 89:26, 1975.
21. Rosen KM, Loeb HS, Gunnar RM, Rahimtoola SH: Mobitz type II block without bundle branch block, *Circulation* 44:1111, 1971.
22. Gupta PK, Lichstein E, Chadda KD: Electrophysiological features of Mobitz type II A-V block occurring within the His bundle, *Br Heart J* 34:1232, 1972.
23. Rosen KM, Loeb HS, Rahimtoola SH: Mobitz type II block with narrow QRS complex and Stokes-Adams attacks, *Arch Intern Med* 1342:595, 1973.
24. Puech P, Grolleau R, Guimond C: Incidence of different types of AV block and their localization by His bundle recordings. In Wellens HJJ, Lie KI, Janse MJ, editors: *The conduction system of the heart: structure, function, and clinical implications,* Philadelphia, 1976, Lea & Febiger.
25. Rosenbaum MB, Nau GJ, Levy RJ: Wenckebach periods in the bundle branches, *Circulation* 40:79, 1969.
26. Friedberg HD, Schamroth L: The Wenckebach phenomenon in left bundle branch block, *Am J Cardiol* 24:591, 1969.
27. Schamroth L: *The disorders of cardiac rhythm,* Oxford, 1980, Blackwell Scientific Publications.
28. Pritchett ELC: *Office management of arrhythmias,* Philadelphia, 1982, WB Saunders.
29. WHO/ISC Task Force: Definition of terms related to cardiac rhythm, *Am Heart J* 95:796, 1978.
30. Josephson ME, Seides SF: *Clinical cardiac electrophysiology: techniques and interpretations,* Philadelphia, 1979, Lea & Febiger.
31. Danzig R, Alpern H, Swan HJC: The significance of atrial rate in patients with atrioventricular conduction abnormalities complicating acute myocardial infarction, *Am J Cardiol* 24:707, 1969.
32. Stock RJ, Macken DL: Observations on heart block during continuous electrocardiographic monitoring in myocardial infarction, *Circulation* 38:993, 1968.
33. Scheinman M, Brenman B: Clinical and anatomic implications of intraventricular conduction blocks in acute myocardial infarction, *Circulation* 46:753, 1972.
34. Langendorf R, Cohen H, Gozo EG: Observations on second degree atrioventricular block, including new criteria for the differential diagnosis between type I and type II block, *Am J Cardiol* 29:111, 1972.
35. Marriott HJL: AV block: an overdue overhaul, *Emerg Med* 13(6):85, 1981.
36. Langendorf R, Pick A: Artificial pacing of the human heart: its contribution to the understanding of the arrhythmias, *Am J Cardiol* 28:516, 1971.

CHAPTER 20

Parasystole

ECG in parasystole 329
Modulated parasystole
  330
Exit block 331
Classic ventricular
  parasystole 333
Classic parasystole without
  exit block 334
Classic parasystole with
  exit block 337
Concealed parasystole 337
Intermittent parasys-
  tole 337
Parasystolic accelerated
  idioventricular rhythm
  338
Fixed coupling in
  parasystole 338
Clinical significance 338
Atrial parasystole 340

PARASYSTOLE IS A FORM OF ABNORMAL AUTOMATICITY OR TRIGGERED ACTIVITY THAT can be present in the atria, AV junction, ventricles, or even the SA node.[1] The parasystolic focus is surrounded by an abnormal (depressed) area that shields it from being discharged or reset but not from being influenced electronically by extraneous impulses. Protection by the surrounding shield may be absolute, intermittent, or modulated by the dominant cardiac rhythm. It may be transient in its manifestation because of exit block, or it may manifest itself at every opportunity.

Whatever form the zone of protection assumes, when it is effective the underlying rhythm (usually sinus) in no way determines whether the parasystolic focus fires (although in the modulated form it influences its timing). Thus parasystolic beats have a random relationship to the underlying rhythm on the surface electrocardiogram (ECG). For the same reason the interectopic intervals in classical parasystole (absolute protection) are simple multiples of a common denominator, reflecting the rate and the undisturbed rhythm of the parasystolic focus, although the impulses themselves need not appear regularly.

In its modulated form the parasystolic focus is protected from being reset but does not necessarily maintain fixed cycle lengths. Since the initial microelectrode studies of Jalife and Moe,[1] many investigators have shown that such an assumption cannot be made. According to Castellanos, Saoudi, Moleiro, and Myerburg,[2] if impulses can exit across such a depressed zone it is likely that the parasystolic focus is subject to some degree of modulation by electrotonic depolarizations arising in the surrounding tissue.

ECG IN PARASYSTOLE
No Fixed Coupling

Ventricular ectopic beats are often exactly coupled to the preceding complex. Except for cases of entrainment, the parasystolic beat is not linked to a preceding beat; it is independent.

Fusion Beats

With a long enough tracing, an occasional fusion beat is also a feature of parasystole. If the parasystole is ventricular, the fusion beats result because the ectopic focus discharges just before or just as the sinus-conducted beat enters the ventricles. If the parasystole is atrial, fusion beats result because the ectopic focus discharges at the same time as or just before the SA node. The fusion beats obviously occur by chance and therefore are not necessary for making the diagnosis of parasystole.

Interectopic Intervals

The parasystolic focus may sometimes beat without being influenced electrotonically by the sinus (or dominant) rhythm. At such times the minimum time interval between interectopic beats is an exact multiple of longer time intervals. After identifying what appears to be the minimum interval in a suspected tracing, the parasystolic rhythm can then be "walked out" (measured). An ectopic complex appears when the ventricles (or the atria in the case of atrial parasystole) are nonrefractory. Failure of the parasystolic impulse to appear when expected is called "exit block."

MODULATED PARASYSTOLE

A parasystolic focus is said to be modulated when its regular rhythm is disrupted by impulses arising in the surrounding tissues. In such a case, subthreshold electrotonic depolarizations are transmitted across the depressed barrier. These depolarizations prolong or shorten the parasystolic cycle depending on the amplitude of the electrotonic event and the relationship of the parasystolic and sinus beats to each other.

Any pacemaker that is in contact with surrounding depressed myocardium that is exhibiting entrance (but not exit) block may experience modulation of its rhythm by the electrotonic effects in the surrounding tissue.[3] A series of studies initiated in Moe's laboratory have demonstrated electrotonic modulation of a protected automatic focus.[3-5] Considering the clinical and experimental observations of the past and the studies from Moe's group, we now know that entrance block may or may not be absolute and is caused by abnormal tissue, not by the normal refractoriness associated with rapid rhythms. That is, the ectopic focus can be totally shielded from the influence of extraneous impulses, or it can be modulated when subthreshold electrotonic depolarizations are transmitted across the depressed barrier. Early studies demonstrating this electrotonic link were accomplished through computer model simulations and were later confirmed in a biologic model. The electrotonic theory is based on the following premises:

1. The cycle length of a pacemaker can be altered by partial depolarization.
2. If the partial depolarization occurs early in phase 4 depolarization of the parasystolic focus, the next discharge is delayed. If the partial depolarization occurs later in phase 4, the next expected discharge from the parasystolic focus is early (captured by the invading impulse) because, with the membrane potential closer to threshold, an additional partial depolarization across the zone of protection causes it to fire prematurely. The ectopic pacemaker may in fact be entrained by the dominant pacemaker. In such a case there would be fixed coupling to the dominant pacemaker over a wide range of frequencies.[1,6-9]
3. In spite of the entrance block, the parasystolic focus is not entirely independent of the electrical influences surrounding it.
4. The parasystolic cycle may be modulated (prolonged or shortened) depending on (a) the amplitude of the electrotonic events, and (b) the relationship of the two cycle lengths (parasystolic and sinus) to each other.

In addition to these findings, experimental studies by Jalife, Moe, and colleagues[1,4,9-12] showed that coupled beats can result from parasystolic rhythms and that the parasystolic focus could be modulated by a slight change in heart rate, ectopic pacemaker rate, level of block, and position of the parasystolic pacemaker relative to the block border. Thus the

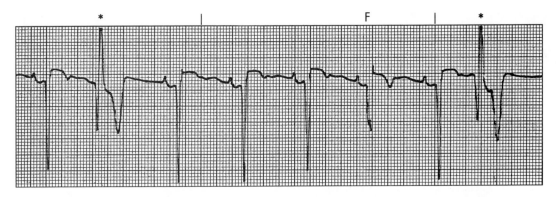

FIGURE 20-1 An example of classic ventricular parasystole. Note the fusion beat *(F)* and the variable coupling intervals of the ectopic beats *(asterisk)*. The interectopic intervals have a common denominator.

premise that the interectopic intervals are simple multiples of a common denominator is clearly not an obligatory feature of a parasystolic rhythm.

Figure 20-1 is an example of classic ventricular parasystole. The ventricular ectopic beats have variable coupling intervals; there is a fusion complex (F), and the interectopic intervals are multiples of a common denominator. However, modulation of the rhythm would probably be demonstrated on a longer tracing.

Figure 20-2 illustrates atrial parasystole, which is less common and more difficult to diagnose than the ventricular variety. In this example, a diagnosis is even more difficult because the parasystolic P waves are almost identical in shape to the sinus P waves. A modulated parasystole originating in the SA node has been described.[4] The atrial parasystole in Figure 20-2 may well be such a case. It fulfills the criteria given: (1) premature P waves having contours identical to sinus P waves, (2) variable coupling intervals, and (3) PP intervals of the parasystolic-sinus pair that are not longer than the PP intervals of the sinus rhythm.

EXIT BLOCK

In the presence of exit block no excitation of the heart from the parasystolic focus can arise. Exit block is therefore present when an expected parasystolic impulse is not propagated, even though the ventricles appear nonrefractory on the surface ECG. The rate of the parasystolic focus with exit block is usually faster than that of the dominant rhythm.[13] The concept of exit block has been experimentally demonstrated time and time again.

Entrance block prevents extraneous impulses from invading and resetting the ectopic focus; exit block limits the number of impulses propagated from the regularly firing ectopic pacemaker. Parasystole cannot exist unless the focus is protected by entrance block, nor can it excite the heart unless exit block is at least transiently absent; persistent exit block results in concealed parasystole.

Exit block should not be confused with normal refractoriness in surrounding tissue. For example, if the ectopic focus discharges just before or during the QRS complex, there may be a fusion beat. If the discharge occurs a little later, it cannot emerge because of normal refractoriness in surrounding tissue. However, this is not exit block.

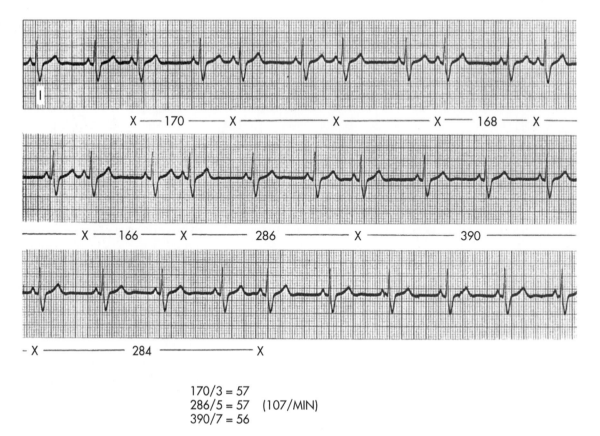

$$170/3 = 57$$
$$286/5 = 57 \quad (107/MIN)$$
$$390/7 = 56$$

FIGURE 20-2 Atrial parasystole (SA nodal). The parasystolic P waves *(X)* are identical in shape to the sinus P waves. There is no exact coupling, the interectopic intervals have a common denominator, and the parasystolic P wave resets the SA node. (Courtesy Alan Lindsay, MD.)

Exit block exists if the parasystolic impulse fires when the ventricles are apparently non-refractory but does not result in a propagated impulse.

Cranefield[14] proposes that the cause of exit block is concealed conduction in that the zone of protection around the parasystolic focus can be incompletely penetrated from both sides (the sinus conducted impulse and the parasystolic impulse). Refractoriness results every time a sinus impulse enters this zone but fails to traverse it; every time a parasystolic impulse enters and is blocked, the same occurs. Therefore the period during which it is possible for an impulse to emerge successfully from the zone surrounding the parasystolic focus may be shorter than appears on the surface ECG. According to Cranefield, exit block can be relieved by a local increase in catecholamines, a local improvement in perfusion, sinus slowing, or summation.

The patterns of exit block are generally type II, but type I may also occur (Wenckebach conduction of the emerging impulse). First- and third-degree blocks would not be detected on the ECG.

CLASSIC VENTRICULAR PARASYSTOLE

Classic ventricular parasystole implies an automatic focus with absolute protection by virtue of entrance block. It is recognized because of the perfect regularity of the ectopic rhythm and the marked variation in the coupling intervals of the ectopic beats (no fixed coupling), with or without fusion. When associated with no fixed coupling, absolute regularity is an indication that the protected focus has not been reset by the dominant rhythm; when the interectopic intervals are multiples of a common denominator, absolute entrance block can be assumed. This type of parasystole may or may not manifest exit block, and it may be intermittent. The rate of the parasystolic pacemaker and the degree of exit block can vary with cardiotropic drugs, electrolyte abnormalities, or autonomic impulses, which makes it difficult at times to determine the precise mechanism of a given arrhythmia.

"No fixed coupling" is recognized by marked variations in the intervals between the ectopic beats and the preceding beats of the dominant rhythm. The term *coupling* is inappropriate in the setting of parasystole, but it shall continue to be used since there is no acceptable alternative. Coupling strictly refers to the interval between the dominant (usually sinus) beat and the coupled beat; a coupled beat is one that is related to (dependent on) the preceding beat to which it owes its existence. Because the quintessence of parasystole is *independence,* there is no coupling, either constant or varying. The ectopic impulse propagates into the ventricular tissue when the ventricles are not refractory at the time of the ectopic discharge. However, it should be realized that, as explained in the section Fixed Coupling in Parasystole, fixed coupling does not preclude a diagnosis of parasystole any more than variable coupling proves parasystole. Exact coupling may occur in arrhythmias assumed to be parasystolic, and variable coupling may be seen in those arrhythmias assumed to be supported by reentry.

Interectopic Intervals as Simple Multiples of a Common Denominator

Interectopic intervals reflect the rate of the parasystolic focus, but the impulses themselves need not appear regularly. The times at which the parasystolic impulses activate the ventricles are not related to the sinus rhythm. They are instead related to each other because the interval between any two parasystolic complexes depends on the firing rate of the ectopic focus and therefore equals that interval or is some multiple of it. A variance of ±0.10 second or more is commonly allowed since the exit of the parasystolic impulse may be delayed occasionally. This delay occurs because of refractoriness of the surrounding ventricular tissue as a result of the preceding sinus-conducted impulse. In such a case the parasystolic impulse would be delayed in evoking a QRS complex because of local slow conduction.

Fusion Beats

Fusion occurs between the dominant and the parasystolic impulses and is a mathematical certainty that is eventually seen if the ECG tracing is long enough. However, fusion beats are not essential to the diagnosis. They occur when the fixed frequency of the parasystolic focus coincides with activation of the ventricles from the sinus impulse.

CLASSIC PARASYSTOLE WITHOUT EXIT BLOCK

Classic parasystole without exit block is most common when the rate of the parasystolic focus is slower than that of the sinus rhythm, which allows all parasystolic beats to fall within the nonrefractory period. With faster parasystolic rates, the diagnosis of parasystole is made when it can be shown that the sporadic appearance of the nonparasystolic rhythm does not reset the ectopic rhythm.

Classic parasystole without exit block may behave exactly like the simplest of all pacemakers—the "fixed-rate" pacemaker. The fixed-rate pacemaker fires regularly regardless of the competitive sinus rhythm because it cannot be shut off by a competing rhythm. As a result, the paced beats show a varying relationship to the sinus beats but are always a constant interval (or a multiple of that constant interval) from each other. The varying relationship to the dominant rhythm attests to one of its two cardinal characteristics: (1) it is *independent,* and (2) the common denominator of the interectopic intervals declares that it cannot be disturbed. There are only two differences in the ECG between artificial (pacemaker) and natural parasystole: (1) the "blip" that precedes and initiates all paced beats and (2) the parasystolic focus that can be modulated (but not actually discharged) by electrotonic potentials transmitted across the region of block.

A fixed-rate artificial pacemaker is shown in Figure 20-3 to illustrate the firing of the parasystolic focus and to plot the interectopic intervals. It is easily appreciated in this tracing that the fusion beats (F) result from simultaneous propagation within the ventricles of an ectopic impulse (paced beat in this case) and a conducted sinus impulse.

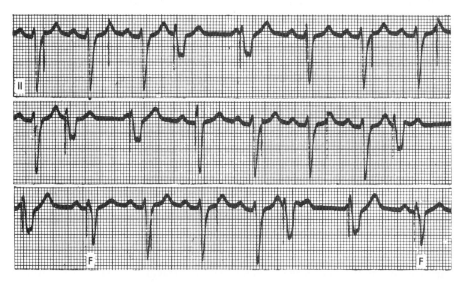

FIGURE 20-3 Strips are continuous. Fixed-rate pacemaker for comparison with ventricular parasystole. The fusion beats *(F)* result from a collision within the ventricles of the paced beat (comparable to the parasystolic focus) and the sinus-conducted beat.

Note the parasystolic behavior of the fixed-rate pacemaker:

1. It is protected in the sense that nothing can shut it off.
2. Whenever its impulse falls at a time when the ventricles are responsive, a QRS complex accompanies the pacemaker blip.
3. Whenever it falls at a time when the ventricles are refractory, the blip appears, but no ventricular complex results.
4. Thus the longer interectopic intervals are multiples of the shortest interectopic interval. In the second strip of Figure 20-3, the long interectopic interval (350 ms) equals four times the shortest interval (87 ms).
5. A fusion beat (F) results whenever the artificial discharge coincides with sinus conduction into the ventricles.
6. Because parasystole represents an independent rhythm and is not beholden to the preceding beat, it will appear at varying intervals after the sinus beats (variable coupling).

These six points are characteristic of parasystole. Parasystole is first suspected in the clinical tracing if ectopic beats show varying coupling intervals, as is seen in the artificially created parasystole of Fig. 20-3, which is an example of classical parasystole without exit block. The eye-catching feature is that the interval between the ectopic beat and the preceding sinus beat is never the same. It is a decided change from the exact coupling of an extrasystole to the sinus beat, which is thought caused by reentry or afterpotentials.

There is then an attempt to demonstrate that the ectopic rhythm cannot be interrupted. This is accomplished by showing that the interectopic intervals have a common denominator.

Figure 20-4 illustrates the special pattern of fusion that occurs when the ectopic focus is on the same side as a bundle branch block (BBB). Note that the third beat in the bottom strip looks remarkably normal because the sinus impulse activated the unblocked left ventricle while the ectopic impulse was simultaneously activating the right side of the blocked branch to produce a normally narrow QRS complex.

In the presence of BBB, the parasystolic beats often arise on the side of the block and therefore have a shape characteristic of a block of the opposite bundle branch (see Figure 20-4). The pathologic condition responsible for the BBB may also provide the conditions necessary for parasystole (i.e., slightly to moderately injured Purkinje fibers with consequent abnormal automaticity).

The apparent relationship between BBB and parasystole might also explain the preponderance of ventricular parasystole over atrial and junctional parasystoles and the common link between parasystole and organic heart disease.

Figure 20-5 illustrates classical ventricular parasystole in the presence of atrial fibrillation. The diagnosis of fusion is made with less assurance in such a case because it is never known exactly when the next fibrillatory impulse will be conducted to the ventricles. However, in Figure 20-5 it is reasonably certain that the third beat from the end of the second strip *(X)* is a fusion beat because, assuming parasystole, this is precisely where an ectopic beat would be expected. It is therefore reasonable to conclude that the beat in question is mainly conducted from the fibrillating atria but contains a small distorting contribution from the ventricular ectopic focus.

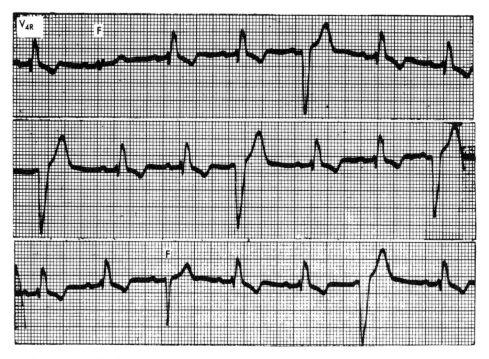

FIGURE 20-4 The three strips are continuous and show a right ventricular parasystole competing with a sinus rhythm with right bundle branch block. Note the presence of no fixed coupling *(F)* and fusion beats.

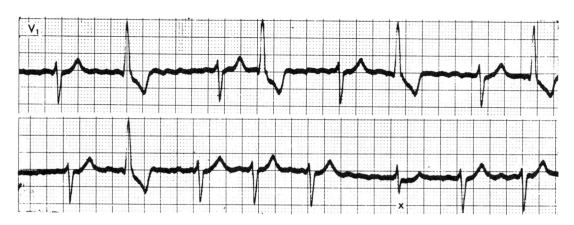

FIGURE 20-5 Atrial fibrillation and parasystole.

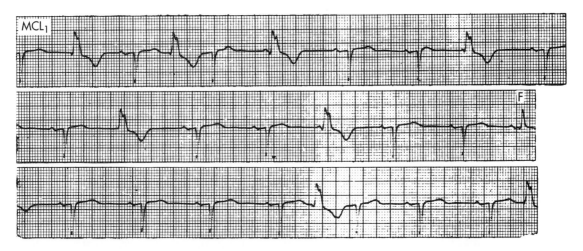

FIGURE 20-6 Strips are continuous. Classic ventricular parasystole with exit block. The exit block is noted in the bottom tracing; a ventricular ectopic beat was due midway between the first two complexes but did not occur even though the ventricles were nonrefractory.

CLASSIC PARASYSTOLE WITH EXIT BLOCK

The exit block in ventricular parasystole is usually of the type II variety. Assuming the usual criteria for ventricular parasystole are also present, it is recognized when an anticipated ectopic beat fails to appear even though the ventricles are nonrefractory. Figure 20-6 is an example of classic ventricular parasystole with exit block. In the bottom strip, an ectopic beat is expected to fuse with the sinus impulse midway between the two complexes, but it does not appear.

CONCEALED PARASYSTOLE

Concealed parasystole is seen only during sinus slowing. The explanation for the concealment of the parasystolic focus with faster rhythm is a refractory period in the area of protection (exit block) that is longer than that of the faster sinus rhythm. Thus the parasystolic focus maintains its fixed rate but does not exit into the surrounding myocardium until the underlying rhythm drops below a critical rate.

INTERMITTENT PARASYSTOLE

Intermittent parasystole may have absolute protection, or the protection may be limited to the initial portions of the cycle (phase 3). It is characterized by long nonparasystolic intervals interspersed with a series of parasystolic beats. In almost all cases of intermittent parasystole the first beat of each series has fixed coupling. The intermittent character of the parasystolic rhythm may be caused either by a cessation of automatic activity or by a periodic loss of protection. Cranefield[15] has postulated that entrance block may be temporarily relieved because of summation (Figure 20-7). Thus if neighboring fibers in the depressed segment of tissue are activated simultaneously and evoke subthreshold action potentials, the two currents summate, reach threshold, and

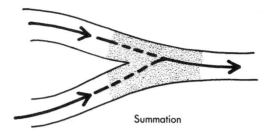

FIGURE 20-7 Summation may occur when two currents from depressed areas, each of which could not be propagated on its own, join to form a current that can be propagated.

evoke an action potential that *can* propagate. If this propagation occurs, the parasystolic focus is reset by the two invading impulses, which causes intermittent parasystole. Electrotonic modulation of the parasystolic focus may also explain some cases of intermittent parasystole.

PARASYSTOLIC ACCELERATED IDIOVENTRICULAR RHYTHM

With faster ventricular ectopic rates and no exit block, the number of ectopic beats may be more than the sinus rhythm and may indeed resemble an accelerated idioventricular rhythm (AIVR) or ventricular tachycardia. In such a case there is no way to recognize the rhythm as parasystolic unless there are interruptions with nonparasystolic beats that do not reset the ectopic focus. Figure 20-8 shows a continuous parasystolic AIVR without exit block. The proof is seen in the bottom tracing when the non-parasystolic beats fail to reset the parasystolic focus.

FIXED COUPLING IN PARASYSTOLE

Fixed coupling may be seen if, by chance, the rates of the parasystolic focus and SA node are mathematically related. For example, there is a fixed relationship (coincidental rather than real) between the sinus beat and the parasystolic one if the sinus rate is 70 beats/min and the rate of the parasystolic focus is 35 beats/min. As a result an ectopic beat will appear and follow every other normal beat at a fixed interval.

Supernormality is also recognized as a mechanism for fixed coupling in parasystole. Fixed coupling may result when the impulse from the parasystolic focus is subthreshold, and it is effective only when it falls during the supernormal phase. An artificial example of fixed coupling caused by supernormality can be seen in Figure 20-9. A subthreshold fixed-rate pacemaker fires at a regular rate throughout the tracing and is effective only when it falls during the supernormal phase of excitability.

Reversed coupling and modulation of the ectopic pacemaker by the dominant pacemaker (electrotonic influences) have already been mentioned as possible causes of constant coupling in parasystole.

CLINICAL SIGNIFICANCE

Ventricular parasystole is generally regarded as a benign rhythm. Because parasystole is an independent, autonomous rhythm that cannot be interrupted, it follows that its

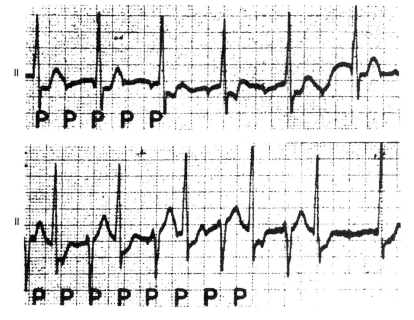

FIGURE 20-8 Parasystolic accelerated idioventricular rhythm without exit block. Protection is demonstrated in the bottom strip by the appearance of nonparasystolic beats that fail to affect the ectopic cycle length. The resulting ECG pattern resembles that of bidirectional tachycardia. (From Castellanos A, Molerio F, Kayden D, Myerburg RJ: Evolving concepts in the electrocardiographical diagnosis of ventricular parasystole. In Josephson ME, Wellens HJJ, editors: *Tachycardias: mechanisms, diagnosis, treatment,* Philadelphia, 1984, Lea & Febiger.)

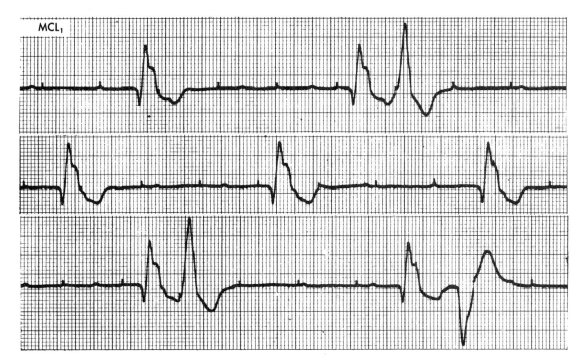

FIGURE 20-9 Fixed coupling resulting from supernormality. In this tracing a subthreshold pacemaker is effective only when it fires during the supernormal period.

impulses (as with the blip of a fixed-rate pacemaker) must sometimes land on the T waves of the competitive sinus beats. Because of this inevitable R-on-T incidence, parasystole may be thought to be dangerous. It is, however, an empirical observation that a parasystolic beat rarely occurs on the T wave because the effective refractory period of nonparasystolic beats is usually equal to or slightly longer than the QT interval. Moreover, there is no acceptable evidence that parasystolic (automatic) beats arriving in the vulnerable period would provoke ventricular tachycardia or ventricular fibrillation, even in the setting of acute myocardial infarction.

The benign nature of ventricular parasystole may result because the parasystolic rhythm is usually not fast or sustained and is easily suppressed by antiarrhythmic drugs. For example, lidocaine slows the rate of the focus and walls it off by compounding the depression in the area of entrance block surrounding the focus. Ventricular parasystole also occurs in apparently healthy individuals.

ATRIAL PARASYSTOLE

Atrial or junctional parasystole is less common than ventricular parasystole and is more difficult to diagnose. This difficulty arises because the anomalous ventricular complex is easier to identify and because an atrial and, possibly, a junctional parasystolic discharge interrupts and resets the sinus rhythm to produce what is called *reversed coupling*. Because the SA node is reset by the ectopic impulse, the interval between the atrial or junctional parasystolic beat and the sinus P wave is the same each time (exact coupling). However, instead of the usual situation in which the ectopic beat is coupled to the preceding sinus beat, the reverse is true—the sinus beat is coupled to the ectopic beat.

Figure 20-10 provides examples of atrial parasystole. In Figure 20-10, *A*, the parasystolic P waves are very similar to the sinus P waves. Note that the coupling interval between the atrial parasystolic beat and the preceding sinus P wave varies but that the interval between it and the following sinus P wave is constant (reversed coupling). In this tracing the common denominator of the interectopic intervals is 57, making this a parasystolic tachycardia at a rate of 107 beats/min. Fusion beats can be seen in Figure 20-10, *B*; the coupling interval becomes longer and longer until the two impulses fuse within the atria.

SUMMARY

Parasystole is usually ventricular but may also be atrial or, less commonly, junctional or SA nodal. The ECG characteristics of parasystole are variable intervals between ectopic beats and the preceding normal beats and, in its classic form, interectopic intervals that have a common denominator (i.e., the focus is never reset, thanks to a zone of protection surrounding it [entrance block]). Microelectrode studies have further shown that entrance block is caused by one-way block in depressed tissue. Thus the protection associated with a parasystolic focus is an abnormal mechanism. This protection can be continuous or intermittent, with or without exit block, producing the classic form of parasystole in which the cycle length of the ectopic focus is not influenced at all by extraneous impulses. Parasystole may also be concealed and may demonstrate a classic form when it emerges. The parasystolic focus can be modulated by electrotonic sub-

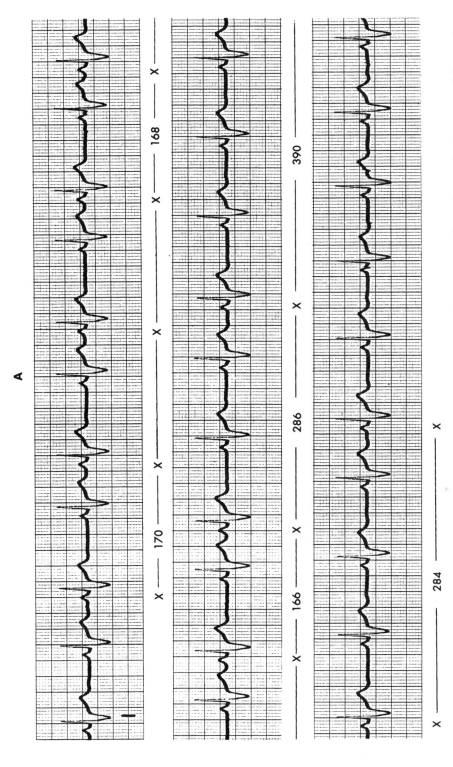

FIGURE 20-10 A, Atrial parasystole with reversed coupling. Note that the atrial ectopic beats (very similar in shape to the sinus P waves) have an inconsistent relationship with the preceding sinus P wave but are precisely linked to the sinus P wave that follows. Because the common denominator for the interectopic intervals is 57, the rate of this atrial parasystolic focus is 107 beats/min. (Courtesy Alan Lindsay, MD.)

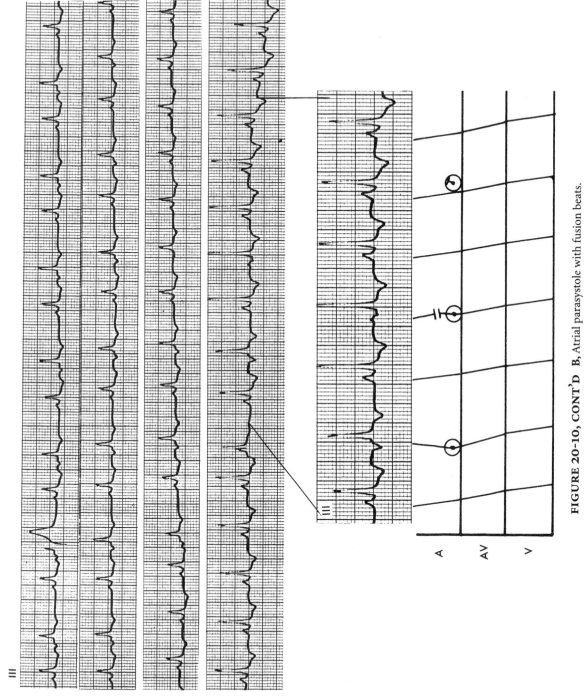

FIGURE 20-10, CONT'D B, Atrial parasystole with fusion beats.

threshold currents that traverse the band of depressed tissue and produce the nonclassic form of parasystole. Although the parasystolic focus is never actually reset by the extraneous rhythm, its cycle length can be altered in that early beats cause a delay in parasystolic discharge and late beats cause an acceleration of the discharge. Exit block exists when an expected parasystolic impulse does not appear in spite of a nonrefractory ventricle.

REFERENCES

1. Jalife J, Moe GK: Effects of electrotonic potentials on pacemaker activity of canine Purkinje fibers in relation to parasystole, *Circ Res* 39:801, 1976.
2. Castellanos A, Saoudi N, Moleiro F, Myerburg RJ: Parasystole. In Zipes DP, Jalife J, editors: *Cardiac electrophysiology from cell to bedside,* ed 2, Philadelphia, 1995, WB Saunders.
3. Moe GK, Antzelevitch C, Jalife J: Premature contractions: reentrant or parasystolic? In Harrison DC, editor: *Cardiac arrhythmias,* Boston, 1981, GK Hall.
4. Antzelevitch C, Jalife J, Moe GK: Electrotonic modulation of pacemaker activity: further biological and mathematical observations on the behavior of modulated parasystole, *Circulation* 66:1225, 1982.
5. Jalife J, Antzelevitch C, Moe GK: The case for modulated parasystole, *Pacing Clin Electrophysiol* 5:811, 1982.
6. Wit AL: Cellular electrophysiologic mechanisms of cardiac arrhythmias, *Ann NY Acad Sci* 432:1, 1986.
7. Ferrier GR, Rosenthal JE: Automaticity and entrance block induced by focal depolarization of mammalian ventricular tissues, *Circ Res* 47:238, 1980.
8. Wennemark JR, Bandura JP, Brody DA, Ruesta VJ: Microelectrode study of high grade block in canine Purkinje fibers, *J Electrocardiol* 8:299, 1975.
9. Jalife J, Moe GK: A biologic model of parasystole, *Am J Cardiol* 43:761, 1979.
10. Moe GK, Jalife J, Mueller WJ, Moe B: A mathematical model of parasystole and its application to clinical arrhythmias, *Circulation* 56:968, 1977.
11. Moe GK, Jalife J: An appraisal of "efficacy" in the treatment of ventricular premature beats, *Life Sci* 22:1189, 1978.
12. Antzelivitch C, Bernstein MJ, Feldman HN, Moe GK: Parasystole, reentry and tachycardia: a canine preparation of cardiac arrhythmias occurring across inexcitable segments of tissue, *Circulation* 68:1101, 1983.
13. El-Sherif N: The ventricular premature complex: mechanisms and significance: an update. In Mandel WS, editor: *Cardiac arrhythmias, their mechanisms, diagnosis and management,* Philadelphia, 1987, JB Lippincott.
14. Cranefield PF: *The conduction of the cardiac impulse,* Mt Kisco, NY, 1975, Futura.

CHAPTER 21

Supernormal Conduction

The supernormal
period 345
Concealed supernormal
conduction 346
Mimics of supernormal
conduction 348

SUPERNORMAL CONDUCTION IS DEPENDENT ON SUPERNORMAL EXCITABILITY, A CONdition that exists during a brief period of repolarization during which time excitation is possible in response to an otherwise subthreshold stimulus; that same stimulus does not elicit a response proximal or distal to the supernormal period.[1] Electrocardiographically, supernormal conduction is not better than normal conduction, only better than expected. Conduction is better earlier in the cycle than later and occurs when block is expected.

Supernormal excitability was first described in 1938 for heart muscle.[2] With the advent of the microelectrode, supernormal excitability was demonstrated in 1953 in isolated Purkinje fibers from sheep and calves.[3] Since that time intracellular stimulation methods have demonstrated supernormal excitability in the bundle branch–Purkinje system and in Bachmann's bundle but not in the AV node, bundle of His, or working myocardium.[4-6]

THE SUPERNORMAL PERIOD

The supernormal period occurs at the end of phase 3. During this period a stimulus of less than the normally required intensity can initiate an action potential that can be propagated.

Supernormal excitability is diagnosed when the myocardium responds to a stimulus that is ineffective when applied earlier or later in the cycle. During the supernormal period the cell has recovered enough to respond to a stimulus; because the membrane potential is still reduced, it requires only a little additional depolarization to bring the fiber to threshold. Thus a smaller stimulus than is normally required elicits an action potential during the supernormal phase of excitability.

The shaded areas in Figure 21-1 illustrate the supernormal period and its relationship to the total refractory period. There is a point within this time that the current requirement for excitation is at its minimum. This point is indicated by an *X* within the shaded areas. Spear and Moore[7] have found that the duration of the supernormal phase remains the same in spite of changes in the action potential duration. Thus as the action potential shortens, the supernormal period occupies more of it. Electrocardiographically, the supernormal period falls at the end of the T wave, and evidence of its presence is arrived at by deductive reasoning.

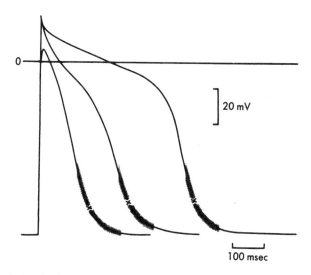

FIGURE 21-1 Relationship between the supernormal period and the total refractory period. (*X* indicates the moment of maximal supernormality and the point of minimum current requirements. Shaded areas delineate the boundaries of the period of supernormal excitability.) Above are shown superimposed action potentials. The longest duration action potential was evoked at a basic cycle length of 800 ms. The shorter action potentials were successively evoked premature beats at cycle lengths of 460 and 251 ms. (From Spear JF, Moore EN: The effect of changes in rate and rhythm on supernormal excitability in the isolated Purkinje system of the dog, *Circulation* 50:1174, 1974.)

Figure 21-2 is an example of supernormal excitability. In this tracing a failing pacemaker is ineffective except when the pacing stimulus lands between the nadir and the end of the T wave.

Spear and Moore[7] have demonstrated the relationship between supernormal excitability and supernormal conduction. The mechanism is as follows: The propagation of a conduction wave relies on local currents flowing across the membranes just in front of the propagating action potential. If the downstream cells can be brought to threshold faster because of reduced current requirements for excitation during late repolarization, then conduction velocity is improved over that expected at a later time in diastole, when current requirements to reach threshold are greater.

Supernormal conduction can be seen in Figure 21-3. Most of the sinus impulses are conducted with right bundle branch block (RBBB). However, two early beats are conducted normally, which suggests supernormal conduction in the right bundle branch (RBB). This is also an example of critical rate RBBB because the sinus impulses following the atrial premature beat (APB) end a longer cycle (overdrive suppression) and are conducted normally.

CONCEALED SUPERNORMAL CONDUCTION

In Figure 21-4 there are two instances of manifest supernormal conduction (fifth beat in each tracing) and two instances of concealed supernormal conduction (after the

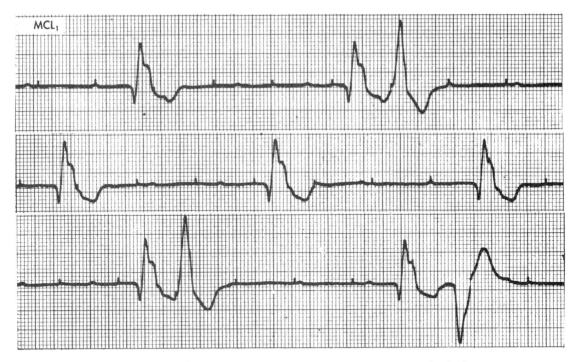

FIGURE 21-2 Strips are continuous. Complete AV block with very slow left idioventricular rhythm. The implanted pacemaker is ineffective except on two occasions in which the stimulus lands in the "supernormal" phase of excitability (toward the end of the T wave).

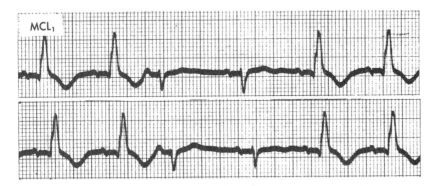

FIGURE 21-3 Strips are not continuous. Supernormal conduction in the right bundle branch. The third beats in the two tracings are atrial premature beats with normal conduction in the face of an underlying right bundle branch block with much longer cycles.

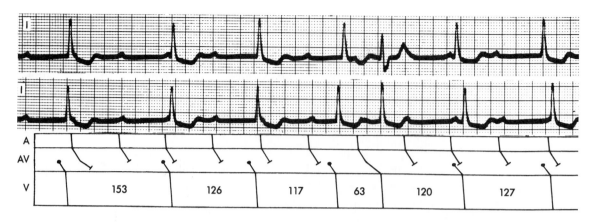

FIGURE 21-4 Strips show a significant degree of AV block with a junctional escape rhythm at a rate of 48 beats/min. The first cycle in each strip is longer than the other cycles because the atrial impulse immediately following the first QRS complex is conducted into the AV junction and resets the junctional pacemaker (see laddergram). The fifth beat in each strip is conducted from the somewhat later atrial impulses, deforming the ST segment or T wave of the preceding beat. These atrial impulses may be considered examples of supernormal conduction because they occur much earlier in the cycle than many that are not conducted at all. Because the impulses after the first QRS complex do not reach the ventricles and their conduction is only inferred, they are examples of concealed supernormal conduction.

first beat in each tracing). Supernormal conduction is evident just beyond the middle of each strip. The sinus P waves that deform the ST segment in the top strip and the T wave in the bottom represent impulses that are conducted; later sinus impulses, with an expected better chance of conduction, are blocked.

Concealed supernormal conduction is not quite as easy to recognize. Apart from the two instances of capture caused by manifest supernormal conduction, notice in Figure 21-4 the irregularity of the junctional escape rhythm in the face of a significant degree of AV block. The following principle often facilitates a diagnosis: When an independent rhythm (in this case junctional) manifests two cycle lengths, subtract the shorter cycle length from the longer, *starting from the end of the long cycle*. At that point look for possible clues that may explain what has lengthened this cycle beyond the shorter ones. Applying this principle to Figure 21-4, note that a sinus P wave just precedes the spot measured to in the longer cycle. Clearly this sinus P wave is causally related to the lengthened cycle and implies penetration of that sinus impulse into the AV junction, thus discharging and resetting the junctional pacemaker. The postponement of the next expected junctional beat earmarks this as concealed conduction.

MIMICS OF SUPERNORMAL CONDUCTION

Supernormality is certainly a possibility when conduction is better earlier than later. However, other mechanisms should also be considered, some of which are listed as follows.[8-10] Keep in mind that the mechanism may not always be proven conclusively:

1. Concealed junctional extrasystoles
2. Phase 4 (paradoxical critical rate)

3. Reentry with ventricular echo
4. The gap phenomenon

Concealed Junctional Extrasystoles

In Figure 21-5 the underlying sinus rhythm is regular at 68 beats/min. Note that each shorter RP interval is complemented by a shorter PR interval, suggesting supernormal conduction of these alternate beats. A much more likely explanation postulated by Langendorf[11] in 1948 is that the longer PRs are the result of concealed junctional extrasystoles, as illustrated in the laddergram in Figure 21-5.

Phase 4 (Paradoxical Critical Rate)

Enhanced phase 4 depolarization within the bundle branch system may result in bundle branch block (BBB) (phase 4 block; see Chapter 15). In such a case the maximum diastolic potential immediately follows repolarization, from which point the membrane potential is steadily reduced. Thus an action potential initiated early in the cycle (immediately after repolarization) would have a steeper and higher phase 0 and consequently better conduction than would an action potential initiated later in the cycle.[12-15]

In Figure 21-6 the underlying rhythm is a sinus bradycardia at 50 beats/min, with a faster junctional escape rate of 56 beats/min producing AV dissociation. If the fibers of the RBB have enhanced automaticity, late-arriving impulses resulting from the bradycardia find a reduced membrane potential, and conduction is blocked. Because diastolic depolarization begins immediately after repolarization, the membrane potential is maximum early in the cycle; in fact, the earlier the better. Note that all of the beats except two early ones are conducted with RBBB. When ventricular capture occurs (fifth beat), there is much less evidence of BBB, which suggests that conduction occurred either before the membrane potential could be reduced or because the impulse arrived during the phase of supernormal excitability in the RBB.

Concealed Reentry

Figure 21-7 is another example of simulated supernormal conduction. A shorter PR interval (fourth beat) unexpectedly interrupts what starts as a Wenckebach sequence. Because the P wave of this impulse is close to the preceding T wave, supernormal conduction might be suspected. A more likely explanation is that, after the lengthened PR interval of the third beat, there is reentry with retrograde conduction (see laddergram). The descent of the next atrial impulse thwarts this attempt at an atrial echo. However, further (anterograde) reentry produces a ventricular echo as the impulse returns to the ventricles, making it appear that the atrial impulse was conducted during a period of supernormality.

The Gap Phenomenon

The gap phenomenon was originally described by Moe, Mendez, and Han[16] in 1965 as a zone in which premature atrial stimuli encountered AV block, whereas AV conduction was accomplished if the stimulus occurred earlier or later. Since that time as many as six types of gaps have been described for anterograde conduction.[17]

The more commonly encountered gaps are thought to be functional in nature and depend on a difference in refractoriness between the cells at two different levels in the AV conduction system so that an APB is blocked in the His-Purkinje system but not in

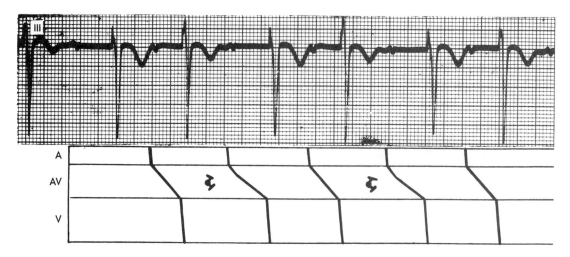

FIGURE 21-5 Concealed junctional extrasystoles mimicking supernormal conduction.

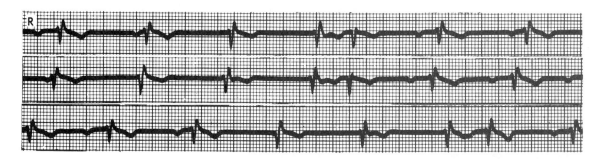

FIGURE 21-6 Strips are continuous. A junctional rhythm with right bundle branch block aberration is dissociated from a slightly slower sinus rhythm. The three early beats are ventricular captures. The first two are conducted with much less evidence of RBBB, which suggests conduction during the "supernormal" phase of the RBB or conduction before reduction of the membrane potential.

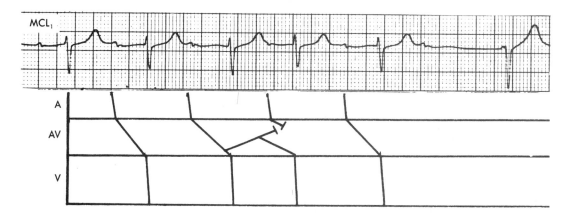

FIGURE 21-7 Concealed reentry as a mimic of supernormal conduction.

the AV node. This apparently selective block occurs because the shortest time between two atrial impulses needed for the AV node to conduct (functional refractory period) is less than the effective refractory period of the His-Purkinje system.

Figure 21-8 diagrammatically illustrates the mechanism of the gap phenomenon. In Figure 21-8, *A*, an APB is not conducted to the ventricles because the impulse traverses the AV node rapidly enough to arrive while the His-Purkinje system is still in its effective refractory period. With a shorter coupling interval, the impulse travels more slowly through the AV node, which is in its relative refractory period (Figure 21-8, *B*). By the time this impulse traverses the AV node, the His-Purkinje system has completed its effective refractory period and conduction is possible. Ventricular activation results.

Figure 21-9 diagrammatically illustrates another level of the gap phenomenon, in which the effective refractory period of the His-Purkinje system exceeds both the functional and the effective refractory period of the AV node so that the His-Purkinje

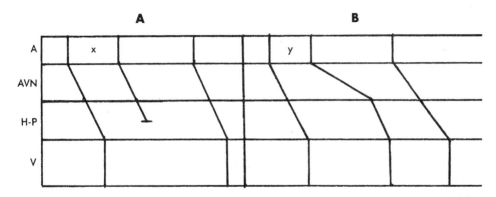

FIGURE 21-8 Diagrammatic representation of the mechanism of the gap phenomenon. **A,** The initial block is in the His-Purkinje system. **B,** The required conduction delay is in the AV node.

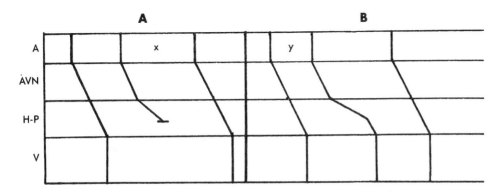

FIGURE 21-9 Diagrammatic representation of the mechanism of another type of gap phenomenon. **A,** The initial block is low in the His-Purkinje system. **B,** The required conduction delay is in the bundle branches.

system and not the AV node is the site of conduction delay. In Figure 21-9, *A*, an APB is blocked within the His-Purkinje system. At a shorter coupling interval an APB is delayed in the proximal His-Purkinje system, probably in the bundle branches, which gives the distal portion time to recover. Ventricular activation results (Figure 21-9, *B*).[15]

Figures 21-8 and 21-9 illustrate that the gap phenomenon depends on conduction delay in fibers activated during their relative refractory period, when conduction velocity is slower than it would have been if activation had occurred later in the cycle. Other types of gap phenomenon are described in which the required conduction delay is in the His bundle, the proximal AV node, or the atria.[17,18]

The gap phenomenon has also been described in a retrograde direction and in fact is thought to occur more commonly during retrograde than during anterograde conduction.[19] The site of retrograde block is the AV node or upper reaches of the His-Purkinje system, whereas the gap-produced retrograde delay in conduction is lower in the His-Purkinje system.

SUMMARY

During the supernormal period of the action potential (the end of phase 3), a stimulus occurs that could not elicit a propagated action potential before or after that time. In other words, a stimulus of less-than-normal intensity can result in a propagated action potential if it occurs during the supernormal period. Two factors are responsible for this phenomenon: (1) the availability of fast sodium channels, and (2) the proximity of the membrane potential to threshold potential. The same mechanism is responsible for supernormal conduction. Faster conduction results if the downstream cells can be brought to threshold potential more easily because the stimulus arrives during that point of repolarization when enough fast sodium channels are available for a propagated action potential.

REFERENCES

1. Fisch C: "Supernormal" conduction. In Zipes DP, Jalife J, editors: *Cardiac electrophysiology from cell to bedside*, ed 2, Philadelphia, 1995, WB Saunders.
2. Cranefield PE, Hoffman BE, Siebens AA: Anodal excitation of cardiac muscle, *Am J Physiol* 190:383, 1957.
3. Weidmann S: Effects of calcium ions and local anesthetics on electrical properties of Purkinje fibers, *J Physiol* 129:568, 1955.
4. Spear JF, Moore EN: The effect of changes in rate and rhythm on supernormal excitability in the isolated Purkinje system of the dog: a possible role in re-entrant arrhythmias, *Circulation* 50:1144, 1974.
5. Childers RW, Merideth J, Moe GJ: Supernormality in Bachmann's bundle: an in vivo and in vitro study, *Circ Res* 21:363, 1968.
6. Puech P, Guimond C, Nadeau R et al: Supernormal conduction in the intact heart. In Narula OS, editor: *Cardiac arrhythmias: electrophysiology, diagnosis, and management*, Baltimore, 1979, Williams & Wilkins.
7. Spear JF, Moore EN: Supernormal excitability and conduction. In Wellens HJJ, Lie KI, Janse MJ, editors: *The conduction system of the heart: structure, function and clinical implications*, Philadelphia, 1976, Lea & Febiger.

8. Moe GK, Childers RW, Merideth J: An appraisal of "supernormal" A-V conduction, *Circulation* 38:5, 1968.

9. Damato AN, Wit AL, Lau SH: Observations on the mechanism of one type of so-called supernormal A-V conduction, *Am Heart J* 82:725, 1971.

10. Gallagher JJ, Damato AN, Varghese PJ et al: Alternative mechanisms of apparent supernormal atrioventricular conduction, *Am J Cardiol* 31:362, 1973.

11. Langendorf R: Concealed A-V conduction: the effect of blocked impulses on the formation and conduction of subsequent impulses, *Am Heart J* 35:542, 1948.

12. Singer DH, Lazzara R, Hoffman BF: Interrelationships between automaticity and conduction in Purkinje fibers, *Circ Res* 22:537, 1967.

13. Rosenbaum MB, Elizari MV, Levi RJ, Nau GJ: The mechanisms of intermittent bundle branch block: relationship to prolonged recovery, hypopolarization, and spontaneous diastolic depolarization, *Chest* 63:666, 1973.

14. Pick A, Fishman AP: Observations in heart block: supernormality of A-V and intraventricular conduction and ventricular parasystole under the influence of epinephrine, *Acta Cardiol* 5:270, 1950.

15. Hoffman BF: Physiology of A-V transmission, *Circulation* 24:506, 1961.

16. Moe GK, Mendez C, Han J: Aberrant A-V impulse propagation in the dog heart: a study of functional bundle branch block, *Circ Res* 16:261, 1965.

17. Damato AN, Akhtar M, Ruskin J et al: Gap phenomena: antegrade and retrograde. In Wellens HJJ, Lie KI, Janse MJ, editors: *The conduction system of the heart: structure, function, and clinical implications*, Philadelphia, 1976, Lea & Febiger.

18. Wu D, Denes P, Dhingra R, Rosen KM: Nature of gap phenomenon in man, *Circ Res* 34:682, 1974.

19. Akhtar M, Damato AN, Caracta AR et al: The gap phenomenon during retrograde conduction in man, *Circulation* 49:811, 1974.

CHAPTER **22**

An Approach to Arrhythmias

Principles of moni-
  toring 355
  Monitor according to the
  clinical setting 355
  One lead is not
  enough 356
  Electrode positions for
  MCL₁ and MCL₆ 356
A systematic approach 358
  Know the causes 358
  Milk the QRS 359
  Cherchez le P 359
  Who's married
    to whom? 363
  Pinpoint the primary
    disturbance 363

MANY DISTURBANCES OF RHYTHM AND CONDUCTION CAN BE RECOGNIZED AT FIRST glance. For example, atrial flutter with 4:1 conduction, atrial fibrillation with rapid ventricular response, or sinus rhythm with right bundle branch block (RBBB) can usually be spotted immediately. There are, however, a significant number of dysrhythmias that defy immediate recognition and require a systematic attack. The five-point approach discussed in this chapter evolved after analyzing the reasons for mistakes made in diagnosing arrhythmias. It is therefore designed to avoid the common errors of omission and commission. Before outlining this systematic approach, it is worth making some observations about the principles of monitoring.

PRINCIPLES OF MONITORING
Monitor According to the Clinical Setting

Providing multiple lead monitoring systems and tailoring the lead selection to each patient's individual clinical condition is important. Although V₁ clearly supplies much information, it is hardly the appropriate lead for a patient admitted with unstable angina; in fact this lead can mask critical proximal left anterior descending stenosis with alarming results.[1,2] On the other hand, when a patient is admitted for paroxysms of narrow QRS tachycardia, the main purpose of hospitalization is to obtain a record of the tachycardia in at least five leads (I, II, III, V₁, and V₆). Monitoring in all five leads is ideal; if only two leads are available, leads I and II are good choices.

Lead II is an appropriate monitoring lead in other clinical settings (e.g., for a patient in sinus rhythm who is taking digitalis) (see Chapter 13). For atrial fibrillation in patients who are taking digitalis, lead V₁ is the required monitoring lead so that toxicity (junctional tachycardia or fascicular ventricular tachycardia) can be recognized. Lead V₁ is also an excellent choice when evaluating for bundle branch block and for the differential diagnosis between ventricular tachycardia and aberration. Many times in a right chest lead an ectopic P wave can easily be differentiated from a sinus P wave because of its shape. When it is diphasic, the sinus P wave is usually + / − (∿); the ectopic or retrograde P wave, when diphasic, is usually − / + (∿).

Under no circumstances should there be one "standard" monitoring lead for the unit—not lead II, and not lead V₁. For many years a counterfeit lead II was used for everyone in some critical care units—a lead in which left bundle branch block (LBBB), RBBB, and left and right ventricular ectopics *can* look identical and a lead in which the

355

onset of critical proximal left anterior descending coronary artery stenosis is completely missed. For these reasons, lead II is one of the least satisfactory leads for constant monitoring. What is the virtue of a monitoring lead that can look similar in these four conditions and can let a mortal condition go undetected?

One Lead is Not Enough

It is important to appreciate the limitations of a single lead and to know when to obtain additional leads and which to obtain. Another reason a single lead may be inadequate is that it may fail to reveal inconspicuous items in the tracing such as P waves or pacemaker spikes.

More than one lead is helpful when the distinction between ectopy and aberration is uncertain in a right chest lead. In Figure 22-1 the pattern of the tachycardia in MCL_1 could be either left ventricular or supraventricular with RBBB aberration. A look at MCL_6 indicates with reasonable certainty that the origin of the tachycardia is supraventricular. When V_1 is positive, a small q in V_6 indicates supraventricular tachycardia.

Electrode Positions for MCL_1 and MCL_6

The modified CL_1 (MCL_1) monitoring lead was introduced in 1968.[3] The positive electrode is placed at the C_1 (V_1) position, the negative electrode at the left shoulder, and the ground (which may be placed anywhere) usually at the right shoulder. This pattern leaves a clear platform for emergency cardioversion and an unencumbered precordium for physical examination. In addition, this lead closely imitates V_1 and thus affords several diagnostic advantages:

1. One can immediately distinguish between left ventricular ectopy (QRS mostly positive) and right ventricular ectopy (QRS mostly negative) in most instances.
2. RBBB and LBBB can be recognized with ease.
3. P waves are sometimes best or seen only in a right chest lead.
4. Most important, a right chest lead gives the best opportunity for the differential diagnosis between VT and aberration (see Chapter 16).

The disadvantages of lead MCL_1 are that it fails to recognize the following:

1. Critical proximal LAD stenosis in patients with unstable angina
2. Shifts of axis in patients with acute anterior myocardial infarction who are at risk for developing hemiblock
3. The left-to-right and inferior-to-superior orientation of the P axis

MCL_6 can be obtained by placing the positive electrode at the C_6 (V_6) position to obtain an MCL_6, a reasonable imitation of V_6. To simulate lead III (M_3) for the purpose of recording the polarity of the retrograde P', place the positive electrode low on the left flank below the diaphragm (leaving the negative electrode at the left shoulder). A left chest lead (V_6 or MCL_6) is not reliable for distinguishing between left and right ventricular ectopy because the QRS complex in both may be either positive or negative.

Figure 22-2 illustrates the information that can be derived from a right chest lead and is not usually available in lead II. In Figure 22-2, *A*, the rSR' pattern of the sinus beats is typical of RBBB; the qR pattern with early peak in the first extrasystole is typical of ectopy of left ventricular origin; the rS pattern of the second extrasystole is typical of a right ventricular origin. In Figure 22-2, *B*, the atrial fibrillation is interrupted by

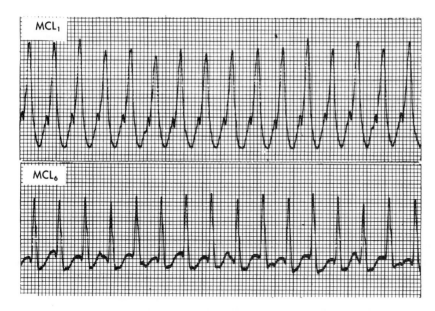

FIGURE 22-1 Supraventricular tachycardia with RBBB aberration. From lead MCL$_1$ alone, left ventricular tachycardia cannot be distinguished from supraventricular tachycardia with RBBB aberration. However, the qRs pattern in MCL$_6$ immediately identifies it as supraventricular.

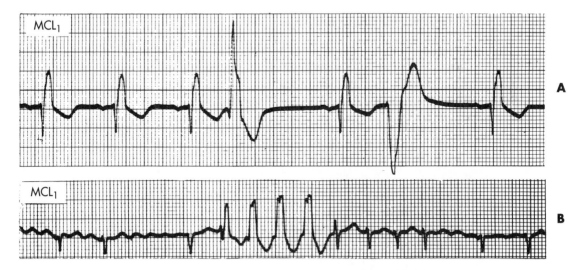

FIGURE 22-2 A, Patterns of RBBB (sinus beats), left ventricular ectopy (fourth beat), and right ventricular ectopy (sixth beat) are readily recognized. **B,** Short run of aberrantly conducted beats during atrial fibrillation. The aberration is recognized by the characteristic triphasic (rSR′) contour of the first anomalous beat.

a burst of bizarre beats that are certain to evoke the "lidocaine reflex"; however, the telltale shape (rSR′) of the first of these wide beats shows that it is a run of aberrantly conducted beats rather than a run of ventricular tachycardia.

A SYSTEMATIC APPROACH

Failing a diagnosis that is obvious, the following systematic five-point approach is necessary:

1. Know the causes
2. Milk the QRS
3. Cherchez le P
4. Who is married to whom?
5. Pinpoint the primary disturbance

Know the Causes

Knowing the possible causes is the first step in any medical diagnosis. It is part of the equipment that a clinician carries and is prepared at a moment's notice to use when faced with an unidentified arrhythmia.

The eight basic arrhythmias are early beats, unexpected pauses, tachycardias, bradycardias, bigeminal rhythms, group beating, total irregularity, and regular nonsinus rhythms at normal rates. The most common causes of most of these basic arrhythmias are discussed in the following sections.

Causes of early beats

- Extrasystoles
- Parasystole
- Capture beats
- Reciprocal beats
- Better conduction interrupting poorer conduction
- Supernormal conduction during AV block
- Rhythm resumption after inapparent bigeminy

Causes of pauses

- Nonconducted atrial extrasystoles
- Second-degree AV block
- Second-degree SA block
- "Sick sinus" variants
- Concealed conduction
- Concealed junctional extrasystoles
- Pacemaker pauses

Causes of bradycardia

- Sinus bradycardia
- SA block
- Nonconducted atrial bigeminy
- AV block

Causes of bigeminy (skeleton classification)

- Extrasystoles
- Parasystole
- 3:2 conduction
- Reciprocal beating
- Fortuitous pairing in atrial fibrillation

Common causes of group beating

- Supraventricular tachycardia with Wenckebach periods
- Atrial flutter with 2:1 "filtering" at the upper level in the junction and Wenckebach periodicity below
- Sinus rhythm with two or more consecutive extrasystoles
- Recurrent bursts of ventricular or supraventricular tachycardia
- Every third beat an interpolated ventricular extrasystole

Common causes of chaotic irregularity

- Atrial fibrillation
- Atrial flutter with varying AV conduction
- Chaotic (multifocal) atrial tachycardia
- Shifting (wandering) pacemaker with atrial extrasystoles
- Sinus rhythm with multifocal extrasystoles
- Mixed ventricular rhythms

Milk the QRS

In arrhythmia detection, give priority to ventricular behavior. In general, it matters little what the atria are doing as long as the ventricles are behaving themselves.

When measuring the QRS duration, be sure to check at least two leads because initial or terminal forces may be isoelectric in a particular lead and cause the QRS complex to appear narrow in that lead only.

If the QRS is of normal duration, the rhythm is supraventricular; if it is wide and bizarre, it must be decided whether it is supraventricular with ventricular aberration or ectopic ventricular. A knowledge of the ECG in the distinction between aberrancy and ectopy allows one to get the most out of the QRS milking process (see Chapter 16).

Cherchez le P

If the shape of the QRS complex does not help in making a diagnosis, turn to the P wave for help. In the past the P wave, as the key to arrhythmias, has certainly been overemphasized. However, there are times when it holds the diagnostic clue and must be given the starring role. In searching for P waves, there are several clues and caveats to bear in mind.

The S_5 lead

The S_5 lead is obtained by placing the positive electrode at the fifth right interspace close to the sternum (just below the C_1 position) and the negative electrode on the manubrium of the sternum. This placement sometimes greatly magnifies the P wave, rendering it readily visible when it may have been virtually indiscernible in other leads. Figure 22-3 illustrates

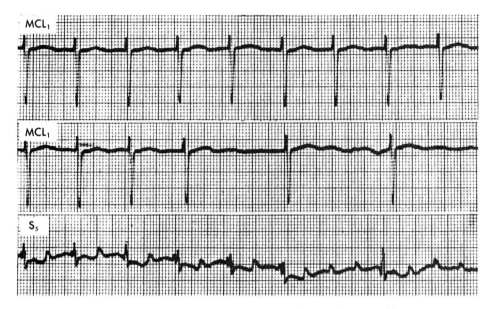

FIGURE 22-3 Top strip of MCL₁ shows barely perceptible P′ waves of an atrial tachycardia. Second strip shows the effect of carotid sinus stimulation: the ventricular rate halves because of increased AV block, and additional P′ waves become barely visible through the artifact. In contrast, the strip of lead S₅ has prominent P waves.

this amplifying effect and makes the diagnosis of atrial tachycardia with 2:1 block immediately apparent. If it succeeds, this technique is certainly preferable to invasive ones (atrial wire or esophageal electrode).

The Bix rule

Whenever P waves of a supraventricular tachycardia occur exactly halfway between the ventricular complexes, it should always be suspected that additional P waves are hiding within the QRS complex—a point emphasized by the late Harold Bix of Vienna and Baltimore. In the top strip of Figure 22-4 the P′ wave is midway between the QRS complexes. Moments later the conduction pattern alters (middle strip) and exposes the lurking P′ waves. It is clearly important to know if there are twice as many atrial impulses as are apparent; if there are, there is the ever present danger that the ventricular rate may double or almost double, especially if the atrial rate should decrease. It is better to be forewarned and take steps to prevent such potentially disastrous acceleration.

The haystack principle

If searching for a needle in a haystack, a small haystack is obviously preferable to a large one. Therefore whenever an elusive P wave or pacemaker spike cannot be found, give the lead with the least baseline disturbance (the smallest ventricular complexes) a chance to help. There are some leads that no one would think of looking at to solve an arrhythmia (e.g., aV_R). The patient whose tracing is illustrated in Figure 22-5 died

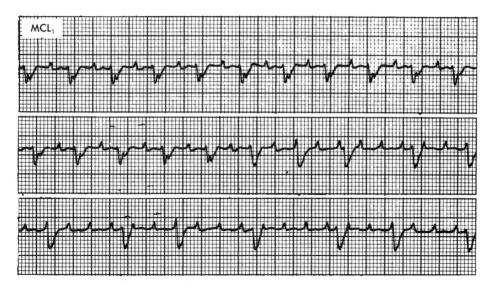

FIGURE 22-4 Bix rule *(top strip)*. The P waves are midway between the ventricular complexes, making one suspect a hidden P′ wave.

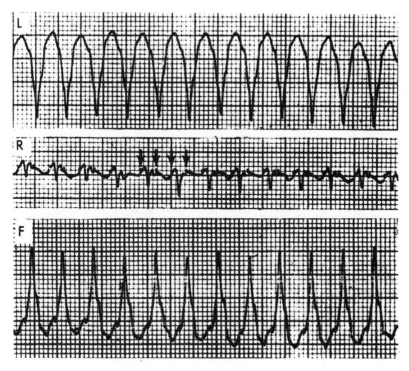

FIGURE 22-5 Haystack principle. Patient's runaway pacemaker is recognizable only in the lead with the least disturbance of the baseline, in this case aV_R.

because no one thought to apply the haystack principle and look in aV_R. He had a runaway pacemaker at a discharge rate of 440 beats/min with a halved ventricular response of 220 beats/min. Lead aV_R was the lead with the smallest ventricular complex, and it was the only lead in which the pacemaker "blips" were plainly visible (arrows). The patient went into shock and died because none of the attempted therapeutic measures affected the tachycardia; all that was needed was to disconnect the wayward pulse generator.

Mind your Ps

"Mind your *Ps*" means to be wary of things that look like P waves and particularly applies to P-like waves that are adjacent to the QRS complex; they may actually be part of the QRS complex. This is a trap for unwary sufferers of the "P-preoccupation syndrome," to whom anything that looks like a P wave *is* a P wave. For example, the strips of V_1 and V_2 in Figure 22-6 would be diagnosed by many as supraventricular tachycardia for the wrong reasons. In V_1 the QRS complex does not seem to be very wide and appears to be preceded by a small P wave. In V_2 an apparently narrow QRS complex is followed by what appears to be a retrograde P wave. In fact, the P-like waves in both leads are part of the QRS complex. If the QRS duration is measured in V_3, it is found to be 0.14 second. To attain a QRS complex of that duration in V_1 and V_2, the P-like waves must be included in the measurement.

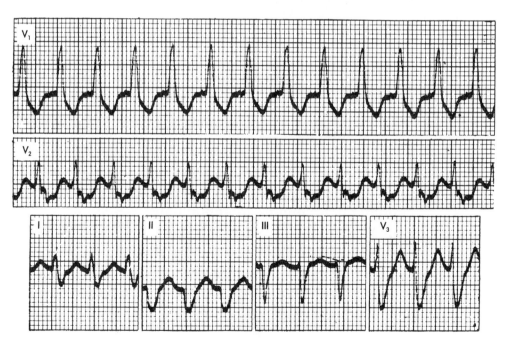

FIGURE 22-6 Mind your *Ps*. The QRS duration in leads I and V_3 measures 0.14 second. Therefore the P-like waves in the other leads must be part of the QRS complex.

Find a break

A solution is most likely to be spotted at a break in rhythm. At the beginning of the strip in Figure 22-7, the rhythm is regular at a rate of 200 beats/min; it is impossible to know whether the tachycardia is ectopic atrial, ectopic junctional, or reciprocating in the AV junction. A fourth possibility is that the little peak is part of the QRS complex and not a P wave at all. Farther along the strip there is a pause in the rhythm. The most common cause of a pause is a nonconducted atrial extrasystole; and, sure enough, there at the arrow in Fig. 22-7 is the culprit — in this situation a diagnostic ally. As a result of the pause, the P wave can be seen in front of the next QRS complex, and therefore the mechanism is atrial tachycardia.

Who's Married to Whom?

Establishing relationships is often the crucial step in arriving at a firm diagnosis. This principle is illustrated in Figure 22-8, in which a junctional rhythm is dissociated from sinus bradycardia. On three occasions there are bizarre early beats of a qR configuration that is nondiagnostic. The fact that they are seen *only* when a P wave is emerging beyond the preceding QRS complex shows that they are "married to" the preceding P waves and establishes them as conducted (capture) beats with RBBB aberration rather than ventricular extrasystoles.

Pinpoint the Primary Disturbance

Never be content to let the diagnosis rest with a phenomenon such as AV dissociation, escape, or aberration. These phenomena are always secondary to some primary disturbance.

In Figure 22-9 there is a junctional rhythm with retrograde conduction at a rate of 31 beats/min. If this strip is shown to most observers to obtain a *diagnosis,* almost certainly the answer will be "junctional rhythm." However, this is not a diagnosis. No junc-

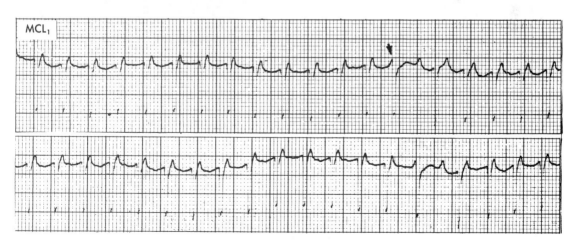

FIGURE 22-7 Focus on the break in rhythm *(arrow)*, and it provides the answer: the P' wave precedes rather than follows the QRS complex.

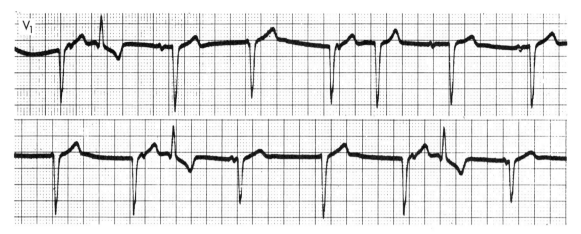

FIGURE 22-8 Who is married to whom? Strips are continuous. Early beats are consistently preceded by a sinus P wave emerging just beyond the QRS complex and are therefore conducted (capture) beats. The underlying rhythm is sinus bradycardia producing AV dissociation.

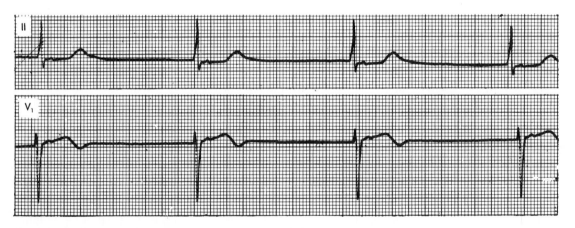

FIGURE 22-9 Pinpoint the primary condition, which is sick sinus syndrome with resulting AV junctional escape (rate = 31 beats/min) with retrograde conduction.

tional rhythm could possibly hold sway in the presence of a normal SA node. The diagnosis—the primary disturbance—is a sick SA node; junctional rhythm is a secondary escape mechanism.

Figure 22-10 presents a chance to review several of the points discussed in the section entitled A Systematic Approach (see p. 358). This tracing was sent thousands of miles with note asking, "This patient needed a pacemaker for this funny sort of block—what is it?"

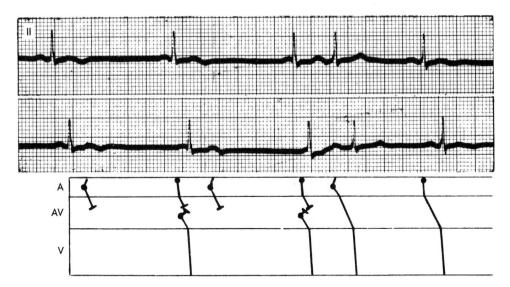

FIGURE 22-10 Strips are continuous. Sinus rhythm with atrial bigeminy; most of the APBs are not conducted, with resulting junctional escape.

After observing the presence of bradycardia and two premature supraventricular beats, probably the first things noticed are AV dissociation and the different shapes of the T waves. The P′ wave is a common reason for such distortion, and the diagnosis falls into your lap: conducted and nonconducted bigeminal APBs with junctional escape beats.

Failing this approach, the diagnosis could have been reached by any of the following methods:

1. Review the causes of bradycardia. Nonconducted atrial bigeminy is third on the list and elicits a careful examination of the T waves, in which are found the nonconducted APBs.
2. A motivation by the injunction to "find the break," would lead to concentrating on the early beats because they represent the "break" in the otherwise regular rhythm. Attention would then be directed to the T waves and the hidden P waves.
3. Reciting the causes of early supraventricular beats would have led to thinking first of atrial extrasystoles.

REFERENCES

1. Thorne D, Gozensky C: Rabbit ears: an aid in distinguishing ventricular ectopy from aberration, *Heart Lung* 3:634, 1974.
2. Wellens HJJ, Bär FW, Lie KI: The value of the electrocardiogram in the differential diagnosis of a tachycardia with a widened QRS complex, *Am J Med* 64:27, 1978.
3. Marriott HJL, Fogg E: Constant monitoring for cardiac dysrhythmias and blocks, *Mod Concepts Cardiovasc Dis* 39:103, 1970.

Historical background 367
Clinical application of the signal-averaged ECG 367
Problems in analyzing small ECG signals 368
Signal averaging 368
Spatial averaging 369
Ensemble averaging (signal averaging) 369
Time domain analysis of the signal-averaged ECG 369
Interpreting the time domain signal-averaged ECG 370
Frequency domain analysis of the signal-averaged ECG 372
Limitations 376
Other analytic methods 376

HISTORICAL BACKGROUND

It is doubtful that eighteenth-century mathematician Jean Baptiste Joseph Fourier (1768-1830) had in mind the welfare of patients with coronary artery disease when he developed the mathematics that (among other things) allows time domain signals to be transformed to the frequency domain and back again. For decades this pure mathematic process, the continuous Fourier transform (CFT), was of little use outside the abstract world of mathematicians. In 1903 Runge[1] described a computational technique for sampling the time domain signal at 12 or 24 points and determining the Fourier transform, thus providing the discrete Fourier transform (DFT). Although the DFT allowed practical use of the CFT, the large number of complex calculations required strained the computational resources of that time (i.e., graduate students). Research continued, and in 1965 Cooley and Tukey[2] developed the fast Fourier transform (FFT) algorithm. The FFT algorithm vastly reduced the number and complexity of the calculations required to evaluate the DFT. It is highly probable that the first computer program to evaluate the FFT was written at this time. This high-speed method of calculating the DFT launched the modern era of the Fourier transform as an analytic tool.

The FFT is used extensively in radar, air traffic control, image enhancement, communications, oceanography, character recognition, and system simulation. The relatively recent availability of low-cost computers has allowed researchers to use this powerful diagnostic tool to evaluate patients with coronary artery disease.

CLINICAL APPLICATION OF THE SIGNAL-AVERAGED ECG

Sophisticated techniques from the radar and communication disciplines—signal averaging, filtering, and FFT—are applied to the analysis of the electrocardiogram (ECG). These techniques allow the examination of portions of the ECG previously obscured by noise and artifacts. In the evaluation of late potentials, the filtered signal-averaged ECG (SAECG) is an important tool.[3]

Patients surviving acute myocardial infarction may be at risk for developing life-threatening arrhythmias. In patients with a history of myocardial infarction, certain low-level, high-frequency ECG signals have been observed and correlated with an increased risk for developing spontaneous arrhythmias.[4-7] These distinctive signals, called *late potentials,* are high-frequency, low-amplitude events that occur late in and are continuous with the QRS complex. They apparently arise from delayed and disorganized activity in areas of the myocardium at the interface of fibrous scar tissue and normal tissue.[8,9] Because these late potentials are very low-level phenomena, special techniques and equipment have been developed to record them.

367

The American College of Cardiology has published an expert consensus document regarding SAECG.[10] The consensus is that SAECG has an established value in determining a patient's risk for developing sustained ventricular arrhythmias in two clinical settings:

1. Postmyocardial infarction patients with sinus rhythm and no ECG evidence of bundle branch block or intraventricular conduction delay
2. Ischemic heart disease and unexplained syncope

There are also two clinical settings in which SAECG is valuable for determining risk for development of sustained ventricular arrhythmias but in which further evidence is desirable:

1. Nonischemic cardiomyopathy
2. Assessment of successful surgery for ventricular tachycardia

SAECG is not indicated in the following clinical settings:

1. Ischemic heart disease and documented sustained ventricular arrhythmias
2. Asymptomatic patients without detectable heart disease

PROBLEMS IN ANALYZING SMALL ECG SIGNALS

Although presenting the ECG of the electrical cardiac cycle in a noise-free manner is a demanding task, it is a much greater challenge to record and analyze ECG signals at the microvolt level. Noise from skeletal muscle movement, amplifier and instrumentation noise, power frequency and its harmonics, and tissue electrode interface can interfere with the recording of the electrical cardiac cycle. The small signals of late potentials are largely masked by noise and larger, low-frequency signals (e.g., the ST segment).[11]

Tissue-electrode artifacts can be minimized by lightly sanding the skin with fine sandpaper (220 grit), wiping the skin with alcohol, and using silver–silver chloride electrodes. Shielding and twisting input cables reduces power frequency noise. For investigations that require extremely low noise levels, the patient and equipment are enclosed in a Faraday cage. Muscle noise can be reduced by the use of muscle relaxants or spatial-averaging techniques.[12]

Further reduction of noise requires the use of sophisticated techniques that have been developed to separate low-amplitude and high-frequency signals from noise and low-frequency signals. These techniques are based on enhancing the characteristics of the desired signals while repressing the undesired signals.

SIGNAL AVERAGING

The objective of signal averaging is to reduce the noise that contaminates the ECG. Signal averaging can be accomplished with either spatial averaging or ensemble averaging; both of these techniques have unique advantages and disadvantages and are used according to the situation. Both are based on the assumption that noise is random and the signal of interest is coherent and repetitive. Consequently, when several inputs representing the same event are added together, the coherent signal is reinforced and the noise cancels itself. The degree of noise reduction obtained is proportional to the square root of the number of inputs averaged. The key lies in maintaining coherence and in obtaining multiple inputs that represent the ECG.

SPATIAL AVERAGING

With spatial averaging, multiple electrodes are averaged over a single complex; with ensemble averaging, a single vector electrode is set over multiple complexes. The advantage of spatial averaging is its ability to provide an SAECG from a single beat, thereby allowing beat-to-beat analysis of transient events and complex arrhythmias.[12]

With spatial averaging, 4 to 16 electrodes are used to obtain the necessary multiple inputs.[13] These inputs are averaged to provide noise reduction. The amount of noise reduction available with spatial averaging is restricted by several factors: (1) the practical limit on the number of electrodes that can be placed, (2) the possibility that closely spaced electrodes will respond to a common noise source and not cancel effectively, and (3) the theoretical limit of a twofold to fourfold reduction in noise.

ENSEMBLE AVERAGING (SIGNAL AVERAGING)

Ensemble averaging as applied to cardiology is commonly referred to as *signal averaging;* other terms are *temporal averaging* and *serial averaging.*

The multiple inputs necessary for signal averaging are gathered from standard orthogonal bipolar X, Y, and Z leads over a series of ECG cycles. Because the average can be taken over a large number of beats (typically 100 or more), the noise can theoretically be reduced by a factor of 10 or more. The tacit assumptions underlying signal averaging are that the waveform is repetitive and can be captured without losing beat-to-beat synchronization.

Signal averaging is a computer-based process in which each electrode lead input is amplified. The voltage of each lead is measured, or sampled, at intervals of 1 ms or less; each sample is converted into a digital number with at least a 12-bit precision.[14] The ECG is thereby converted from an analog voltage waveform into a series of digital numbers that are, in essence, an ECG of at least 100 QRS complexes. These digital QRS complexes are aligned and averaged by a computer with a recognition template to reject ectopic or excessively noisy beats.

Fundamental to signal averaging is the establishment of a starting, or fiducial, point (usually a point on a fast-moving portion of the QRS complex) to use in aligning each of the series of QRS complexes. If the fiducial point is unstable (jitter) or if the portion of the waveform of interest does not have a stable time relationship to the starting point, the waveform will be smoothed and high-frequency components will be lost.[15] To ensure that the analysis uses valid data, the equipment often provides outputs regarding the correlation coefficient and jitter. These signal-averaged data can be presented and analyzed in the time domain, frequency domain, or both.

TIME DOMAIN ANALYSIS OF THE SIGNAL-AVERAGED ECG

Time domain analysis, also referred to as high-pass filtering, presents the ECG as a function of time. After the individual lead signals have been signal averaged, they are filtered and combined to form the composite SAECG. Filtering removes the large, low-frequency components that would obscure the low-level, high-frequency late potentials. Two types of filters are commonly used in processing SAECG signals:

1. High-pass filters, which emphasize the high frequencies and minimize the low frequencies

2. Band-pass filters, which emphasize the midrange and high frequencies and minimize the low frequencies and the very high frequencies

High-pass filters typically reject frequencies below 25 to 40 Hz, whereas the band-pass filters reject frequencies below 25 to 40 Hz and above 250 Hz.[12,14,16-19] The work of Vatterott, Bailey, and Hammill[16] and El-Sherif, Restivo, and Craelius et al[12] investigates the use of different filter frequency bounds. A bidirectional four-pole Butterworth filter usually is used to minimize ringing and artifacts. After the X, Y, and Z leads have been signal averaged and filtered, the vector magnitudes are combined $(X^2 + Y^2 + Z^2)^2$ to form the composite SAECG. Studies have also evaluated the filtered X, Y, and Z leads.[12,20]

INTERPRETING THE TIME DOMAIN SIGNAL-AVERAGED ECG

A typical filtered SAECG for a normal subject is shown in Fig. 23-1. Because very high gain is required to display the late potentials, the main portion of the complex exceeds the vertical range and is cut off or clipped. The investigation of late potentials centers around the magnitude and duration of the signals generated by the delayed depolarization of a portion of the myocardium.

The following areas are of interest in the SAECG:

1. Duration of the filtered QRS complex (QRSD), which is indicative of how long the completion of the QRS complex is delayed by late potentials.[14]

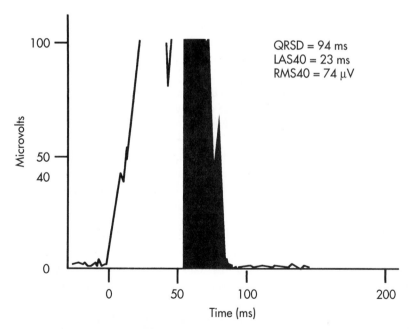

QRSD = 94 ms
LAS40 = 23 ms
RMS40 = 74 μV

FIGURE 23-1 Signal-averaged ECG depicting a normal subject. *QRSD,* Duration of the high-frequency QRS complex; *LAS40,* duration of low-amplitude signals less than 40 μV; *RMS40,* the root mean square voltage of the last 40 ms of the complex *(shaded area).*

2. Amount of energy in the late potentials as given by the root mean square (RMS) voltage in the terminal 40 ms of the QRS complex (RMS40).[14]
3. Duration of the late potentials as indicated by the duration of the low-amplitude signals (LAS) less than 40 μV in the terminal QRS region (LAS40).[14,16]

These values can either be read from the SAECG itself or derived by the computer system.

In Figure 23-1, the time base starts at the onset of the filtered QRS, and the QRSD is 94 ms. The shaded portion defines the final 40 ms of the complex. RMS40 is computed from this portion of the complex. The duration of LAS40 is the interval from the intersection of the 40 μV line and falling edge of the QRS complex to the termination of the filtered QRS complex. Defining a late potential and scoring an SAECG as normal or abnormal are highly dependent on technique. Although a consensus among investigators has yet to emerge, there are representative criteria for 40 Hz filtering: late potentials exist when the filtered QRS complex is longer than 114 to 120 ms, there is less than 20 μV RMS of signal in the terminal 40 ms of the filtered QRS, or the terminal portion of the filtered QRS remains below 40 μV for longer than 38 ms.[4,9,14,21] Different criteria are used to enhance sensitivity or specificity, usually one at the expense of the other.[22] The criteria are altered if bundle branch block is present, and frequency domain analysis may be preferred.[23,24] Figure 23-2 depicts an abnormal SAECG with late potentials.

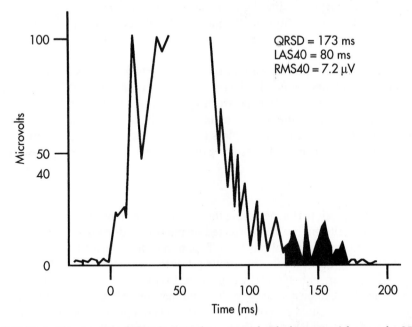

QRSD = 173 ms
LAS40 = 80 ms
RMS40 = 7.2 μV

FIGURE 23-2 Signal-averaged ECG depicting late potentials. The late potentials cause the QRSD to be lengthened, with a substantial portion of the increase caused by the slowly decaying low-level signals in LAS40. The energy level in RMS40 is now composed of low-level signals and contains much less energy. *QRSD,* Duration of the high-frequency QRS complex; *LAS40,* duration of low-amplitude signals less than 40 μV; *RMS40,* the root mean square voltage of the last 40 ms of the complex *(shaded area).*

FREQUENCY DOMAIN ANALYSIS OF THE SIGNAL-AVERAGED ECG

In the same manner in which a rainbow spreads the component color spectrum of sunlight across the sky, a frequency domain ECG spreads the constituent frequencies along the horizontal axis. Frequency domain plots are often referred to as *spectral plots* and are the spectrum of the time domain waveform. As would be expected, there is a certain mirror relationship between the time domain and the frequency domain.

With the time domain ECG, it is easy to distinguish events happening at different times. However, it is very difficult to distinguish events occurring at the same time at different frequencies. The time domain SAECG attempts to compensate for this shortcoming through the use of filters, which tend to eliminate the undesired frequencies. These filters introduce artifacts that must be understood when reading the SAECG.

In the frequency domain, SAECG events of different frequencies that occur at the same time are easily discriminated. Events that are of the same frequency but occur at different times pose a problem. Just as a filter is used in the time domain to reject signals occurring at unwanted frequencies, a "window" is used in the frequency domain to reject part of the waveform that occurs at unwanted times and select those occurring in the desired time slot. Figure 23-3 depicts an arbitrary waveform, a unity data window, and the portion of the waveform selected by the window. Unfortunately, just as the filter introduces some distortion in the time domain, so does the window in the frequency domain.

Analysis of the SAECG using the frequency domain offers a different way of displaying the ECG. This technique mathematically breaks down the ECG into its component frequencies, which allows examination of the contributions of the individual frequencies.

Any continuous time domain waveform (e.g., an idealized ECG) is composed of a series of sinusoidal components. This series consists of a fundamental frequency and a series of harmonics whose frequencies are integer multiples of the fundamental. FFT is usually used to accomplish the transformation from the time domain to the frequency domain. Frequency domain analysis plots the amplitude of the fundamental and its harmonics against frequency. The resulting display of information offers new insights into the SAECG.

Method

Frequency analysis is performed using the signal-averaged inputs derived from Frank X, Y, and Z leads, although other corrected or uncorrected leads are used. Sampling rates of 1 kHz or greater are typically used. To eliminate filtering artifacts, the inputs are either unfiltered or filtered only to remove extremely low (less than 0.5 Hz) and extremely high (greater than 450 Hz) frequencies. Existing as an array of numbers in a computer, the ECG can be displayed, scaled, and manipulated. By positioning the cursor window over the desired part of the waveform, spectral plots of the entire QRS complex or any part of it can be made. The terminal 40 ms of the QRS complex and the ST segment are of greatest interest. Once the window is positioned and its length set (either manually or by computer), the computer calculates the FFT and displays the frequency domain tracing. Because the degree of late potential activity is indicated by the energy in the high-frequency components, the frequency domain tracing often shows the mag-

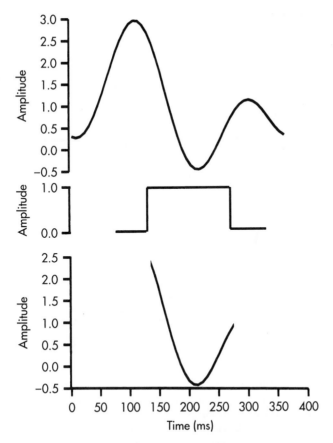

FIGURE 23-3 A unity gain window used for selecting a section of a waveform. The top tracing is an arbitrary waveform, the middle is a unity data window positioned to select a segment of the top waveform, and the lower trace is the selected result. The window can be lengthened or shortened and moved in time to select the desired portion of the waveform.

nitude squared (power is proportional to the square of the voltage), giving the power spectrum. A representative FFT tracing is illustrated in Figure 23-4.

One of the basic assumptions made in using the FFT on a portion of any waveform is that the signal is continuous—the start point and endpoint of the signal are at the same level. If this is not the case, false frequency responses will be produced in the FFT. To reduce these errors, window-shaping functions such as Blackman-Harris are used to smooth the data to zero at the boundaries and reduce the false side lobes. Figure 23-5 depicts the use of a shaped window to reduce edge discontinuities. Unfortunately, these shaped windows can reduce the high frequencies in the ECG and, if the sloped edge of the window is positioned over the late potentials, severely attenuate them.

The spectral resolution is related solely to the reciprocal of the window length. A window length of 100 ms provides a frequency resolution of 1/0.100 s or 10 Hz. The fun-

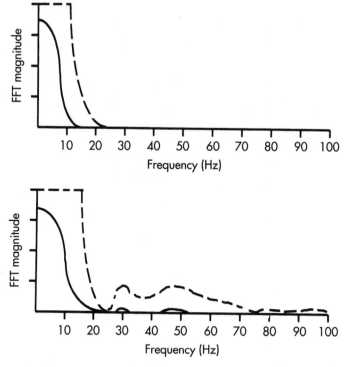

FIGURE 23-4 Representative frequency domain tracings. The top tracing is a normal subject, and the lower tracing demonstrates the presence of high-frequency potentials. The dashed curve is a 10 × magnification of the solid curve. Evaluation of the fast Fourier transform *(FFT)* of an ECG is based on the areas or ratio of areas under the curve for different frequency ranges and on the frequency and magnitude of peaks.

damental will be 10 Hz and the harmonics will be integer multiples of this fundamental (e.g., 20, 30, 40 Hz). Longer windows will provide greater resolution and conversely. However, it must be kept in mind that short windows not only have poorer resolution but also attenuate more of the signal with the sloped sides of the window. Each point in the FFT algorithm accepts one point (one sample) of the ECG complex. A commonly used FFT is one of 512 points, which will accommodate up to a 512-ms window at a 1-kHz sample rate. However, the windows chosen are usually much shorter, and the remaining unfilled points are filled with zeros. The selection of the length and position of the window can have a great effect on the results of tests on the same data. In the example of a patient with anterior wall myocardial infarction and recurrent ventricular tachycardia, Kelen, Henkin, and Fontaine et al[25] have shown that a small change in the boundary of the analyzed segment on the order of 10 ms can result in changes in the area ratio of several hundred percent. Some researchers have conducted FFT analysis over the entire cardiac cycle.[26]

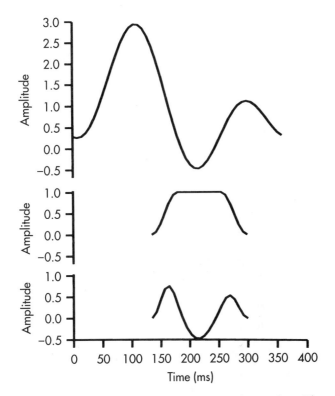

FIGURE 23-5 A shaped window used for selecting a portion of a waveform. The top tracing is the same waveform shown in Figure 23-3, and the middle tracing is a shaped window. (The slope of the sides is exaggerated for illustration; usually each slope is only approximately 10% of the total window length.) The lower tracing is the result of a sample-by-sample multiplication of the top waveform by the window. Portions of the top tracing that fall under the sloped sides are severely attenuated.

Interpreting the Frequency Domain Signal-Averaged ECG

The interpretation of the frequency domain ECG is highly subject to technique. However, a common thread runs through the evaluation criteria in that they evaluate the amount of high-frequency energy present, usually by means of an area ratio. An area ratio is calculated by dividing the area of the high-frequency portion of the spectrum by the total area of the spectrum. The definition of what comprises the high-frequency spectrum varies according to the individual researcher.[27] Pierce, Easley, Windle, and Engel[17] used the ratio of the area between 60 and 120 Hz to that of 0 to 120 Hz, whereas Cain, Lindsay, and Arthur et al[28] relied on the ratio of the 20- to 50-Hz region to the 10- to 50-Hz area. The area ratio of the 40- to 120-Hz to the 0 to 120 Hz regions was used by Kinsohita et al.[29] In addition to the area ratios, some researchers also consider the frequency peaks.[28]

LIMITATIONS

The inherent underlying mathematic principles of the techniques described in this chapter pose limitations that the diagnostician should consider when interpreting the tracings:

1. Sampling and filtering can introduce artifacts or distortions of their own, which must be considered in any diagnosis.
2. The ability of the FFT to accurately transform the time domain SAECG into the frequency domain depends on how well the FFT of the selected portion of the SAECG relates to the CFT. The window width, shape, and position can have a drastic effect on the repeatability of the resulting frequency domain ECG.

OTHER ANALYTIC METHODS

The analytic methods previously described can be combined in various configurations to improve screening accuracy. Among these methods are the following:

1. **Spectral temporal mapping.** Spectral temporal mapping displays both time and frequency information in a three-dimensional plot. The plot is generated by dividing the ST segment into 20 to 30 segments. Each of the segments is of the same length (typically 80 ms) but starts a few milliseconds later. By stepping the window through each of these segments, the frequency components of each segment are computed using FFT. The data are then displayed as a three-dimensional surface map with amplitude on the vertical axis, frequency on the horizontal axis, and time on the Z axis.[30,31]
2. **Large electrode arrays.** Studies have been made using ensemble-averaging techniques on body map arrays of electrodes.[32-34] In these studies 28 to 87 body leads were used to gather ECG data. The data were signal averaged to reduce noise and then evaluated. Tests in canines have shown that the results of the body map array SAECG correlate more closely to the epicardial measurements than to the standard three-lead SAECG.[33]
3. **Multivariate analysis.** Multivariate analysis statistically combines several factors that may affect the accuracy with which risk factors are determined. The factors combined are time domain SAECG, frequency domain SAECG, age, infarct location, number of diseased coronary vessels, left ventricular ejection fraction, infarct-related coronary artery patency, treatment received, delay between admission and SAECG recording, and delay between admission and coronary angiography.

SUMMARY

Sophisticated techniques from the radar and communication disciplines such as signal averaging, digital filtering, and fast Fourier transform are being applied to the analysis of the ECG. These tools allow the researcher and diagnostician to examine portions of the ECG that were previously obscured by noise and artifacts. As the subject of the bulk of the clinical studies, the time domain signal-averaged ECG has emerged as an important tool in the evaluation of late potentials. Although the techniques and standards are still evolving,[35-37] the time domain and frequency domain signal-averaged ECG alone or in combination with other tests and factors provide noninvasive tests by which to identify myocardial infarction patients who are at risk for sustained ventricular tachycardia or sudden death.

REFERENCES

1. Runge CZ: *Math Phys* 48:443, 1903.
2. Cooley JW, Tukey JW: An algorithm for the machine calculation of complex Fourier series, *Math Comput* 19:297, 1965.
3. Couderc JP, Fareh S, Chevalier P et al: Stratification of time-frequency abnormalities in the signal-averaged high-resolution ECG in postinfarction patients with and without ventricular tachycardia and congenital long QT syndrome, *J Electrocardiol* 29(suppl):180, 1996.
4. Simson MB: Signal-averaged electrocardiography. In Zipes DP, Jalife J, editors: *Cardiac electrophysiology from cell to bedside,* ed 2, Philadelphia, 1995, WB Saunders.
5. Steinberg JS, Regan A, Sciacca RR et al: Predicting arrhythmic events after acute myocardial infarction using the signal-averaged electrocardiogram, *Am J Cardiol* 69:13, 1992.
6. Simson MB: Noninvasive identification of patients at risk for sudden cardiac death, *Circulation* 85(suppl I):I-145, 1992.
7. Lindsay BD, Ambros HD, Schechtman KB et al: Noninvasive detection of patients with ischemic and nonischemic heart disease prone to ventricular fibrillation, *J Am Coll Cardiol* 16:1656, 1990.
8. Klein H, Karp RB, Kouchoukos NT et al: Intraoperative electrophysiologic mapping of the ventricles during sinus rhythm in patients with previous myocardial infarction: identification of the electrophysiologic substrate of ventricular arrhythmias, *Circulation* 66:847, 1982.
9. Simson MB, Untereker WJ, Spielmann SR et al: The relationship between late potentials on the body surface and directly recorded fragmented electrograms in patients with ventricular tachycardia, *Am J Cardiol* 51:659, 1983.
10. Cain ME, Anderson JL, Arnsdorf MF et al: Signal-averaged electrocardiography, *J Am Coll Cardiol* 27:238, 1996.
11. Christiansen EH, Frost L, Molgaard H et al: Effect of residual noise level on reproducibility of the signal-averaged ECG, *J Electrocardiol* 29:235, 1996.
12. El-Sherif N, Restivo M, Craelius et al: The high-resolution electrocardiogram: technical and basic aspects. In El-Sherif N, Samet P, editors: *Cardiac pacing and electrophysiology,* ed 3, Philadelphia, 1991, WB Saunders.
13. Flowers NC, Shvartsman V, Kennelly BM et al: Surface recording of His-Purkinje activity on an every-beat basis without digital averaging, *Circulation* 63:948, 1981.
14. Breithardt G, Cain ME, El-Sherif N et al: Standards for analysis of ventricular late potentials using high-resolution or signal-averaged electrocardiography: a statement from a task force committee of the European Society of Cardiology, the American Heart Association, and the American College of Cardiology, *J Am Coll Cardiol* 17:999, 1991.
15. Ros HH, Koeleman ASM, Akker TJ: The technique of signal averaging and its practical application in the separation of atrial and His-Purkinje activity. In Hombach V, Hilger HH, editors: *Signal averaging technique in clinical cardiology,* New York, 1981, FK Schattauer Verlag.
16. Vatterott PJ, Bailey KR, Hammill SC: Improving the predictive ability of the signal-averaged electrocardiogram with a linear logistic model incorporating clinical variables, *Circulation* 81:797, 1990.
17. Pierce DL, Easley AR, Windle JR, Engel TR: Fast Fourier transformation of the entire low amplitude late QRS potential to predict ventricular tachycardia, *J Am Coll Cardiol* 14:1731, 1989.
18. Nalos PC, Eli SG, Mandel WJ et al: Utility of the signal-averaged electrocardiogram in patients presenting with sustained ventricular tachycardia or fibrillation while on an antiarrhythmic drug, *Am Heart J* 115:108, 1988.
19. El-Sherif N, Ursell SN, Bekheit S et al: Prognostic significance of the signal-averaged ECG depends on the time of recording in the postinfarction period, *Am Heart J* 118:256, 1989.
20. Leor MD, Hod H, Rotstein Z et al: Effects of thrombolysis on the 12-lead signal-averaged ECG in the early postinfarction period, *Am Heart J* 120:495, 1990.

21. Hood MA, Pogwizd SM, Peirick J et al: Contribution of myocardium responsible for ventricular tachycardia to abnormalities detected by analysis of signal-averaged ECGs, *Circulation* 86:1888, 1992.

22. Lander P, Berbari EJ, Rajagopalan CV et al: Critical analysis of the signal-averaged electrocardiogram, *Circulation* 87:105, 1993.

23. Buckingham TA, Lingle A, Greenwalt T et al: Power law analysis of the signal-averaged electrocardiogram for identification of patients with ventricular tachycardia: effect of bundle branch block, *Am Heart J* 124:1220, 1992.

24. Fontaine JM, Rao R, Henkin R et al: Study of the influence of left bundle branch block on the signal-averaged electrocardiogram: a qualitative and quantitative analysis, *Am Heart J* 121:494, 1991.

25. Kelen GJ, Henkin R, Fontaine JM et al: Effects of analyzed signal duration and phase on the results of fast Fourier transform analysis of the surface electrocardiogram in subjects with and without late potentials, *Am J Cardiol* 60:1282, 1987.

26. Cain ME, Dieter A, Markham J et al: Diagnostic implications of spectral and temporal analysis of the entire cardiac cycle in patients with ventricular tachycardia, *Circulation* 83:1637, 1991.

27. Malik M, Kulakowski P, Poloniecki J et al: Frequency versus time domain analysis of signal-averaged electrocardiograms, I. Reproducibility of the results, *J Am Coll Cardiol* 20:127, 1992.

28. Cain ME, Lindsay BD, Arthur RM et al: Noninvasive detection of patients prone to life-threatening ventricular arrhythmias by frequency analysis of electrocardiographic signals. In Zipes DP, Jalife J, editors: *Cardiac electrophysiology,* Philadelphia, 1990, WB Saunders.

29. Kinoshita O, Kamakura S, Ohe T et al: Spectral analysis of signal-averaged electrocardiograms in patients with idiopathic ventricular tachycardia of left ventricular origin, *Circulation* 85:2054, 1992.

30. McClements BM, Adgey AAJ: Value of signal-averaged electrocardiography, radionuclide ventriculography, Holter monitoring, and clinical variables for prediction of arrhythmic events in survivors of acute myocardial infarction in the thrombolytic era, *J Am Coll Cardiol* 21:1419, 1993.

31. Steinberg JS, Prystowsky E, Freedman RA et al: Use of the signal-averaged electrocardiogram for predicting inducible ventricular tachycardia in patients with unexplained syncope: relation to clinical variables in a multivariate analysis, *J Am Coll Cardiol* 23:99, 1994.

32. David SW, Denniss RA, Uther JB et al: Signal-averaged electrocardiogram: improved identification of patients with ventricular tachycardia using a 28-lead optimal array, *Circulation* 87:857, 1993.

33. Freedman RA, Fuller MS, Greenberg GM et al: Detection and localization of prolonged epicardial electrograms with 64-lead body surface signal-averaged electrocardiography, *Circulation* 84:871, 1991.

34. Shibata T, Kubota I, Ikeda K et al: Body surface mapping of high-frequency components in the terminal portion during QRS complex for the prediction of ventricular tachycardia in patients with previous myocardial infarction, *Circulation* 82:2084, 1990.

35. Sierra G, Fetsch T, Reinhardt L et al: Multiresolution decomposition of the signal-averaged ECG using the mallat approach for prediction of arrhythmic events after myocardial infarction, *J Electrocardiol* 29:223, 1996.

36. Reinhardt L, Mäkijärvi M, Fetsch T et al: Predictive value of wavelet correlation functions of signal-averaged electrocardiogram in patients after anterior versus inferior myocardial infarction, *J Am Coll Cardiol* 27:53, 1996.

37. Mehta D, Goldman M, David O, Gomes JA: Value of quantitative measurement of signal-averaged electrocardiographic variables in arrhythmogenic right ventricular dysplasia: correlation with echocardiographic right ventricular cavity dimensions, *J Am Coll Cardiol* 28:713, 1996.

Index

A

Aberrancy vs ectopy, **237-260**
  AV dissociation in, 240
  axis in, 247, 251-252
  baseline ECG in, 238
  differential diagnosis in, 238
  ECG signs in **245-251**
  history in, 238-239
  misdiagnosis in, 237
  procainamide in, 237-238
  QRS configuration in, **243-252**
  what not to use in, 238
Aberrant ventricular conduction, **215-
      236**
  alternating, 233
  atrial fibrillation and, 230-231
  atrial tachycardia and, 231-233
  clinical implication of, 233
  concealed retrograde conduction in,
      74-75
  ECG patterns in, **223-225**
  ectopy vs, **237-260**
  frequency of, 216
  hemiblock in, 223
  initial deflection in, 227
  left bundle branch block and, 215, **223,**
      228, 231, 232, 233, 234
  mechanisms of, **215-220**
  phase 3, **215-217,** 219, 222, 235
  phase 4, 215, **217-220,** 233, 235
  preceding atrial activity in, 227, 228
  QRS configuration in, 243-253
  QRS duration in, 226

Aberrant ventricular conduction—cont'd
  right bundle branch block and, 74, 75,
      215, **223,** 228, 231, 232, 233,
      234, 350
  second-in-the-row anomaly in, 229-230
Ablation
  chemical, 126
  radiofrequency catheter, 911, 120-121,
      132, 142, 155, 160, 171, 173, 279
Accelerated idiojunctional rhythm, 191
Accelerated idioventricular rhythm, 48,
      197, 338, 339
Accessory pathway, 155, 204, 252, 256,
      261-276
  atrial fibrillation with, **262-269**
    differential diagnosis in, 265
    ECG features of, 262
    emergency treatment of, 267
    mechanism of, 266-277, 269
  concealed, 163, 261
  latent, 163, 261
  location, 261
  multiple, 269, 272, 274
  overt, 261
Acetylcholine-activated K$^+$ current, **23,** 42
N-acetylprocainamide (NAPA), 53
Aconitine, 53
Action potential, **29-39,** 64, 217, 219
  digitalis and, 181
  fast- and slow-response, 29-30
  ischemia's effect on, 64
  phases of, 33-36

Entries in **boldface** refer to main discussions.

Action potential—cont'd
  plateau-prolonged, 20, 29, 35, 39
  recording of, 30-32
  SA nodal, **32-33**
Action potentials compared, 30
Adenosine, 23, 17, 89
Adenosine triphosphatase (ATPase), 13,
    14, 15, 16, 20
Adenosine triphosphate (ATP), 15, 16, 17,
    23, 155, 272
Adenosine triphosphate-activated potas-
    sium current, **23**
Adenosine triphosphate-dependent cal-
    cium pump, **16-17**
β-adrenergic blockade and stimulation,
    41-42
β-adrenergic receptor-effector coupling
    system, 41-42
Afterdepolarizations
  definition of, 49
  delayed, **55-57**, 180, 181
    arrhythmias of, 55
    causes of, 55
    mechanisms of, 54-55
    vulnerable parameter of, 56
  early, **53-54**
    arrhythmias of, 53
    causes of, 53
    distinguishing features of, 53
    mechanisms of, 53
    vulnerable parameter of, 54
Allorhythmia defined, 145
Alternating aberrancy, 233
Amiodarone, 182, 203, 206
Anatomic reentry, 57
Angina, 91
Anisotropic conduction, 60
Anisotropic reentry, 58, 59
Antiarrhythmic drugs and arrhythmias,
    203-214
Anticoagulation, 126
Antidromic circus movement tachycardia
    (CMT), **269-274**
  ECG features of, 272
  emergency treatment of, 272-274
  mechanism of, 272

Antidromic defined, 153
Antihistamines, 44, 297
Aprindine, 206
Arrhythmias
  ischemia-induced, **63-66**
  reperfusion, 53
  systematic approach to, **358-365**
  warning, 101-102
Arrhythmogenic mechanisms, **47-68**
  ischemia-induced, 63-66
Arterial pulse, 104
Ashman's phenomenon, 230-231
Astemizole, 44
Asystole, ventricular, 320
Atherosclerosis, coronary, 95-96
ATP; *see* Adenosine triphosphate
ATPase; *see* Adenosine triphosphatase
ATP-dependent Ca^{2+} membrane pumps,
    16-17
Atrial fibrillation, **99-108;** *see also* Fibrilla-
    tion, atrial
Atrial flutter, **109-130;** *see also* Flutter, atrial
Atrial parasystole, **340-342**
Atrial premature beats, nonconducted,
    82, 83
Atrial stunning, 106
Atrial tachycardia, 48, 126, **131-143**, 186,
    189, 190
  aberrancy in, 231-233
  ablation of, 126
  carotid sinus massage for, 156
  chaotic, 135, 137
  classification of, 131
  clinical implications of, 131-132
  cure of, 142
  differential diagnosis in, 138
  focal, 134-135, 139-140
  incessant, 135, 136, 156
  incidence of, 142
  incisional reentrant, 124, **132**
    treatment of, 132
    mechanism of, 132
  mechanisms of, 131
  multifocal, 135, 137
  nonparoxysmal, 135, 138
  nonsustained paroxysmal, 138

Atrial tachycardia—cont'd
    P′ wave in, 139-140
    paroxysmal, 156
    pediatrics in, 140
    postoperative, 140-142
    treatment of, 142
    warning arrhythmias of, 140-142
Atrioventricular; *see* AV entries
Atypical circus movement tachycardia,
        173-174
Automaticity, 15
    abnormal, **48-49,** 51, 52, 329
        arrhythmias of, 48-49
        vulnerable parameter of, 49
    altered, **47-49**
        differential diagnosis in, 49, 50-53
    enhanced, 218, 220
    enhanced normal, **47-48,** 49, 50, 220
        arrhythmias of, 48
        vulnerable parameter of, 48
Autonomic nervous system, **41-45,** 87, 95
    tests for, 88
AV block; *see* Block, AV
AV dissociation, 80, 82, **240-241,** 259
    ECG signs of, 240-241
    first heart sound in, 240
    jugular pulse in, 240
    P waves in, 241
    physical signs of, 240
    systolic blood pressure in, 240
AV junction, 3
AV nodal reentrant tachycardia, 57, 138,
        157-161, 171-173
    atrial anatomy in, 157
    atypical, 171-173
        clinical implications of, 173
        definition of, 171
        distinguishing features of, 171
        ECG recognition of, 171
        mechanism of, 171
        treatment of, 173
    clinical implications of, 160
    definition of, 157
    differential diagnosis in, 174-176
    distinguishing features of, 160
    ECG recognition of, 160

AV nodal reentrant tachycardia—cont'd
    mechanism of, 158, 159
    treatment of, 160
AV node, **3-7**
    action potential of, 32-33
    activation of, 33
    atrial approaches to, **6-7**
    compact, 4-5, 7
    membrane channels in, 18
    transitional, 6
Axis, 247, 251-252, 259

B

Bazett's formula, 295
Beats
    capture, 253, 254, 255, 259
    early, causes of, 358
    fusion, 253, 254, 255, 259, **329,** 331,
        333, 335, 340
    reciprocal, **145-152**
Bifascicular ventricular tachycardia,
        192-194, 196
Bigeminy
    causes of, 359
    concealed ventricular, **197-198**
    rule of, 230
    ventricular, 76, 77, 195-197
Bix rule, 360, 361
Blackman-Harris window shaping, 373
Block
    AV, 185, 187, 197, **311-328,** 348
        acute complete, 319
        complete, 50, **319-320**
        definitions of, 320-321
        first-degree, 311
        high-grade, 318-319
        level of, 314
        misconceptions of, 323-326
        nonconducted beats in, 311-312
        nondegrees of, 321-323
        PR interval in, 311, 315
        reclassification of, 326-327
        RP-dependent PR intervals in,
            315-316
        RP/PR reciprocity in, 315-316
        second-degree, 311-312

Block—cont'd
AV—cont'd
skipped P waves in, 317
2:1, 316-317
type I and II, 76, 78, **312-314**
anatomy versus behavior in, 312-314
characteristics of, 314
exit, **331-332**
rate-dependent and critical rate, **220-222**
right bundle branch, 10
SA, 69
sinus exit, **92-94,** 185
systolic, 216
β-blockers, 100, 203, 304
Blood pressure, systolic, 240
Bradycardia, 218, 220
causes of, 358
sinus, 94, 185, 358
Bradycardia-dependent bundle branch block, 218
Bradycardia-tachycardia syndrome, 94, 95
Broad QRS tachycardia, **215-310**
aberrancy in, **215-260**
accessory pathways and, **261-276**
axis in, 247, 251-252
baseline ECG in, 238
capture beats in, 253
differential diagnosis in, 223-230, **238-259**
fusion beats in, 253
history taking in, 238-239
initial deflection of, 227, 228
misdiagnosis in, 237
nodoventricular fibers in, 274-276
procainamide in, 237-238
QRS width in, 253
V_1-negative, 247-252
V_1-positive, 245-247
Bundle branch block, 259, 335, 336, 346, 347
aberrancy in, 215, 216, 217, 218, 220, **223,** 225, 227, 228, 230, 231, 232, 233, 234
bradycardia-dependent, 218
critical rate, 346

Bundle branch block—cont'd
phase 3, **215-217,** 219
preexisting, 252, 256
rate-dependent, **220-222**
tachycardia-dependent, 216
Bundle branch reentrant tachycardia; *see* Tachycardia, bundle branch reentrant
Bundle branches, **7-10**
left, 7-9
right, 9-10

C

Calcium, intracellular, 20, 21
Calcium channels (I_{Ca}), **19-20,** 29, 42
Calcium-induced calcium release (CICR), 19, 20
Capture beats, 253, 254, 255, 259
Cardiac Arrhythmia Suppression Trial, 204-205
Cardiac cell microstructure, 29, 31
Cardiac death, risk stratification for post-MI, 89
Cardiac output, 104
Cardiomyopathy, 245, 285, 368
Cardiomyopathy, tachycardia-induced, 104
Cardioversion, direct current, 106, 119, 155, 272
Carotid sinus massage, 86, 112, **156-157**
caution with, 157
procedure for, 157
CAST; *see* Cardiac Arrhythmia Suppression Trial
Catecholamines, 41-42, 53, 55, 66, 100
"Causes of pauses," 358
Cell function, normal, 13-14
Cerebral oxygen supply, 104
Cesium, 53
Channels, membrane, **17-24,** 207-208
blockade of, 208-210
calcium (I_{Ca}), **19-20,** 29, 42
disease and, 44
L- and T-type calcium, **19-20,** 35, 53
pH and blockade of, 209, 210
potassium blockade of, 44

Channels, membrane—cont'd
  potassium rectifying, **21-23**
  receptor-operated, 17
  sodium (I_{Na}), **17-19**, 29, 44, 208-211
  voltage-operated, 17
Chaotic atrial tachycardia, 135, 137
Chaotic irregularity, causes of, 359
Chemical ablation, 126
"Cherchez le P," **359**
Circus movement reentry, 56
Circus movement tachycardia (CMT), 138,
        151, **163-171, 173-174,** 274, 275
  aberration and, 165, 166
  antidromic, **269-274**
    ECG features of, 272
    emergency treatment of, 272-274
    mechanism of, 272
  clinical implications of, 165
  differential diagnosis in, 174-176
  distinguishing features of, 163
  ECG recognition of, 163-165
  left-sided pathway in, 165, 167
  long RP′ type, 173-174
  mechanism of, 163, 164
  orthodromic
    fast accessory pathway in, **163-171**
    slow accessory pathway in, **173-174**
  QRS alternans in, 165, 168
  sinus tachycardia initiation of, 165, 170
  treatment of, 171
  ventral premature beat initiation of,
        165, 169
Classic parasystole, **329-343**
CMT; *see* Circus movement tachycardia
Compact AV node, 4, 7
  blood supply to, 5
  location of, 4
  structure of, 5
Compartment surgery, 107
Complete AV block, 50, **319-320**
Concealed accessory pathway, 163
Concealed conduction, **72-84,** 92, 215,
        230, 348
  aberrancy and, 74-75
  in atrial fibrillation, 73-74

Concealed conduction—cont'd
  history of, 73
  impulse formation and, **81-83**
  interpolated ventricular extrasystoles
        with, 75-76
  of junctional extrasystoles, **76-79**
  retrograde, 74-76
Concealed junctional extrasystoles, **76-79,**
        80, 348, 349
Concealed parasystole, 337
Concealed reentry, 349
Concealed supernormal conduction, 346-348
Concealed ventricular bigeminy, **197-198**
Concordant precordial patterns, 238, **253,**
        254, 256, 257, 258, 259
Conduction
  aberrant, **215-236**
  abnormal and drugs, 210-213
  concealed, 72-84; *see also* Concealed
        conduction
  concealed supernormal, 346-348
  retrograde Wenckebach, 243, 246
  slow, 206
  supernormal, **345-353**
  velocity of, **36-37**
  ventricular-atrial (VA), **241-243**
  Wenckebach, 112, 114, 115, 186
Conduction system
  activation of and ECG, 72
  components of, 1
  development and functions of, 1-11
  innervation of, 11
Conduction time, sinoatrial, 69-70, 88
Contraction, 14, 17, 19, **20,** 21
Coronary artery bypass grafting, 105
Coronary artery disease, chronic, 303
Coronary atherosclerosis, 95-96
Coronary sinus ostium, **111,** 116
Corridor surgery, 107
Coupling
  excitation-contraction, 14
  reversed, 338, 340, 341
Coupling system
  β-adrenergic receptor-effector, 41-42
  muscarinic receptor-effector, 42-43

Crista terminalis, 89, **110-111,** 115, 116, 120
"Cristal tachycardias," 89, 139
Critical rate, 337
Critical rate, paradoxical, 218, 221, 349
Critical rate block, 220-222
Currents, membrane, **17-24,** 207-208;
        see also Channels, membrane
    acetylcholine-activated K$^+$ [I$_{K(ACh)}$;
        I$_{K(Ado)}$], **23,** 42
    adenosine triphosphate-activated
        potassium (K$_{ATP}$), 23
    delayed rectifier (I$_K$), **22,** 29, 44
    inward K$^+$ rectifier (I$_{K1}$), 22-23
    pacemaker, (I$_f$), **23,** 29, 42
    sodium (I$_{Na}$), **17-19,** 29, 44, 208-211
    transient outward K$^+$ (I$_{to}$), 21-23

D

Deficit, pulse, 104
Delayed afterdepolarizations, **55-57,** 180,
        181
Delayed rectifier current, **22,** 29, 44
Delta wave, 162
Depolarization, **14-15,** 17, 18, 20, 22, 23,
        24, 63
    phase 4, **33,** 34
    rapid, 14, 16, 17, 18, 22, 23
    slow diastolic, 13, 14, 24, 220
Diastole, electrical, 13, 208, 210
Differential diagnosis
    of atrial flutter, 124
    of atrial tachycardia, 138
    of broad QRS tachycardia, 223-230,
        238-259
Digibind, 198-199
Digitalis, 20, 55, 100, 180-182, 203, 205, 319
    and potassium derangements, 180-182
Digitalis dysrhythmias, **179-201**
    atrial tachycardia, 186
        ECG recognition of, 186-188
    AV block, 185-186
    bifascicular ventricular tachycardia,
        192-194
        ECG recognition of, 194

Digitalis dysrhythmias—cont'd
    cellular electrophysiology of, 179-180
    double tachycardia, 194
    ECG recognition of, **185-198**
    fascicular ventricular tachycardia,
        192
    junctional tachycardia, 185, 188
        ECG recognition of, 188-191
    mortality from, 179
    SA block, 185
    sinus bradycardia, 185
    systematic approach to ECG and,
        183-184
    treatment of, 198-199
        early stages, 198
        Fab fragments, 199
        life-threatening, 198
    ventricular bigeminy, 195-197
        concealed, 197, 198
Digitalis glycosides, 179, 232
Digitalis toxicity, 55, 245
    clinical alert to, **184-185**
    systematic approach to the ECG in,
        183-184
        atrial evaluation in, 183
        AV conduction evaluation in, 184
        monitoring of, 184
    treatment of, **198-199**
Digoxin
    ECG effects of, 183
    factors interacting with, **182**
    serum concentration of, **182-183**
    specific antibody Fab fragments of,
        198-199
Diltiazem, 182
Direct current cardioversion, 155, 272
Disease
    chronic coronary artery, 303
    heart, 91, 245, 368
    membrane channels and, 44
    organic, 220, 259
Disopyramide, 206
Dissociation, AV, **240-241,** 259; *see also*
        AV dissociation

Double tachycardia, 194, 196

Drug-channel interactions, 43

Drugs; *see also* individual drug names

   arrhythmias and antiarrhythmic, **203-214**

   cardiac function and, **43-44**

   class I, 203, 204, 210

   class Ia, 206

   class Ib, 206

   class Ic, 205, 206, 252

   class III, 204, 206

   classes of, 206

   competition and potentiation of, 44

   conduction-slowing, 245, 256

   coronary vasodilators, 206

   frequency-dependent, 209

   inotropics, 206

   local anesthetic antiarrhythmic, 208-210

   proarrhythmic, 206

   prolonged repolarization and, 43

   rate-dependent, 43

   tonic-blocking action, 209

   use-dependent, 43, 209

   voltage-dependent antiarrhythmic, 43

dV/dt, 217

Dysrhythmia vs arrhythmia, 47

E

Early afterdepolarizations, **53-54**

ECG

   signal-averaged, 88, 370, 371

      clinical application of, **367-368**

      frequency domain analysis of, **372-375**

      time domain analysis of, **369-371**

   silent zones of, 69

ECG monitoring, 184, **355-358**

ECG recording, ambulatory, 88

Edrophonium, 203

Ejection fraction, left ventricular, 89, 205

Electrical diastole, 13, 208, 210

Electrical remodeling, 104

Electrocardiogram; *see* ECG entries

Electrode arrays, large, 376

Electrogenic pump, 16

Electrogram

   His bundle, **70-72**

      deflections of, 71

      indications for, 71-72

      intervals and normal values of, 71

   SA nodal, **69-70**

      clinical value of, 69

      SA conduction time in, 69-70

Electrophysiologic testing, 88

Electrophysiology, study of, 13

Electrotonic modulation, 329, **330**, 334, 338, 340-343

Endocrine system, 95

Ensemble averaging, 369

Entrance block, 330, 331, 333, 337, 340

Erythromycin, 44, 297

Eustachian ridge and valve, **111**, 115, 116, 117, 120

Excitability, 16, 218

   supernormal, **345**, 346, 349

Excitable gap, 56

Excitation-contraction coupling, 14

Exercise testing, 88

Exit block

   in parasystole, 329, 330, **331-332**, 333, 334-337, 338, 340

   SA, **92-94**, 185

Extrasystoles, interpolated ventricular, 75, 76

F

Fab fragments, digoxin specific antibody, 198-199

   oleander poisoning and, 199

   renal failure and, 199

Fascicles, 7-9

Fascicular ventricular tachycardia, 192, 193, 194, 195, 226, 245, **286-287**

Fasciculo-ventricular fibers, 262

Fast pathways, 6-7, 157, 158

Fast response action potential, 29-30
Fast sodium channels, **17-19,** 29, 44
  blockade of, 203, 206, 208-211
Fibers, Purkinje, 10
Fibrillation, atrial, 94, **99-108,** 189, 191,
          193, 194, 204, 230-231, 232, 336
  aberrancy in, 230
  accessory pathways in, **262-269**
    differential diagnosis of, 265
    ECG features of, 262
    emergency treatment of, 267
    mechanism of, 266-277, 269
  atrial stunning post-cardioversion, 106
  block in, 100
  bundle branch block in, 265
  cardiomyopathy in, 104
  carotid sinus massage effect on, 156
  classification of, 99
  concealed conduction in, **73-74,** 104
  controlled, 100
  differential diagnosis in, 138
  ECG in, 99-100
  electrical remodeling in, 104
  fibrillatory line of, 101
  heart rate in, 99-100
  incidence of, 105
  initiation of, 100
  mechanism of, 102-104
  multiple accessory pathways in, 269
  in pediatrics, 106
  physical findings in, 104-105
  post–myocardial infarction, 102
  postoperative, 101, 105
  QRS complexes in, 101
  rhythm in, 101
  surgery for, 106-107
  symptoms of, 104
  terminology of, 99
  thromboembolism in, 106
  treatment of, 106-107
  uncomplicated, 102
  uncontrolled, 100
  ventricular response in, 100
  warning arrhythmias of, 101-102
Fibrillation, ventricular, 63, 204
Fibrillatory line, 101

"Find a break", **363**
First-degree AV block, 311
Fixed coupling, 338
Flutter, atrial, **109-130**
  accessory pathway and, 125, 258, 269
  acute treatment of, 119-120, 121, 123
  antiarrhythmics and, 112, 113
  anticoagulation for, 126
  atrial structures involved in, 110-112
  atypical (type II), 110, **122-124**
    ECG recognition of, 123
    genesis of flutter waves in, 122
    mechanism of, 122
    treatment of, 123-124
  carotid sinus massage in, 112
  chronic, 125
  classification of, 110
  clinical setting of, 125
  clockwise, 110, **121-122**
    ECG in, 121
    genesis of flutter waves in, 120-121
    mechanism of, 120
    treatment of, 121
  conduction ratio in, 112
  counterclockwise, 110, 112, 114, **115-
          121**
    ECG in, 118
    genesis of flutter waves in, 117-118
    mechanism of, 115-116
    treatment of, 121
  differential diagnosis in, 124, 138
  ECG in, 112-113, 118, 121, 123
  history of, 109-110
  incidence of, 125
  incisional reentrant, 110
  isthmus of slow conduction in, **116-
          117,** 120
  long-term treatment of, 120
  mechanism of, 115-117
  in pediatrics, 113
  pertinent atrial structures in, 110-112
  physical signs of, 124
  propranolol in, 114
  recurrences of, 120
  treatment of, 119-121
  types and features of, 126

Flutter, atrial—cont'd
  typical (type I), 110, **115-122**
  ventricular rate and rhythm in, 112
  Wenckebach conduction in, 112, 115
Flutter waves, 117-118, 121, 122
Focal atrial tachycardia, 134-135, 139-140
Fossa ovalis, 111
Fourier, 367
Fourier transform
  continuous (CFT), 367
  discrete (DFT), 367
  fast (FFT), 367, 372, 373, 374, 376
Frank leads, 373
Frequency domain analysis, 367, 369, 371, **372-376**
Frequency-dependent drugs, 209
"Frog sign", 157
Functional reentry, 57
Fusion beats, 253, 254, 255, 259, 329, 331, 333

G

Gap, excitable, 57
Gap junctions, **24-25**
Gap phenomenon, 349-352
Gating, 17
Group beating, 184, 185
  causes of, 359

H

"h" gate, 18-19
"Haystack principle," **360-362**
Heart disease, 91, 245
Heart failure, 104
Heart rate
  acetylcholine and, 23, 24
  increase in, 89
Heart rate variability, **88-89**
  clinical value of, 88
  evaluation of, 88-89
  fetal distress and, 88
  history of, 88
Heart sound, first, 104, 240
Hemiblock, left anterior, 9
High-grade AV block, 317-319

His bundle, 3, 4, **7**
  blood supply to, 7
  location of, 7
His bundle electrogram, **70-72**
  deflections of, 71
  indications for, 71-72
  intervals and normal values of, 71
His bundle intervals, 71
History taking, 238-239, 243
Horseshoe sinus node, 3
Hypercalcemia, 55
Hyperkalemia, 181-182
Hyperpolarization, 22, 23
Hyperthermia, 88
Hypokalemia, 180-181, 297
Hypothermia, 88
Hypoxia, 53

I

I_{Ca}, **19-20**, 29, 42
I_f, **23**, 29, 41, 42
$I_{K(ACh)}$, 23, 42
$I_{K(Ado)}$, **23**, 42
I_K, **22**, 29, 41, 44
I_{K1}, 22-23
I_{Na}, **17-19**, 29, 42, 44, 208-211
I_{to}, 21-23
Idiojunctional rhythm, 82, 191
Idiopathic ventricular tachycardia; *see*
      Ventricular tachycardia, idio-
      pathic
Idioventricular rhythm
  accelerated, 50, 197, 335
  slow, 347
Incessant atrial tachycardia, 135, 136
Incessant junctional tachycardia, **173-174**
  clinical implications of, 174
  definition of, 173
  distinguishing features of, 173-174
  ECG recognition of, 173
  mechanism of, 173
  treatment of, 174
Incisional reentrant atrial tachycardia,
      110, 124, **132**
Infarction, myocardial, 42, 245, 252, 259
Inhibition, **62-63**

Innervation, conduction system, 110
Interfascicular reentrant ventricular
    tachycardia, 284
Intermittent parasystole, 337-338
Interpolated atrial premature beat, 86
Interpolated ventricular extrasystoles,
    75, 76
Interval
    PR, 311
    QT, 43, 44, 54, 205, 295
Intervals, His bundle, 71
Inward K$^+$ rectifier current, 22-23
Irregularity, chaotic, 359
Ischemia-induced arrhythmias, 63-66
Isotropic conduction, 60

J

Jugular pulse, 104, 124, 157, 240
Junction, gap, **24-25**
Junctional escape, 93, 348
Junctional extrasystoles, concealed, 76-80,
    349, 350
Junctional rhythm, accelerated, 80, 81,
    350
Junctional tachycardia, 48, 49, 188, 191

K

K$_{ATP}$, 23
Koch, triangle of, 4, 5, 7

L

Latent accessory pathway, 163
Lead I value, 155, 280
Leads MCL$_1$ and MCL$_6$, **356-358**
Left bundle branch block
    aberrancy, 215, **223**, 228, 231, 232, 233,
        234
    pattern, 225
Lewis, 234
Lidocaine, 43, 233
Long QT syndrome, **294-303**
    acquired, 294-300
        corrected QT in, 295
        QT prolongation in, 294-295

Long QT syndrome—cont'd
    congenital, 300-302
        corrected QT in, 302
        ECG recognition of, 300, 301
        screening for, 302
        T waves in, 302
        treatment of, 302
    emergency treatment of, 298-299
    latent, 298
Long-short sequence, 295, 296, 230, 231, 232
LQTS (long QT syndrome), **293-302**
L-type calcium channels, **19-20,** 35, 41, 53

M

"m" gate, 18-19
Magnesium, 20, 299
Mahaim fibers, 261, 262, 274-276
Mapping, pace, 280
Mayer, 57, 154
Maze surgery, 107
MCL$_1$ and MCL$_6$, **356-358**
Mechanisms
    of aberrancy, **215-220**
    arrhythmogenic, **47-68**
    of proarrhythmic drugs, 206-207
    of tachycardia, 65
Membrane channels, **17-24,** 29, 35, 53, 42,
        44, 207-211
    closed-state, 208
    inactivated-state, 208
    open-state, 208
Membrane potential, 13, 14, 15, 21, 22
    resting, 13, **14,** 16
Membrane pumps, **15-17**
Membrane responsiveness, 220
Mexiletine, 206
"Milk the QRS," **359**
"Mind your Ps," **362**
Mitral stenosis, 102, 103
Mobitz, 312
Modulated parasystole, 330-331
Modulation, electrotonic, 330
Monitoring, ECG, 184, **355-358**
    best leads for, 356-358

Monitoring, ECG—cont'd
  clinical setting and, 355-356
  systematic approach to, 358-365
Monomorphic ventricular tachycardia, 277
Monophasic complex, 245
Moricizine, 206
Multifocal atrial tachycardia, 135, 137
Multivariate analysis, 376
Muscarinic receptor-effector coupling
      system, 42-43
Myocardial contraction, 20
Myocardial infarction, 42, 88, 89, 252,
    259, 367
Myocardial ischemia, acute, 304-307
Myocardium, cell function of, **13-25**

N

Narrow QRS tachycardia, **153-177**
Nervous system
  autonomic, 41-45
  sympathetic, 44
Node, AV, **3-7**
  approaches to, **6-7**
  compact, 4, 7
  membrane channels in, 18
  transitional, 6
Nodoventricular fibers, 262, **274-276**
Nonparoxysmal atrial tachycardia, 135,
  138

O

Oleander poisoning, 199
Orthodromic circus movement tachycar-
    dia (CMT), **163-171, 173-174**
Orthodromic defined, 153
Overdrive suppression, 16, **37-39**, 49, 50-
  52, 346

P

P waves
  in AV dissociation, 241
  different shapes of, 86, 87
  skipped, 317
Pace mapping, 280

Pacemaker
  fixed rate, 334-335
  therapy, 96
  wandering atrial, 86
Pacemaker cells, 13
  latent, 218
Pacemaker current, **23,** 29, 41, 42
Pacemaker therapy, 96
Pacing, rapid, 55
Palpitation, 104
Paradoxical critical rate, 218, 349
Parasystole
  atrial, 332, **340-342**
  ventricular, **329-343**
    accelerated idioventricular rhythm
      in, 338
    classic
      with exit block, 337
      without exit block, **334-336**
    clinical significance of, 338-340
    concealed, 337
    ECG in, 329-330
    electrotonic modulation in, 329, **330,**
      334, 338, 340-343
    entrance block in, 330, 331, 333, 337,
      340
    exit block in, 329, 330, **331-332,** 333,
      334-337, 338, 340
    fixed coupling in, 329, 338
    and fixed rate pacemaker, 334-335
    fusion beats in, **329,** 331, 333, 335,
      340
    interectopic intervals of, 330
    intermittent, 337-338
    modulated, 329, **330-331**
    protected zone in (entrance block),
      329, 330, 331, 332, 333, 335,
      337, 340
    zone of protection in, 329
Paroxysmal supraventricular tachycardia
    (PSVT); *see* Tachycardia, par-
    oxysmal supraventricular
Pathways, slow and fast, 6-7, 157, 158
Pauses, causes of, 358

Pediatrics
    atrial fibrillation in, 106
    atrial flutter in, 113
    atrial tachycardia in, 140
    idiopathic ventricular tachycardia in,
        277-278
    paroxysmal supraventricular tachycar-
        dia in, 176
    sick sinus syndrome in, 94-95
Periodicity, Wenckebach, 314-316
Permeability, selective, 13, **14**
Phase 0, 33-35
Phase 1, 35
Phase 2, 35
Phase 3 aberration, **215-217,** 219, 222, 235
Phase 4 aberration, 215, **217-220,** 233, 235
Phase 4 depolarization, **33,** 44
Phenomenon
    Ashman's, 230-231
    gap, 349-352
    long-short, 295, 296, 230, 231, 232
"Pinpoint the primary," **363**
Polymorphic ventricular tachycardia; *see*
        Tachycardia, polymorphic ven-
        tricular
Polyuria, 104
Potassium blockade, 44
Potassium channel blockers, 203, 296-298
Potassium derangements, 180-182
Potassium rectifying channels, **21-23**
Potential, membrane, 13
    action, **29-39**
    resting, 13, **14,** 16
    threshold, 13, **15**
Potentials, late, 367
PR interval, 311
Precordial concordance, 238, 253, 254,
        256, 257, 258, 259
Preexcitation, 163
    exercise and, 262
    intermittent, 262
Proarrhythmia, **203-214**
    clinical manifestations of, 205
    defined, 203
    drugs in, 206

Proarrhythmia—cont'd
    history of, 204-205
    mechanisms of, 206-207
    predictors of, 205
    prolonged refractory period in,
        206-207
    slow conduction in, 206
Proarrhythmic drugs, 206
    membrane channels and, 207-211
Procainamide, 56, 57, 155, 206, 233, 259,
        272, 262
Propafenone, 206
Propranolol, 114
PSVT; *see* Paroxysmal supraventricular
        tachycardia
Pulse deficit, 104
Pumps, membrane, **15-17**
    ATP-dependent Ca^{2+}, **16-17**
    electrogenic, 16
    sodium-potassium ATPase, 13-14, **15-
        16**
Purkinje fibers, 10

Q
Q in V_6, 249
QR complex, 256
QRS width, 226, 253, 259
QRSD, 370
QT interval, 43, 54, 229, 205, 295
QT interval, corrected (QTc), 295, 302
Quinidine, 53, 182, 206, 232, 233
"Quinidine syncope," 203

R
R, wide, 249, 250
"Rabbit ear" sign, 245, 246, 259
Radiofrequency catheter ablation, 91,
        120-121, 126, 132, 142, 155,
        160, 171, 173, 279
    complications following, 279
Rapid depolarization, 14
Rate, paradoxical critical, 218
Rate-dependent bundle branch block,
        220-222
Rate-dependent drugs, 43

Reciprocal beats,
    AV junctional, 145, 146
    A-V-A sequence, 147-148
    V-A-V sequence, 145, 147
    ventricular, 145, 146
Reciprocating defined, 153
Reciprocating supraventricular tachycardia, 174-176
Rectifying channels, potassium, 21-23
Reentry, **56-61,** 63, 210, 280, 349
    anatomic, 57
    anisotropic, 58, 59, 60
    circus movement, 56
    concealed, 349, 350
    functional, 57
    SA nodal, **89-92,** 174-176
    termination of, 60-61
    types of, 58
    vulnerable parameters of, 60
Reflection, 58-60
Refractory period, 36, 206-207, 211
Remodeling, electrical, 104
Renal failure, 199
Reperfusion arrhythmias, 53, 55
Repolarization, 15
    prolonged, 43
Responsiveness, membrane, 220
Resting membrane potential, 13, **14,** 16
Retrograde concealed conduction, 215, 230
Right bundle branch block, 10
    aberrancy, 215, **223,** 228, 231, 232, 233, 234
    pattern of, 223
RP/PR reciprocity, 314-316
R:S ratio, 245
Ryanodine receptor (RyR), 19

S

S downstroke, 249, 250
S$_5$ lead, 359-360
S nadir, 249, 250
SA block, 69, 94
SA conduction time, 69-70, 87, 88
SA exit block, **92-94,** 185
    first-degree, 92

SA exit block—cont'd
    second-degree, 92-93
    third-degree, 93
    type I, 92-93
    type II, 93
SA nodal reentrant tachycardia; *see*
        Tachycardia, SA nodal reentrant
SA node
    action potential of, **32-33**
    anatomy of, 85
    blood supply to, **2,** 87, 95
    conduction velocity within, 86
    depolarization within, 87
    development of, **1-3**
    diagnostic tests for function of, 88
    dysfunction of, 3, **89-98**
    electrogram of, 69-70
    horseshoe, 2, 3
    hyperthermia and hypothermia and, 88
    location of, 1-2
    membrane channels in, 18
    nerve supply of, 87
    pacemaker shifts within, 86, 87
    physiology of, 85-86
    temperature of, 88
    threshold potential of, 15
    structure of, 2
Sarcoplasmic reticulum, 17, 19, 20, 21
Second-degree AV block, 311-312
Second-in-the-row anomaly, 229-230
Shaped window, 373, 375
Sick sinus syndrome, 91, **94-96**
    causes of, 95
    disease processes of, 95-96
    drugs implicated in, 95
    ECG in, 94
    history of, 94
    mechanisms of, 95
    in pediatrics, 94-95
    treatment of, 96
Signal-averaged ECG, 88, 370, 371
    clinical application of, **367-368**
    frequency domain analysis of, **372-375**
    time domain analysis of, **369-371**
Signal averaging, 368

Sinoatrial; *see* SA entries
Sinus arrest, 69, 94
Sinus bradycardia, 94, 185, 358
Sinus node; *see* SA node
Sinus node electrogram, **69-70**
Sinus tachycardia, 156
Sinus Wenckebach, 92-93
Slow calcium channels, **19-20**, 35, 41, 53
Slow diastolic depolarization, 13, 14, 203, 220
Slow pathways, 6-7, 157, 158
Slow response action potential, 29-30
Sodium (I_{Na}) channels, **17-19**, 29, 42, 44, 208-211
　blockade of, 210-211
Sodium gradient, 16, 20, 21
Sodium-calcium exchanger, 20-21
Sodium-potassium ATPase membrane pumps, **15-16**
Sotalol, 53, 206
D-sotalol, 44, 204
Spatial averaging, 369
Spectral temporal mapping, 376
SSS; *see* Sick sinus syndrome
Stunning, atrial 106
Sulcus terminalis, 111
Summation, **61-62,** 337-338
Supernormal conduction, 335, 338, 339, **345-353**
　concealed, **346-348**
　mimics of, 348-352
Supernormal excitability, 216, 345, 346, 349
Supernormal period, 216, 345-346
Supernormality, **345-353**
Suppression, overdrive, 16, **37-39**
Supraventricular tachycardia; *see* Tachycardia, supraventricular
Surgery
　compartment, 107
　corridor, 107
　maze, 107
　valvular, 105
Syncope, 91
Syndrome
　bradycardia-tachycardia, 94, 95

Syndrome—cont'd
　long QT, **293-302;** *see also* Long QT syndrome
　Wolff-Parkinson-White, 56, 155, 162, 163, **261-276**
Systole, electrical, 208, 210

T
T waves, in torsades de pointes, 302
Tachycardia
　antidromic circus movement; *see* Antidromic circus movement tachycardia
　atrial; *see* Atrial tachycardia
　atypical circus movement, 173-174
　AV nodal reentrant; *see* AV nodal reentrant tachycardia
　bifascicular ventricular, 192-194, 196
　broad QRS; *see* Broad QRS tachycardia
　bundle branch reentrant, 226, 245, **282-286**
　　clinical presentation of, 285
　　ECG in, 282-283
　　ECG signs of, **245-247, 249-251**
　　idiopathic, 226, 252, **276-282**
　　interfascicular reentrant, 284
　　limitations of ECG signs in, 250
　　long-term treatment of, 286
　　mechanism of, 284
　　mimicking supraventricular tachycardia by, **276-287**
　　monomorphic idiopathic, 277
　　new diagnostic findings for, 256
　　pathophysiology of, 285
　　prognosis in, 286
　cardiomyopathy induced by, 104
　catecholamine-dependent, 55
　chaotic atrial, 135, 137
　circus movement; *see* Circus movement tachycardia
　delayed rectifier current (I_K) and, 22
　double, 194, 196
　fascicular ventricular, 192, 193, 194, 195, 226, 245, **286-287**
　focal atrial, 134-135, 139-140

Tachycardia—cont'd
  idiopathic ventricular; *see* Ventricular
    tachycardia, idiopathic
  incessant atrial, 135, 136
  incessant junctional; *see* Incessant junc-
    tional tachycardia
  incisional reentrant atrial, 124, **132**
  interfascicular reentrant ventricular,
    284
  junctional, 48, 49, 188, 191
  monomorphic ventricular, 277
  multifocal atrial, 135, 137
  narrow QRS, **153-177**
  nonparoxysmal atrial, 135, 138
  orthodromic circus movement, **160-171**
    anatomy involved in, 160-162
    definition of, 160
    mechanism of, 163
  paroxysmal supraventricular (PSVT),
    89, 145, **153-177**, 231, 261
    bedside diagnosis of, 157
    carotid sinus massage for, 156-157
    classification of, 153, 154
    ECG leads during, 155-156
    emergency response to, 155-157
    "frog sign" in, 157
    incidence of, 154
    interruption of, 154-155
    maintenance of, 154-155
    P′ wave in, 175
    pediatrics in, 176
    reentry circuit in, 154-155
    terminology of, 153
    types of, 154
    vagal stimulation for, 156-157
  polymorphic ventricular, **293-310**
    in acquired long QT syndrome, **294-
      300**
    classification of, 293
    in congenital long QT syndrome,
      300-302
    emergency treatment of, 298-299,
      302
    with prolonged QT, 294-303
    without prolonged QT, 303-308

Tachycardia—cont'd
  reciprocating supraventricular, 174-176
  SA nodal reentrant, **89-92**
    ECG of, 90
    ECG documentation of, 90
    differential diagnosis in, 90-91, 174-
      176
    history of, 91
    incidence of, 91
    mechanism of, 91
    symptoms of, 91
    treatment of, 91
  sinus, inappropriate, 48
  summary of mechanisms and charac-
    teristics of, 65-66
  supraventricular, **153-177**, 231, 245,
    247, 261
    ECG signs of aberrancy in, 245, 247
    mimicking of ventricular tachycar-
      dias by, **262-276**
    reciprocating, 174-176
  ventricular, 63, **239-259, 282-286**
    axis in, 247, 251-252
    capture beats and fusion beats in, 843
    concordant pattern in, **253**, 255, 256
    mimicking of supraventricular
      tachycardias by, **276-287**
    post–myocardial infarction, 49
    QRS configuration in, **243-250**
Tachycardia-induced cardiomyopathy, 104
Terfenadine, 44
Threshold membrane potential, 13, **15**
Thromboembolism, 96, 99, 104, 106, 107
Time domain analysis, 367, **369-371**
Tocainide, 206
Todaro, tendon of, 6, 7
Torsades de pointes, 53, 203, 204, 205,
    293, **294-302**
  acquired, 294-300
    antihistamines and, 297
    clinical causes of, 298
    clinical characteristics of, 298
    ECG during, 294
    ECG warning signs in, 294
    erythromycin and, 297

Torsades de pointes—cont'd
　acquired—cont'd
　　hypokalemia and, 297
　　long-short sequence in, 295
　　potassium channel blockers and, 296
　　prevention of, 300
　　QT prolongation before, 294-295
　　summary of mechanisms for, 297-298
　congenital, 300-302
　　ECG recognition of, 300, 301
　emergency treatment of, 298-299
　magnesium for, 299
　possible outcomes of, 299
　symptoms of, 298
Toxicity, digitalis
　clinical alert to, **184-185**
　treatment of, **198-199**
Transient outward K$^+$ current, **21-23**
Treatments
　antidromic circus movement tachycardia, 272-274
　atrial fibrillation, 106-107
　atrial fibrillation with accessory pathway, 267
　atrial flutter, 119-121
　atrial tachycardia, 142
　bundle branch reentrant ventricular tachycardia, 286
　digitalis toxicity, **198-199**
　idiopathic ventricular tachycardia, 278
　paroxysmal supraventricular tachycardia, 155-157
　polymorphic ventricular tachycardia, 298-299, 302
　torsades de pointes, 298-299
Tricuspid annulus, **111-112,** 116
"Triggered," defined, 49
Triggered activity, **49-56,** 180, 280, 329
Triphasic pattern, 245
T-type calcium channels, **19-20,** 35, 53
Type I and II AV block, 312-314

U
Use-dependent antiarrhythmic drugs, 43, 209

V
V_{max}, 217
V_1-negative broad QRS tachycardia, **247-251,** 259
V_1-positive broad QRS tachycardia, **245-247,** 259
Vagal stimulation, **42-43,** 89, 156-157, 272
　carotid sinus massage for, 156-157
Vagotonia, marked, 95
Velocity, conduction, **36-37**
Ventricular asystole, 320
Ventricular bigeminy, 195-197
Ventricular fibrillation, 204
Ventricular parasystole, **329-343**
Ventricular tachycardia; *see* Tachycardia, ventricular
Ventricular tachycardia, idiopathic, 226, 245, 252, **276-282**
　ECG warning of, 277
　emergency treatment of, 278
　history of, 278
　left, **281-282**
　　ECG in, 281-282
　　foci location in, 282
　　mechanism of, 282
　　pathology of, 282
　long-term treatment of, 278
　in pediatrics, 277-278
　prognosis of, 277
　radiofrequency ablation in, 278-279
　right, 55, **279-281**
　　differential diagnosis in, 280
　　ECG in, 279-280
　　foci location in, 280
　　mechanism of, 280
　　pace mapping in, 280
　symptoms of, 277
　warning signs of, 277
Ventriculo-atrial conduction, **241-243**
Verapamil, 100, 182, 203, 238, 239, 259, 282

Voltage-dependent antiarrhythmic drugs, 43
Voltage-dependent gating, 18
Voltage-operated channels, 17
Vulnerable parameter, 48, 49, 55, 56, 60
Vulnerable period, 210

W

Wandering atrial pacemaker, 86
Wenckebach, 312

Wenckebach conduction, 92-93, 112, 114, 115, 186
  retrograde, 145, 146, 243, 246
Wenckebach periodicity, 314-316
"Who's married to whom?", **363**
Window, unity gain, 372, 373
Wolff-Parkinson-White syndrome, 56, 86, 155, 162, 163, 245, **261-276**